EXPLORING THE CONSEQUENCES OF THE COVID-19 PANDEMIC

Social, Cultural, Economic, and Psychological
Insights and Perspectives

EXPLORING THE CONSEQUENCES OF THE COVID-19 PANDEMIC

Social, Cultural, Economic, and Psychological Insights and Perspectives

Edited by
Usha Rana, PhD
Jayanathan Govender, PhD

AAP APPLE
ACADEMIC
PRESS

First edition published 2022

Apple Academic Press Inc.
1265 Goldenrod Circle, NE,
Palm Bay, FL 32905 USA

4164 Lakeshore Road, Burlington,
ON, L7L 1A4 Canada

CRC Press
6000 Broken Sound Parkway NW,
Suite 300, Boca Raton, FL 33487-2742 USA

2 Park Square, Milton Park,
Abingdon, Oxon, OX14 4RN UK

© 2022 by Apple Academic Press, Inc.

Apple Academic Press exclusively co-publishes with CRC Press, an imprint of Taylor & Francis Group, LLC

Library and Archives Canada Cataloguing in Publication

Title: Exploring the consequences of the COVID-19 pandemic : social, cultural, economic, and psychological insights and perspectives / edited by Usha Rana, PhD, Jayanathan Govender, PhD.
Names: Rana, Usha, editor. | Govender, Jay, editor.
Description: First edition. | Includes bibliographical references and index.
Identifiers: Canadiana (print) 20220141177 | Canadiana (ebook) 20220141185 | ISBN 9781774638644 (hardcover) | ISBN 9781774638651 (softcover) | ISBN 9781003277286 (ebook)
Subjects: LCSH: COVID-19 Pandemic, 2020-—Social aspects. | LCSH: COVID-19 Pandemic, 2020-—Economic aspects. | LCSH: COVID-19 Pandemic, 2020-—Psychological aspects.
Classification: LCC RA644.C67 E97 2022 | DDC 362.1962/414—dc23

Library of Congress Cataloging-in-Publication Data

....

CIP data on file with US Library of Congress

....

ISBN: 978-1-77463-864-4 (hbk)
ISBN: 978-1-77463-865-1 (pbk)
ISBN: 978-1-00327-728-6 (ebk)

About the Editors

Usha Rana, PhD
School of Humanities and Social Sciences,
Dr. Harisingh Gour Central University, Madhya Pradesh, India

Usha Rana, PhD, is an Assistant Professor of Sociology and Social Work at the Dr. Harisingh Gour Central University (A Government Central University), Sagar, India. She is an academician in sociology with a specialization in sexual studies and gender studies and has more than 10 years of teaching and research experience. She has published more than 30 articles in reputed national and international peer-reviewed journals/conferences, including SCI/Scopus-indexed journals published by Inderscience, Springer, Elsevier, and Cambridge, respectively. In addition, she also serves as a reviewer for many SCI/Scopus journals. She has delivered lectures as a speaker at various national and international workshops. Dr. Rana is an active member of the International Sociological Association, Indian Sociological Society, and Women's Indian Association, among others. Dr. Rana completed her master's and doctorate in Sociology from Jiwaji University, Gwalior India, and Dr. Harisingh Gour Central University, respectively.

Jayanathan Govender, PhD
School of Social Sciences, University of KwaZulu-Natal, Durban,
South Africa

Jayanathan Govender, PhD, teaches Industrial, Organizational and Labour Studies at the School of Social Sciences at the University of KwaZulu-Natal (UKZN), Durban, South Africa. His interests include civil society, interdisciplinary studies, BRICS sociology, sociological practice, and future research. He has published on topics in public management, participation, higher education, social policy, inequality, and social justice. Dr. Govender completed his master's and doctorate degrees at the University of the Western Cape, Cape Town, South Africa, and the University of KwaZulu-Natal, Durban, South Africa, respectively.

Contents

Contributors

Prachi Agrawal
Department of Mathematics and Scientific Computing, National Institute of Technology Hamirpur, Himachal Pradesh – 177005, India

Jyoti Ahlawat
Post-Doctoral Fellow, University of Victoria, Canada, E-mail: jyotiahlawat@icloud.com

Hongwei Bao
Department of Cultural, Media, and Visual Studies, The University of Nottingham, United Kingdom, E-mail: hongwei.bao@nottingham.ac.uk

William B. Bowes
Department of Humanities and Social Sciences, University of Edinburgh, Edinburgh, United Kingdom, E-mail: W.Bowes@sms.ed.ac.uk

Somdutta Chatterjee
Department of Teacher Education, The West Bengal University of Teachers' Training, Education Planning and Administration (WBUTTEPA), Kolkata, West Bengal, India

Talari Ganesh
Department of Mathematics and Scientific Computing, National Institute of Technology Hamirpur, Himachal Pradesh – 177005, India

Sudaita Ghosh
Department of Political Science, Raiganj University, Raiganj – 733134, West Bengal, India, E-mail: sudaitaghosh@gmail.com

Deepa Gokulsing
Department of Social Studies, University of Mauritius, Mauritius

Lina Gurung
School of Education, Kathmandu University, Dhulikhel, Nepal

Said Ali Hassan
Department of Operations Research and Decision Support, Faculty of Computers and Artificial Intelligence, Cairo University, Egypt

S. S. M. Sadrul Huda
Department of Management, School of Business, North South University, Dhaka, Bangladesh, E-mail: ssadrul@gmail.com

David Jimoh Kayode
Department of Educational Leadership and Management, Faculty of Education, University of Johannesburg, South Africa, E-mail: kayodedj1@gmail.com

Naushad Mamode Khan
Department of Economics and Statistics, University of Mauritius, Mauritius

Pinky Lalthapersad-Pillay
Department of Economics, University of South Africa, South Africa, E-mail: lalthp@unisa.ac.za

Bal Chandra Luitel
School of Education, Kathmandu University, Dhulikhel, Nepal

Chanchal Maity
Bankura University, Bankura, West Bengal, India

Syeeda Raisa Maliha
Re-Think, Re-Search, Dhaka, Bangladesh

Anindya J. Mishra
Full Professor of Sociology, Department of Humanities and Social Sciences,
Indian Institute of Technology, Roorkee, Uttarakhand, India

Neha Mishra
PhD Research Scholar, Department of Humanities and Social Sciences, Indian Institute of Technology,
Roorkee, Uttarakhand, India, E-mail: neha.mishra1293@gmail.com

Ali Wagdy Mohamed
Operations Research Department, Faculty of Graduate Studies for Statistical Research,
Cairo University, Giza – 12613, Egypt; Wireless Intelligent Networks Center (WINC),
School of Engineering and Applied Sciences, Nile University, Giza, Egypt,
E-mail: aliwagdy@gmail.com

Mrinal Mukherjee
Department of Teacher Education, The West Bengal University of Teachers' Training,
Education Planning and Administration (WBUTTEPA), Kolkata, West Bengal, India,
E-mail: dr.mmrinal@gmail.com

Pallav Mukhopadhyay
Assistant Professor, Department of Journalism and Mass Communication,
West Bengal State University, West Bengal, India, E-mail: journalist430@gmail.com

Suraiya Rathankoomar Naicker
Department of Educational Leadership and Management, Faculty of Education,
University of Johannesburg, South Africa

Vannie Naidoo
School of Management, Information Technology and Governance, University of KwaZulu-Natal,
Durban, Westville Campus, Durban, South Africa, E-mail: naidoova@ukzn.ac.za

Debasish Nandy
Kazi Nazrul University, West Bengal, India, E-mail: debasishnandy.kc@gmail.com

Zintle Ntshongwana
Department of Social Work, University of Fort Hare, South Africa

Chandra Lal Pandey
Community Development Program, School of Arts, Kathmandu University, Dhulikhel, Nepal,
E-mail: chandra.pandey@ku.edu.np

Aradhana Ramnund-Mansingh
Human Resource Cluster, MANCOSA Honoris United Universities, Durban, South Africa,
E-mail: raakheemansingh17@gmail.com

Tilottama Raychaudhuri
Assistant Professor of Law, WBNUJS, Kolkata, West Bengal, India

Subir Kumar Roy
Registrar (Addl. Charge) and Associate Professor, Department of Law, Bankura University,
Bankura, West Bengal, India, E-mail: dr.roysubir@gmail.com

Mariam Seedat-Khan
Department of Sociology, University of KwaZulu Natal, Durban, South Africa

Elvin Shava
School of Public Management, Governance, and Public Policy, College of Business and Economics,
University of Johannesburg, South Africa, E-mail: ellyshava@gmail.com

Ashwinee Devi Soobhug
Department of External Trade/Statistics Mauritius, Ministry of Finance,
Economic Planning and Development, Mauritius, E-mail: soobhugn@gmail.com

T. Sowdamini
GITAM Institute of Management, GITAM (Deemed to be) University, Visakhapatnam,
Andhra Pradesh, India, Mobile: + 91-9885532350, E-mail: sthatta@gitam.edu

Magdaline Tanga
School of Further and Continuing Education, University of Fort Hare, South Africa

Pius Tanga
Department of Social Work, University of Fort Hare, South Africa, E-mail: ptanga@ufh.ac.za

Beauty Zindi
Department of Public Administration, Faculty of Management and Commerce,
University of Fort Hare, South Africa

Abbreviations

AHT	abusive head trauma
AIDS	acquired immune deficiency syndrome
ALM	augmented Lagrangian method
ASUU	Academic Staff Union of Universities
BBS	Bangladesh Bureau of Statistics
BCSIR	Bangladesh Council of Science and Industry Research
BEA	Bureau of Economic Analysis
BLS	Bureau of Labor Statistics
BMA	Bangladesh Medical Association
BSMMU	Bangabandhu Sheikh Mujib Medical University
C	contacts
C19 TERS	COVID-19 temporary relief scheme
CARES Act	Coronavirus Aid, Relief, and Economic Security Act
CARMMA	accelerated campaign on reduction of maternal mortality in Africa
CDC	centers for disease control
CERB	Canada emergency response benefit
CSR	corporate social responsibility
D	deceased
DEOs	district education offices
DHET	Department of Higher Education and Training
DIGSK	discrete integer gaining-sharing knowledge-based optimization algorithm
DOE	Department of Education
DRICM	designated reference institute for chemical measurement
EFA	education for all
EiE	education in emergencies
ERL	emergency remote learning
FGN/ASUU	Federal Government of Nigeria/Academic Staff Union of Universities
GoN	Government of Nepal
GSK	gaining-sharing knowledge
HEC	higher education commission
HEOP	health emergency operations plan

HIV   human immunodeficiency virus
I   infected
ICCB   International Convention City Bashundhara
ICESCR   International Covenant on Economic, Social, and Cultural
               Rights
ICT   information communication technology
ICU   intensive care unit
ILO   International Labor Organization
LSGD   local self-government department
MMR   maternal mortality rate
MOE   Ministry of Education
MOO   multi-objective optimization
MOOC   massive open online courses
MoU   memorandum of understanding
MPoA   Maputo platform of action
NAI   nonaccidental injury
NBP   number of benefited people
NBR   National Board of Revenue
NCDC   Nigeria Center for Disease Control
NCW   National Commission for Women
NGOs   non-governmental organizations
NHC   National Human Rights Commission
NHRC   National Human Rights Office
NMU   Nelson Mandela University
O   ordinary
ODEC   open and distance education center
ODL   open distance learning
OFRA   optimum financial resource allocation
OLPC   one laptop per child
PCS   prioritized category status
PG   postgraduate
PGDE   postgraduate diploma in education
PPE   personal protective equipment
PTSD   post-traumatic stress disorder
R   recovered
RU   Rhodes University
SARS   severe acute respiratory syndrome
SARS-CoV   severe acute respiratory syndrome coronavirus
SDGs   sustainable development goals

SRHR	sexual and reproductive health and rights
SSDP	school sector development plan
SSRP	school sector reform plan
STDs	sexually transmitted diseases
STEM	science, technology, engineering, and math
STI	sexually transmitted infections
UCLA	University of California, Los Angeles
UDHR	Universal Declaration of Human Rights
UFH	University of Fort Hare
UG	undergraduate
UIF	Unemployment Insurance Fund
UK	United Kingdom
UN	United Nations
UNESCO	United Nations Educational, Scientific, and Cultural Organization
UNISA	University of South Africa
USA	United States of America
W.A.S.H	water, hygiene, and sanitation
WFH	work from home
WFP	World Food Program
WHO	World Health Organization
WPI	Worcester Polytechnic Institute
WSU	Walter Sisulu University

Acknowledgments

First of all, the authors sincerely acknowledge the support from the publisher during the preparation of this book. The authors would also like to express appreciation to all the contributors for their hard work and interesting research studies.

The authors would like to express their deepest gratitude to Dr. Rupender Singh of the Indian Institute of Technology (Roorkee), who made this book possible. Without his advice and strong support, this book would not be a reality.

Preface

It appears impossible to argue to the contrary, humanity's ultimate capability: The difference between what we do and what we are capable of doing would suffice to solve most of the world's problems. This insightful remark of the human capability by Mahatma Gandhi is observable not only in human history but is axiomatic for the immeasurable future. On the one hand, modern human civilization has experienced vis-à-vis complex sociocultural systems, forged as urban areas, evolving communication technologies, almost fault-less administrative infrastructure, and compound divisions of labor, held together by a seemingly perfect global capitalist system. On the other hand, the 4th Industrial Revolution promises grand egalitarian existentialism, i.e., new human freedom. The revolution merges the material, technological, and biological aspects of what humans use to produce things that make life better, more convenient, and comfortable. The new freedom will replace the modern processes for health, food, housing, transport, and so on, by merging the human capability with artificial and augmented intelligence. Now here is some compelling evidence of that pure human capability identified by Gandhi. That evidence includes those authentic scientific interventions to counter COVID-19, albeit primarily in the world's wealthiest countries.

As good as this latest news about COVID-19 countenance is, it seems that like modernism, global capitalism, the 4th Industrial Revolution, a COVID-19 free world, appears the reserve of the wealthiest countries of the world. This theme will be apparent throughout this collection. It will be the poor who carry the heaviest burdens of this social calamity, not different from those swathes of poor suffering the most and worst from global warming, people who had nothing to do with causing global warming.

Perhaps the most significant focus must come to bear on the interrelation of global capitalism and the state as well as their roles if the world's poor is not to be robbed of their fundamental human rights. This interrelationship is foregrounded in conscience by the *"Universal Declaration of Human Rights (UDHR)"* and it asseverates on "right to life, liberty, and security" to everyone under Article 3. Article 25 sets out the essentials for life during social upheaval:

1. Everyone has the right to a standard of living adequate for the health and well-being of himself and of his family, including food, clothing, and housing and medical care and necessary social services, and the right to security in the event of unemployment, sickness, disability, widowhood, old age or other lack of livelihood in the circumstances beyond his control.
2. Motherhood and childhood are entitled to special care and assistance. All children, whether born in or out of wedlock, shall enjoy the same social protection.

Now, if the state and global capitalism, both abstract independent systems, by the way, and of different political embodiments dispersed in different parts of the world, are tasked with humanity's welfare, should they not be guided by a universal system or convention that is equal for all of humanity, irrespective of where one lives. Where one lives today is a crucial determinant of the reach of opportunities and prospects. The poor have no such reach capability like the rich. Poor people are not appendaged with the material and social devices of either modernism or global capitalism. The poor are flaunted in the boundless outer galaxies of society, hardly recognizable as human beings. It is assumed that they do not know the meaning of self-dignity and suffering under the sparkle of the imminent 4th Industrial Revolution.

The COVID-19 pandemic is a return to the fundamental questions of what it means to be human. Not to be outdone, we humans can choose to be antinomian at the best and worst of times. One such time is now. Without the least grimace, we (the rich) choose to dispense sympathy and aid to the poor in the logical order of last, at best, or not at all, at worst. However, the world (the rich) who incidentally invented the phrase: "With COVID-19, nobody is safe until everyone is safe", understand liberally that their well-being and mortality cannot be safely stashed like money, luxuries, and hedonisms. Still, they persist in doing things the familiar way. Here now is the critical singularity of COVID-19: the old ways of doing things will simply not serve this social calamity.

The holding on to old ways means that we have not as a scientific community yet imagined a meta-methodological approach to social calamities. The historical experience will serve only as a minimal framework for a new and appropriate scientific methodology. The intersections of the ecology, social systems, science, and technology produce a new intellectual capital owned by the people themselves, the rich and poor alike. Frankly, there needs to be a people's science. This line of thinking is evident in versions of development theory. For example, raising the poor's level of health literacy will lead to increased levels of consciousness and better choices related to health issues. Our problem once again is an old one—the polar doctrine of the remedial and the pre-emptive. The economic and moral claims of each of the doctrines are theoretically divergent. Conflicting methodologies frame them. Somehow, the evidence is not evidence because logic (a logic) dictates those polar doctrines are non-referential. By non-referential, two polar doctrines of the remedial and pre-emptive do not form a binary opposition. Each is logical in their own right and are applied independently for meaningful outcomes. The end to this seemingly spurious point, we could say with some hesitation of being reductionist, that a new philosophy of science, embracing a meta-methodology has to be researched and professed to ensure a relevant future human future not enveloped only by the canons of 4th Industrial Revolution.

This book's contributions call for existential and scientific renewal because COVID-19 will surely be followed by another novel organism making the jump from another species to humans. This claim holds because of deforestation, global warming, poverty, and inequality. If food, among the most basic human needs, is not accessible to the poor, they will revert to primitive measures, which, understood or not, is another form of interspecies communication.

Introduction

This collection is a sociological attempt at raising the multiple veils evolving from the COVID-19 pandemic, which in the safest estimation is less than one full calendar year in the making. The multiple veils mysteriously appear, disappear, and transform, with simultaneous effects in the social ecology. COVID-19 is creatively traumatic and transformative for both people and social systems. Embedded in its creative destruction, there appear to be emergence and development exchanges of sorts that feature in open systems. This characteristic is a key property of some living systems, which is not easily understood. Viral life in the form of COVID-19, and supposedly all other life forms, reaches out for novelty. Its interest in human beings is simply to play host to its reproduction, and in the process of physically irritating one host, it travels to several others, creating a complex communicable system. The point, then, of multiple veils is to unravel a key piece of knowledge, i.e., the social effects of the spillover of a minimal life form, *vis-à-vis* human bodies, onto the global existential and social fabrics.

The COVID-19 pandemic's destruction in progress has both known and not yet known linkages, including neo-liberalism, globalization, climate change, destruction of the natural habitat, the culture of comfort and consumption, and so on. Even in the face of disagreement with these linkages, like by some big political names, the COVID-19 pandemic has lifted the veil shielding the unequal and impoverished social relations globally and within states. It also laid bare the racial and racist structures within societies. However, gender relations appeared to suffer the worst, where women have to carry the bigger burden of the multiple impacts of the COVID-19 pandemic.

All societal institutions-politics, culture, and economy have either stalled, or transformed into a new sociality (bluntly termed new normal), but not yet accommodated by vast numbers of people across the globe. It is sometimes accompanied by open resistance, despite the obvious perils posed by the COVID-19 pandemic. This response is typical when people are subjected to distress and disruption of their way of life. The imposition of isolation, as a measure to retard the communicability of the COVID-19 virus, was and remained an existential shock on human sociality.

This period in human history is the worst global experience of destructive destruction. The loss of life, income activities, freedom of self, and distressed public health have severely compounded the material, psychological, and spiritual well-beingness of billions of people. Things that were normal and casual became hyper-organized, military-like protocols, such that people are actors on foreign stages. Mental health among adults and child depression were given new classifications, and in the absence of treatment regimes, gender-based violence, substance abuse, and sexual abuse appeared to rise within intimate spaces.

Amongst the poorer sections of society, those living in squatter and refugee camps and street children, protection against the COVID-19 virus was hardly in evidence. Social distancing was not possible due to crushing living compacts, and since cooperation with others in the vicinity is a norm for their daily needs, formal protocols by local governments were not be observed. The capability of a grandmother with several grandchildren to ensure their safety is greatly reduced by the extent of poor hygiene, lack of running water, and lack of toilet facilities. One new demand on the grandmother is the increased consumption of food when the grandchildren are not at school (since thousands rely on lunches provided at schools).

If the COVID-19 pandemic exposes social inequality, it also crystallizes social inequality. New forms of discrimination and exclusion are strategies by the wealthy á la social distancing. Where poorer people were available for menial jobs, domestic work, childminding, and so on, they are threatened by discrimination and exclusion, job loss, and plain disrespectful treatment. The light on COVID-19 and its ravages is dimmed and displaced for new discriminatory and exclusionary practices. The effect on poor people is not just material, but also on the caveats of human dignity. Breaking down human dignity and losing a sense of self produces feelings of despair, disinterest, and social withdrawal. These conditions, in turn, lead to physical sickness, thereby limiting the ability to pursue the important function of raising an income required for the household. At a broader societal level, the vicious cycle of poverty is reproduced.

Spatial organization, an indicator of the partition of poverty, then has adopted new characteristics, not only serving as signifiers of wealth and enclaves of safety and distance from the other. The connections to places of work, cultural practices, and the taken-for-granted sites of consumption were suddenly disallowed as part of the global response to the spread of the pandemic. Of course, the strategy made sense. However, once again, those who had the capability to isolate as households could do so since they could demand all sorts of goods and services online. Since the burgeoning of online consumerism is a subject matter on its own, the feature that strikes out is how the wealthy are hardly menaced, as compared to other sections of society, by the COVID-19 pandemic. The wealthy are indeed protected by deep layers of comfort.

The workplace was another societal site of overnight transformation. Every economic activity that required people and workers to perform organized work was required to stop without any indication of what the future holds. Income earners and shareholders alike had to endure unprecedented economic shocks. Once governments understood that they had to subsidize these economic losses to companies and individual workers, only wealthy governments could do so. Those experiencing the worst effects of the economic shutdown were the self-employed and entrepreneurs, whose share of the economy is significant and who considerably contribute to economic growth. In the process of this global economic crash, economic policy has also been slated, making such policies that promoted particular sectors redundant and pushing those economic sectors into reverse. The net global effect is spiking public debt, and the reliance on the market to provide capital at very high costs.

The societal domains of spatial organization and workplace saw the necessity of the power of the state intervention and did not produce resistance to that power. It was clear that the state was playing its correct and necessary role. However, the cessation of cultural expression and religious freedom did produce questions about the role of the state, and different forms of resistance were in evidence. In the case of cultural expression, cultural workers who hold dear the idea of freedom of expression on any matter in society, in particular on power relations, were silenced not on the basis that their human rights were being withheld, but on the basis, all gatherings were potent purveyors of the COVID-19 pandemic.

In the case of religions, the contradiction that the state was assuming the higher power presented more complex contradictions between the state and systems of beliefs and canon. There are traditions and legal views that determine the relationship between them. While the emphasis is more towards the Christian Church, the notions of secularism, religious pluralism, and religious liberty also determine the relationship between the entities of state and religion. Crucially the major religious establishments were quick to recognize the need for an end to their practices and gatherings in line with legal requirements. However, the fringe religious movements were guilty of ignoring calls from the state, which led to pockets of consequences that added to the pandemic.

The lessons from the cultural and religious sector concerning their legal rights, are placed in parallel with questions of human rights. Did the response by the state constitute a breach or withdrawal of basic human rights, i.e., the right to movement, the right to earn an income, the right to congregate, and certain personal protection measures made necessary to arrest the spread of the COVID-19 virus, such the compulsory adornment of a face mask in the public space. Of course, the state must strike some acceptable balance between assertive measures to arrest the spread of the COVID-19 virus and to protect lives. The state must also respect human autonomy, dignity, and equality.

The answer is to be found in international law and is deserving of due credit. It recognizes the need for emergency action during pandemics and natural disasters. Accordingly, the *"International Covenant on Civil and Political Rights"* allows for the curbing of the so-called 'liberty of movement' where laws of a state deem it necessary to protect public health and that other rights are treated consistently. Therefore, freedom of expression and association, and the rights to privacy and family life are accorded qualified consideration. However, a limitation must not be arbitrary or discriminate. Restrictions must also be of limited duration and subject to review. This is clearly how people have been experiencing the application of international law in different countries, save where political spats have been exchanged for narrow political interests.

International law in the manner that it regulates pandemics and natural disasters asserts internationalism, which calls for greater political and economic cooperation among the states of the globe. However, internationalism is not neutral. Rather it is framed by interests and ideology, very much evident after World War II. The period lasted until the mid-1970s, which saw the economic expansion and the consolidation of capitalism, making way to globalization. Globalization was driven by advances in international transportation and communication. Globalization saw the integration of peoples of particular nations, the private sector, and governments. The global exchanges through trade, foreign direct investments, and communication led to the expansion of global companies, bringing with it an imbalance in global power relations. The globe developed faults in the structure of the global political economy, where inequality was increased between the most powerful nations, which were few in number, and the remaining nations. The shift towards globalism is an advanced stage of neoliberalism, where the different ideologies and patterns of globalization are establishing their respective flows. Consumerism, social justice, environmentalism, and religion, are seen as the support structures for advancing democracy across the globe. The key contest, though, is the views between a few powerful individuals against organized groups in civil society, indigenous people, and international non-governmental organizations (NGOs) who are highlighting global inequality, unequal relationships, and global warming through the unfair appropriation of the environment. These voices also advocate the 1% argument, where 1% of people of the globe have hegemony over the rest.

The world is encountering severe acute inequalities. The sociologists refer to this condition as "manufactured" uncertainty. This can also be applied to disasters that may appear natural, whereas the underlying causes are actually attributable to deforestation and other forms of encroachment into natural settings. Another example is infrastructure or building collapse, where cost-cutting measures result in weak materials being applied. The costs to the economy accumulate in the form of subsidies, assurance cover, and inflation. The political consequence of "manufactured" uncertainty is not what is being advocated by the powerful, that democracy is enveloping the whole globe, thereby bringing benefits to all people. Rather globalism is making governments unreliable, undemocratic, and incapable of driving the foundation of equality for all.

The best evidence to demonstrate the state of inequality of the globe is the growth of neo-conservative politics. Neo-conservative politics is sustained by authoritarian ideas and leadership. It advocates for certain moral standards, promotes domestic concerns, is anti-migration, denies global warming, and is quick to employ military intervention to assert foreign policy. The media is used as a powerful tool that conveys neo-conservative politics.

Another piece of evidence of inequality is demonstrated by the wealthy themselves, who are turning government towards their favor. The wealthy are seeking the ideal of a safe, protective place in society, to live their lives without interference and assured of a decent life. This effectively means lower taxation, favorable policy approaches supporting their business, and the use of state power to promote their share of the global market. The anxieties of the wealthy are also driving them to seek protection from sectarian religious bodies, who in fact, have no tolerance for the poor and oppressed masses. The notion of society and globalism framed by their ideology is radically opposed to the expectations of the poor, marginalized, and unemployed. Recent advanced research has shown that the *"rich are getting richer, and the poor are getting poorer."* The inequality gap is actually erecting a barrier in the fight against poverty.

Modern capitalism is clearly reshaping the globe in terms of unequal share of wealth, where the global organization of work and production require technology rather than people, where people who did not contribute suffer the effects of global warming to it, and where crushing poverty is the daily experience of the majority of people. The crucial link between the COVID-19 pandemic and modern capitalism, amongst others, is the nature of global production in association with global labor. The experience of compulsory closures of businesses resulted in massive job loss. The opportunity to save jobs was simply not available to labor and its representatives. The informal sector, which retains a large workforce, was the worst off. This sector has no access to credit and savings facilities, putting their lives and that of their households in real danger.

The involuntary reorganization of the workplace caused by the COVID-19 pandemic now exposes the world of work and labor to new vulnerabilities. Instead of absorbing labor, labor will be more and more streamlined, utilized on a contingent basis. Earnings will drop. Virtual working will be both securocratic and multi-layered, demanding a new orientation. Workers will be dehumanized. The drastic reduction of the proportion of workers will reorganize the social means of production. Modern capitalism then is set to reshape itself once again during this generations' advance into the 21st century, which will be shaped by the 4th Industrial Revolution.

The 4th Industrial Revolution brings a compelling set of both advantages and challenges, depending of course, on who is on the side of the 1% and who is on the other side. However, the claim is that the 4th Industrial Revolution is framed along the lines of egalitarianism, where technological advancement is transcended in favor of bringing the *"greatest good for the greatest number of people."* The claim is not very far off from that of modern capitalism, which also advocates for the *"greatest good for the greatest number of people."* Yet in both the 4th industrial revolution and modern capitalism, the reverse to their similar claim is a selected small group of individuals and families or oligarchies, get richer and the majority of poor, get poorer.

The 4th Industrial Revolution will change how humans think about themselves and how they will live their lives. The first three revolutions were based on the changing forms of energy that drove industry and production. In this revolution, while non-fossil forms of energy will be the norm, artificial intelligence is at its center. This means merging the material, technological, and biological aspects of what humans use to produce things that make life better, more convenient, and comfortable. Being human in the future will require merging with artificial and augmented intelligence, that will replace the reliance on those sociologies such as health, food, housing, transport, and so on. The implication for cultural systems is also quite a promise. Importantly as well, how humans negotiate space will be telling on the fortunes of those who take the lead in this next adventure.

However, like in the previous revolutions, there are inherent perils. Previous revolutions did not distribute wealth equitably, rather the capitalist system depended on consumption; neither did they put great effort into environmental sustainability; neither did they eradicate poverty; and neither did they ensure equal public health systems. A rather long list of historical evidence shows that the benefits of capitalism under any of the previous revolutions did not trickle down to everyone or that the rising tide lifted all boats equally. One simple example can eloquently demonstrate capitalism's failure, the internet. If in this epoch people across the globe experience prejudice with internet connection, what then will be those prejudices of the 4th Industrial Revolution? How will the crucial issues of an ever-evolving capitalist system be addressed, i.e., ownership of capital; ownership of the means of production; access to the environment; access to space in the future; access to science and knowledge; access to good health facilities; and of course, access to artificial and augmented intelligence?

Against this backdrop, how are the drivers of modern capitalism placed to explain the COVID-19 pandemic. The seemingly prophetic answer that capitalism is a system, a system that is governed by the so-called invisible hand, simply does not suffice when human life is at the altar of sacrifice. Capitalism is the tension between owners and workers-a class structure that is entrenched *vis-à-vis* evolving stratagems by the powerful who control and direct politics under the guise of democratizing the entire globe; who determine at global fora what is good for themselves first and foremost under the guise that the good of the rest of the world is the concern; and who are making the environment sick under the guise of development.

The COVID-19 pandemic is a consequence of human action in this epoch. Those whose life chances have been compromised by the modern capitalist system drive this human action. The claim that this epoch is the advent of the 4th Industrial Revolution and one of great promise is one of humans' greatest hubris, but also humans' greatest untruth. Humans cannot step into a hygienic revolution of technology and artificial intelligence, without restitution to the environment and end to global warming, because that same revolution will be under threat. Humans have missed the dialectical relationship between the 4th Industrial Revolution and the environment and climate change. The costs to fix the damage to the environment and the costs to cool down the planet is unimaginable. The gains of the 4th Industrial Revolution will be wiped clean by the losses accrued from the doings of the modern capitalist system that is producing great inequality, poverty, and loss of human dignity.

This collection calls for a complex creativity, one that can explain through metaphor, social systems, and the evolution of capitalism, how the social ecology came to be so catastrophically disrupted by the COVID-19 pandemic. The task includes revisiting the history of science, bravely entering into esoteric knowledge areas, and combining reductionist scientific techniques with holistic ones. Western science is valuable, but wholly hinged on reductionism, whereby the properties of a complicated system are understood by the behavior of its component parts. This scientific attitude blocks out novel scientific process that would otherwise be available under these wanting circumstances. Accordingly, there is urgency and necessity of a holistic novel science, or at best, trans-disciplinary scientific techniques, to girdle the study of the COVID-19 pandemic. The approach must expose the underlying reasons for the pandemic; how it is affecting the social ecology; what remedies must be put in place to end its ravages; as well as protocols to prevent new pandemics. It must lay the scientific path for a post-COVID-19 globe.

We are therefore compelled to view the pandemic through the compound eyes, like those of arthropods, which most humans (or sociologists for that matter), have no clue of its structure and functionality. Nature is indeed generous at multiple levels of organization. However, the question is whether social and biomedical scientists are willing to subvert established social theory and scientific method for a novel approach to a novel COVID-19 pandemic. It is clear that a single scientific discipline is ill-equipped to address all of the complexities of the COVID-19 pandemic. It requires all the requisite disciplines to coordinate experimentation; discover interventions; set new public health standards; and provide the fixers for the prevention of a similar outbreak. Some scientists believe that a similar pandemic is inevitable. Such an attitude falls in line with the aphorism that humans do not know a lot more than what they know. That may be true, however, we know that COVID-19 has zoonotic origins, and as such, it is an area that requires more study, which calls for public health investment. There is a clear logical foundation for the argument that public health is an investment, not a costly giveaway.

Sadly, the current approach to the science of the COVID-19 pandemic is fragmented and not contagious from government to government. Each are also in conflict based on philosophy, political will, and standard of public health facilities. There is also the race about who will manufacture the first doses of the vaccine treatments to establish international pride and to assert hegemony over others. The international efforts have also been grainy, but that is only because of the limits applied to international bodies. The pandemic has also been contested for being one. It has received a share of consistory accusations. Not to be undone, the pandemic has acquired a form of denialism, similar to denialisms associated with the HIV/AIDS virus.

In the midst of this disarray, medicine, capitalism, and the social ecology appears to have forged an alliance, promoting a form of medical capitalism. Pandemics require massive investments in therapeutic interventions, including the development of vaccines. States, big pharma, research, and development agencies, as well as universities are motivated to invest significant financial and intellectual capital, in return for shareholder value. This development shows up the contradictions associated with medical capitalism, where the focus is on investor interests, not on safeguarding public health systems in the first place.

So, the project management to the COVID-19 pandemic requires, not just a therapy for the individual inflicted with the COVID-19 virus, but a multi-faceted-trans-disciplinary-global-convention. Every member of every multi-lateral organization must provide the energy, commitment, knowledge, and resources for addressing this and other possible pandemics. There is good reason for this convention becoming a moral obligation in the makings of the 4th Industrial Revolution.

Finally, this collection asks of the social sciences to breach from its familiar settings to socially understand the COVID-19 pandemic, which will assist the scientific endeavors at arresting its transmissibility (across and within species) and attendant fatal consequences. In the end, the global human community must be freed from this cataclysm and potentially others in the future.

The structure of the collection is organized around the complexity, depth, and pervasiveness of the social conditions brought by the COVID-19 pandemic. The underlying aim is to inform a global public health approach and to promote scientific research. The collection is stratified according to social dimensions, or meta-themes that bring analysis and understanding to the multiple phenomena produced by the COVID-19 pandemic. The sub-themes narrow the focus on units of analysis that isolate actual effects on specific population groups.

The editors extend their appreciation and thanks to each of the contributors, listed later in the collection. The contributors are situated across academic institutions in the globe. Their individual research efforts and social commitment will surely converge with other scientific and public health efforts across the globe to what the editors believe to be the *Convention on COVID-19 and Other Pandemics.*

PART I

Community Responses and Social Challenges During COVID-19

CHAPTER 1

'Confronting the Monster': Exploring the Implementation of Social Protection Measures Amid COVID-19 in South Africa

BEAUTY ZINDI[1] and ELVIN SHAVA[2]

[1]Department of Public Administration, Faculty of Management and Commerce, University of Fort Hare, South Africa

[2]School of Public Management, Governance, and Public Policy, College of Business and Economics, University of Johannesburg, South Africa, E-mail: ellyshava@gmail.com

ABSTRACT

The COVID-19 pandemic triggered severe social and economic effects in South Africa, resulting in many people losing their jobs. This had a negative bearing on household income. Accompanied by long-existing social-economic disparities in South Africa, COVID-19 has adversely affected impoverished South African households that rely on government social protection programs to sustain their livelihoods. In response to the unanticipated effects of COVID-19, the government of South Africa quickly implemented social protection measures, including COVID-19 Social Relief of Distress Grant, Social Support Grants, the National Disaster Benefit, and the COVID-19 Temporary Relief Scheme, compensation fund, and the unemployment insurance fund (UIF). These measures were aimed at lessening the burden of the pandemic on poor households in both urban and rural communities. Utilizing a constructivist paradigm that adopts a qualitative approach, the chapter uses document analysis to explore the implementation of social protection measures during COVID-19 in South Africa. The chapter further assesses the challenges faced by the government of South Africa in rendering relief aid as a response to the effects of COVID 19. The findings of the chapter revealed that the distribution of COVID-19 aid was characterized by corruption. Lack of capacity among local municipalities was also noted; these struggled to deal with homeless people. Alleviating household poverty was also a challenge experienced by the government, as the money and food hampers were not enough to support the many hungry families. We conclude that apart from government support, stakeholder intervention was required to assist struggling families and unemployed people, as COVID-19 has uprooted the livelihoods of many citizens. We recommend that the government of South Africa should increase its role as a welfare provider as well as collaborate with stakeholders towards easing the brunt of COVID-19 in communities.

1.1   INTRODUCTION

The COVID-19 pandemic has so far infected over 14 million people and triggered over 600,000 fatalities globally. It has proved to be one of the major challenges of the 21st century; hence, it has been declared a global pandemic so that countries globally can adopt measures to mitigate its spread [1]. Several countries were caught unaware, and therefore struggled to withstand the shocks triggered by this pandemic on the economies, social, and political lives of the people. Most research conducted ever since the outbreak of COVID-19 indicates that the pandemic is already wreaking havoc by disrupting social and economic functions and subjecting people to lives of misery and poverty [2]. Experts have indicated that although COVID-19 infections are indiscriminate, there are some profound and significant demographic variations in its impacts [3]. The burdens triggered by the pandemic created devastation among poor individuals and communities. To contain the effects of this pandemic, some governments, including South Africa, implemented some drastic social and economic strategies to slow the spread of the pandemic [4].

In South Africa, which is one of the countries affected the worst by this global pandemic, early actions that range from large economic stimulus packages and the lowering of interest rates have been initiated as social safety nets for millions of their citizens [5]. Apart from socio-economic measures taken by many countries globally, lockdown restrictions were imposed to minimize the spread of the virus, which resulted in people staying at home [6]. This chapter responds to the following questions:

Which social protection measures did the South African government implement to assist citizens affected by the COVID-19 pandemic?

What are the challenges faced by the South African government in offering relief support to citizens who fell victim to COVID-19 pandemic?

This chapter is structured as follows. After the introduction, the first section offers an overview of the COVID-19 situation in South Africa. The second describes the theoretical and empirical perspectives guiding the chapter, and this is followed by a section on the social protection measures undertaken by the government of South Africa in response to the COVID-19 pandemic. The 4th section discusses the role of the local government amid COVID-19 in South Africa. The 5th section focuses on presentation, analysis, and discussion of findings. The last section concludes and offers recommendations, including direction for further research for the South African government to respond to the effects of COVID-19 effectively.

1.2   OVERVIEW OF THE COVID-19 SITUATION IN SOUTH AFRICA

South Africa is currently facing huge challenges in controlling the COVID-19 pandemic that is spreading very fast with various levels of fatalities across the globe [7]. The virus, which started in Wuhan, China in late 2019, has become a worldwide epidemic within a very short time [1]. Countries such as Italy, Spain, United Kingdom (UK), France, and the United States were severely attacked in terms of infections and deaths regardless of their highly improved and well-equipped health service systems [9]. This has raised great concern for the African continent, which has relatively weak health systems compared to Europe and the Global North, and for the wide expanse of areas on the continent with no health services or health systems in place [10]. While Africa is among the regions that were affected last by the virus, the first case of COVID-19 was reported in Egypt on February 14, 2020, and more than 34,000 cases were confirmed by the end of April [11].

South Africa announced its first case of COVID-19 on March 5 in 2020, and currently has one of the highest confirmed cases on the African continent. Available data shows that as of 15 September 2020, South Africa had recorded 650,749 confirmed COVID-19 cases, of which 579,289 had recovered while 15,499 had died of the pandemic [12]. Global data also reveals that in terms of infections, South Africa is now ranked 5th among the COVID-19 worst affected countries [1]. However, based on mathematical models that help to predict the trends of the pandemic, experts have noted that South Africa has now reached the zenith of the pandemic [14]. Indications are that, increasingly, health care institutions are becoming overwhelmed and unable to cope with treatment and care demands of the pandemic [14]. For Wadvalla [16], the pandemic is indiscriminately affecting all provinces in South Africa, with Gauteng and Western Cape provinces becoming the dual epicenters of the pandemic in the country. In anticipation of a spiraling COVID-19 death toll, authorities in Gauteng and Western Cape provinces have reportedly prepared more than 1 million graves [17]. Although this has attracted criticism from the public, media, and other social analysts, the move was strategic in preparing for the inevitable as the COVID-19 pandemic was ravaging citizens, especially those already suffering from chronic diseases.

Following the outbreak of the COVID-19 pandemic, the government of South Africa outlined and implemented several strategies designed to slow the spread of the pandemic [2]. Among the range of COVID-19 control strategies adopted by South Africa is the imposition of a national lockdown, social distancing, self-isolation/quarantine, practicing self-hygiene, massive testing and treating of the infected as well as cultivating awareness through education and communication programs [10, 17]. Inopportunely, the implementation of these strategies is reportedly accompanied by severe and multifaceted social and economic impacts that are negatively impacting on livelihoods [10]. In many instances, poor people who cannot readily withstand the impacts of the COVID-19 pandemic are in many ways the major reason why the COVID-19 containment strategies are being implemented [2].

While the implementation of the above-mentioned COVID-19 containment and prevention strategies have immensely helped to slow down the spread of the pandemic [23], indications are that these strategies have exposed serious gaps in the country's social protection system. Measures such as social distancing have been noted to be impractical in densely populated communities in which people share basic resources such as water sources, bathrooms, toilets, and public transport [24]. Furthermore, the mandatory national lockdown has been noted to expose people to serious and deepening poverty [24]. Of great concern is that under conditions of a national lockdown, many people involved in the informal sector, including vendors, self-employed, and contract workers, found themselves without incomes and thus unable to afford basic goods and services [26]. As a result, observing, and practicing high levels of hygiene becomes unrealistic due to inefficient and erratic service delivery by local authorities regards the provision of clean water and refuse collection [23].

1.3   THEORETICAL AND EMPIRICAL PERSPECTIVES

The chapter draws from the principal-agent theory, which is commonly used in public administration to explain various problems related to management and administration. The theory was propounded in the 1970s by Ross and Mitnick, and it focuses on contractual relationships between principal and agents [28]. It specifies that one person or entity can arrive at making and taking decisions that will affect another person. According to this theory, the principal has the authority to give instructions and responsibilities to the principal [29]. As research indicates [30], an agent carries his or her work as a steward of the principal and works towards accomplishing the set goals. Relating to the study, principal refers to the government while agents are government arms such as the Department of Social Development and local municipalities that execute government programs and offer social protection assistance such as food hampers and social and relief grants to the communities on behalf of the government. The principal assigns duties and responsibilities to agents to execute, and it is in the best interest of agents to accomplish the objectives set by the principal (government) by providing relief support during stressful times such as the COVID-19 pandemic [31]. The theory emphasizes that the principal (government) and agent (munici-palities) should work collectively towards providing basic services to the citizens effectively and efficiently.

This theory is very crucial in this chapter as it encourages collectiveness and interdependence of the national, provincial, and local governments in the distribution of relief and social protection assistance amid COVID-19 pandemic in South Africa. However, the principal-agent assumptions are made difficult if any of several following conditions exist goal incongruity, uncertainty, information asymmetry, agent risk and interdependence [32]. Therefore, provision of social protection assistance during COVID-19 demands collaborative and mutual understating between the government and implementing agencies, which is essential to minimize corruption and diversion of relief support to struggling communities.

1.4   SOCIAL PROTECTION MEASURES IMPLEMENTED BY THE SOUTH AFRICAN GOVERNMENT

Social protection can generally be understood as constituting various poli-cies and programs designed to reduce the impact of poverty and vulnerability through increasing people's accessibility and participation in the labor market, diminishing their exposure to risks and building their capacities to withstand economic and social volatilities [33]. According to Jha and Acharya [34], the concept of social protection is premised on the view that there are certain situations that elevate people's vulnerability to social and economic injustices. Among other factors [35] singled out old age, unemployment, exclusion, sickness, and disability as key factors responsible for creating and sustaining social and economic inequalities and exacerbating people's vulnerability to poverty and other undesirable social and economic ills. In lieu of these vulnerabilities, governments design and implement various social protection measures to protect people against adverse social and economic outcomes [33]. Given the foregoing analysis, in this chapter, social protection measures can be construed as the various strategies employed by a government or entity of government designed to protect citizens against both anticipated and unanticipated social and economic shocks and or disruptions.

Indications are that social protection measures are important not only because of their ability to protect individuals and families against poverty and its attendant impacts, but they also provide requisite stimulation for economic growth and enhancing social solidarity and stability [35]. As research indicates [38], sustainable social protection measures are crucial as they relay the message that the authorities care about citizens or residents. Recent research revealed that social protection is increasingly becoming an important and indispensable component of good governance [34, 39]. Therefore, efficient, accountable, and accessible social protection programs and policies amid COVID-19 are a strategic instrument in public administration systems [41]. Drawing from this background, the government of South Africa implemented various social protection programs that were a response to the COVID-19 pandemic. These are discussed in subsections.

1.4.1   UNEMPLOYMENT INSURANCE FUND (UIF)

In response to the effects of COVID-19, the South African government announced a set of economic mitigation and relief measures, including an extension of the Unemployment Insurance Fund (UIF) to stipulate paid sick leave and income support to the affected employees [9]. Besides, the government created a Solidarity Fund to offer economic support to individuals, companies, and foundations. The UIF is one of the major social protection measures that have proved efficient and critical in South Africa during the COVID-19 pandemic [36]. The UIF is a contributory social protection strategy that is largely available to people in formal employment [44]. People who are formally employed are statutorily required to make monthly contributions to the fund through deductions from their monthly incomes [36]. Upon losing incomes due to illness, reduced work time and unemployment, contributors can make claims to sustain themselves during the period of having no income [44]. Notably, the UIF is not specifically designed to cushion people against COVID-19 but has been instrumental in helping many people overcome economic challenges associated with loss of income due to the COVID-19 pandemic.

1.4.2   COMPENSATION FUND

South Africa is also providing social protection to employed people through the Compensation Fund [36]. According to Ref. [40], the Compensation Fund in South Africa is a special social protection scheme that provides compensation to employees who are hurt on duty or become sick due to a disease contracted at work or for death that happens because of these injuries or diseases. Furthermore, the Compensation Fund is availed to employees by the employer and is mainly covering permanent employees, domestic workers in a boarding house, an apprentice or trainee farmworker and workers who are paid by a labor agency [36]. While the Compensation Fund is a generic social protection scheme, it (the fund) assumed an important role of availing social protection cover to employees who are vulnerable to contracting COVID-19 in the line of their work [40].

1.4.3   NATIONAL DISASTER BENEFIT AND THE COVID-19 TEMPORARY RELIEF SCHEME (C19 TERS)

Social protection during the COVID-19 pandemic in South Africa has also been provided through the National Disaster Benefit [21]. This scheme is a COVID-19 specific relief that was designed to provide respite during the national lockdown [45]. The scheme, which is closely linked to the UIF, provides financial assistance to help in cases where the employer is unable to pay his/her employees because of the impacts of the pandemic [46]. The scheme is a temporary measure that specifically caters for employers who, due to forced closure, are not able to remunerate their employees [40]. The

National Disaster Benefit scheme has proved to be invaluable during the national lockdown [40].

1.4.4   SOCIAL SUPPORT GRANTS

Social protection in South Africa is also provided within the precincts of several non-contributory social support grants, including the child support grant, care dependency grant, disability grant, war veterans grant, old age grant and Social Relief of Distress grant [37]. These grants constitute the backbone of South Africa's social protection system and are a major social protection shield during the COVID-19 turbulence. The government has increased the child support grant from R440 to R740 per child and caregivers received an additional R500 for the period May 2020 to December 2020 [5]. The government of South Africa mobilized R50 billion towards social support grants to improve the social and economic measures to address the impacts of the COVID-19 pandemic [13]. This amount has been used to increase the value of existing social grants, start a new grant, and allow the delivery of food parcels to the poorest households.

1.4.5   COVID 19-SOCIAL RELIEF OF DISTRESS GRANT

As part of social protection, the South African government implemented the COVID-19 Social Relief of Distress Grant. This grant assisted citizens in vulnerable people in communities to alleviate hunger during the lockdown period. The grant amounted to R350 per month for those who were not benefitting from either social grants or UIF [9]. Nevertheless, this grant is not adequate to alleviate household poverty, hence COVID-19, exposed some weaknesses and deficiencies in the social welfare system of South Africa. Furthermore, the social relief programs were aimed at eradicating hunger in many households by expanding the UIF. Unfortunately, about 45% of the workforce were not eligible for the fund as they earned way above the gazetted R350 monthly salary [20, 36]. The majority were excluded from benefiting from the UIF and only a mere percentage receives social support through the child support grant [20]. This exclusion left more than 8 million people without any source of income and therefore struggling to put food on the table [16]. The increase of social grants alongside the new COVID-19 grants provided relief to most poor households who were adversely affected by the total lockdown.

1.5   ROLE OF LOCAL GOVERNMENT AMID COVID-19 IN SOUTH AFRICA

As enshrined in Ref. [43], local government is the closest sphere to the communities, and it must render quality services. With COVID-19 outbreak, local government became the government-implementing agent, as it helped with water sanitation and information, among other services. Whereas the responsibility of ensuring social protection of citizens during an emergency such as the ongoing COVID-19 in South African is mainly of the central government, analysts have noted that local authorities constitute the vehicles through which the government delivers specific social protection benefits and services to citizens [47]. According to Ref. [16], the proximity of local authorities to communities positions them as the main conduits through which the central government and provincial governments can provide vital social protection and other COVID-19 control services to the public.

1.6   CHALLENGES ENCOUNTERED BY THE SOUTH AFRICAN GOVERNMENT IN THE IMPLEMENTATION OF SOCIAL PROTECTION MEASURES

The following subsections offer an extensive analysis of data drawn from expansive and extant literature sources. Through a qualitative thematic analysis, many challenges that were experienced by local municipalities as agents of government are discussed.

1.6.1   WATER, HYGIENE, AND SANITATION (W.A.S.H) IMPEDIMENTS

Due to the burgeoning population, especially in many urban areas of South Africa, the provision of clean water and sanitation was poor. This increased the risk of residents of informal settlements contracting the coronavirus. Since the outbreak of COVID-19, many people could not access essential goods and services needed to ensure high-quality hygiene to survive the ongoing pandemic [23]. Research indicates that a sustainable supply of clean water is one of the key services in the fight against COVID-19 [36]. In addition, reliable water supply is a critical ingredient needed in maintaining high standards of personal hygiene towards ensuring the prevention of the spread of COVID-19 [18]. Following the World Health Organization (WHO) standard COVID-19 prevention strategies [1], people are encouraged to wash their hands regularly and to keep their bodies well hydrated. Nevertheless, the shortage of clean water supply in some municipalities in South Africa triggered vulnerability as citizens were exposed to the COVID-19 pandemic. Apart from the challenges that confronted local municipalities as agents of the government, social protection inspired responses for COVID-19 were strategic and aimed at improving the supply of clean water services to local communities [23]. Notable efforts of providing clean water were witnessed in the Western Cape Province in which the City of Cape Town rolled out a fleet of 28 water trucks to supply water to over 200,000 households in informal settlements [27]. The strategic intervention of the Western Cape government was not matched by Eastern Cape and Gauteng municipalities, as these took long to unblock water meters for defaulting residents [13]. Further social protection measures were noted in the Valley Municipality in the Western Cape Province, where a debt relief program that targets indigents was implemented to assist households struggling to settle municipal accounts [27].

Similarly, municipalities in Eastern Cape provinces that include Chris Hani, Blue Crane, Route, Makana, Kouga, OR Tambo, Amathole, Alfred Nzo, and Joe Gqabi embarked on borehole drilling and water tank installation programs for water-stressed communities, including informal settlements [18]. Efforts of these municipalities to fulfill the principal-agent theory where municipalities as agents of the government (principal) acted honestly by assisting communities with clean water supplies required to survive the ravaging COVID-19 pandemic were observed.

1.6.2 *INADEQUATE CAPACITY TO ACCOMMODATE HOMELESS PEOPLE*

After President Ramaphosa declared a lockdown in South Africa, the plight of homeless people in many urban areas became an issue of concern, and local municipalities were tasked to find shelter for these vulnerable people to stop the spread of COVID-19. As revealed by a study [9], settling the homeless people and in proper shelter was a challenge, as many resisted despite the danger of spreading the virus in illegal settlements that were not connected to any service delivery systems. In another study [10], researchers lament the failure by homeless people to abide by the requisite COVID-19 prevention strategies such as social self-quarantine; this was a ticking time bomb for the spread of COVID-19.

Apart from lack of capacity to cater for the homeless groups, research affirms that some urban municipalities in the Western Cape, Gauteng, and Mpumalanga provinces successfully accommodated the homeless in protective shelter [23]. In a recent study [11], have highlighted the example of Western Cape Province, in which the local authority designated a local municipal park to accommodate homeless people from Knysna and Sedgefield. Concurrently, local municipalities in the North West, Limpopo, Gauteng, and Mpumalanga Provinces also provided the homeless with shelter, which was a commendable step towards containing the spread of COVID-19 [9]. As agents of the government, local municipalities played a collaborative role, which was strategic to alleviate the impacts of COVID-19.

1.6.3   FOOD INSECURITY CHALLENGES

The devastating effects of COVID-19 in South Africa include severe food insecurity among rural and urban households. A study conducted by Arndt et al. [21], attests to this sentiment as it revealed that COVID-19 pandemic triggered food insecurity among low-income households in South Africa. Observations from Ref. [1] corroborate the food insecurity challenges, as low-income households in developing countries have been exposed to severe household food insecurity amid COVID-19 pandemic Household food security during the ongoing COVID-19 was exacerbated by market speculations that resulted in panic buying [1], thus prompting increases in the prices of basic food staffs [21]. In South Africa, local authorities, as agents acting on behalf of the principal (government), provided social protection through the establishment of soup kitchens and running residential nutrition programs in the established emergency shelters [11]. Reports show that local authorities responsible for Knysna and Sedgefield are running a successful soup kitchen program, which is mainly benefiting homeless and other indigent individuals and households that are food insecure [20]. Furthermore, towards ameliorating food insecurity in and around Gauteng, local governments embarked on food hamper distribution programs targeting food-insecure households [20]. These programs proved essential in alleviating hunger and promoting livelihoods of many households that were affected by the pandemic and its attendant mitigation strategies [11].

1.6.4   INCREASED PRESSURE TO PROVIDE PRIMARY HEALTH CARE SERVICES TO COVID-19 PATIENTS

One of the devastating impacts of the ongoing COVID-19 pandemic in South Africa is that it exerts excessive pressure on the primary health care system of the country [2]. Analysts have indicated that increasingly, the public health care system of the country is becoming overwhelmed by the exponentially rising number of people seeking medical treatment and care [18]. One of the fundamental social protection virtues relates to the provision of high-quality primary health care services [1]. In accordance with the requirements of the Municipal Structures Act, which mandates local authorities to contribute towards the provision of primary health care services, many local authorities in South Africa have played significant roles [22]. Accordingly, local author-ities across the country have been active in providing deep cleaning and fumigation of contaminated surfaces and facilities [11]. In the Eastern Cape, local authorities in partnership with the provincial government have been noted to be undertaking massive testing of suspected cases and conducting contact-tracing exercises [15]. Furthermore [18], elevated contributions of local authorities in rolling out mass screening, targeted tracing and testing of contacts of victims of the pandemic, vulnerable individuals and those with symptoms More so, as already indicated, local authorities across the country have been noted to be seized with the task of establishing, operating, and funding the operations of quarantine and isolation centers for those whose home situations do not allow for effective self-isolation and quarantining [15]. Towards promoting healthy lifestyles, local authorities in the country have also been noted to be closely involved in rolling out massive education and awareness campaigns [11].

1.6.5   LIMITED CAPACITY TO RESPOND TO COVID-19

The analysis of expansive literature sources indicated that local authorities in South Africa could not deliver effective and sustainable social and economic services to enhance the livelihoods of the people. A study conducted by Swanepoel and Labuschagine [25] indicates that more than 55% of the population is struggling to make ends meet Reality is that the municipalities are failing to deliver quality services to enhance the lives of the majority. Indications are that when faced with the COVID-19 pandemic and after receiving directives from the central and provincial governments, many local authorities around the country managed to deliver water services to some communities that had been facing water problems since independence. Assessing the ongoing social protection focused responses by local authorities to the impacts of COVID-19 in South Africa, one can suggest there is a need to continue situating post-COVID-19 recovery and reconstruction agendas on the same human rights inspired trajectory. The current crisis has proved that while the mandate of local authorities revolves around service delivery, to deliver on this mandate effectively, authorities need to adopt a human right thinking for interventions to be inclusive.

1.6.6   CORRUPTION IN THE DISTRIBUTION OF COVID-19 PARCELS

Upholding accountability and transparency in the distribution of food parcels for COVID-19 and Personal Protective Clothing (PPEs) was a challenge among various agencies in South Africa [19]. The provision of food parcels during the COVID-19 period was characterized by high levels of corruption and political interference [42]. As noted by Ref. [13], the delivery of food parcels to vulnerable communities was marred by corruption, which led the President of South Africa to call for the arrest of people who misused the $26 billion economic relief package of the COVID-19 aid. Recently, the Public Protector's office complained of the many cases of misconduct related to COVID-19 grants. Many of these cases were related to the R350 COVID-19 relief scheme, in which the systematic exclusion of citizens was rife. Many people were systematically disqualified over unreasonable grounds, which may relate to corrupt activities of those at the helm of these relief programs [8]. Further analysis of the reports indicates that accessing the UIF was a challenge for many people as their applications were declined on the ground that they earned some income. It can be noted from these assertions that corruption in the COVID-19 relief grants was rampant, which diminished the government's efforts of providing social protection to vulnerable citizens amid the COVID-19 pandemic.

1.7   CONCLUSION AND RECOMMENDATIONS

Drawing from the Principal Agency Theory, the chapter revealed the challenges that confronted the South African government in rendering social protection programs to vulnerable people in communities amid the COVID-19 pandemic. The analyzes of literature sources highlighted corruption as an impediment in the distribution of food parcels for COVID-19 in communities. Unscrupulous leaders hijacked the distribution program, with some diverting the relief funds and resources to their personal use. This is in contrary to the Agency Theory, which requires agents (municipalities, social workers, community development workers) to adhere to the principal (government). Further analysis pointed to extended impoverishment of the citizens in communities, as lockdown regulations prevented the informal sector from thriving. This is an income-generating sector for many people in the country. The provision of social protection assistance in the form of the UIF, for instance, was not enough to curb the deep poverty among South Africans who reside in informal settlements. Whereas the role of government in assisting the vulnerable is emulated, more must be done to ensure that stakeholders combine resources to assist the needy. Based on the findings, therefore, the researchers recommend that the government of South Africa decentralize COVID-19 support offices and channel more resources to grassroots agents such as municipalities and the Department of Social Development. This is fundamental for quick decision-making and effective intervention in households affected by the COVID-19 pandemic. Further empirical research in social protection can be conducted to assess the relationship between social protection and poverty reduction in rural municipalities in South Africa.

KEYWORDS

- **COVID-19**
- **local government**
- **poverty alleviation**
- **social protection measures**
- **South Africa**
- **unemployment insurance fund**
- **water, hygiene, and sanitation**

REFERENCES

1. World Health Organization, (2020). *Water, Sanitation, Hygiene and Waste Management for COVID-19: Technical Brief (No. WHO/2019-NcOV/IPC_WASH/2020.1)*. World Health Organization.

2. Dalufeya, G., (2020). Social and emergency assistance ex-ante and during COVID-19 in the SADC region. *The International Journal of Community and Social Development, 2*(2), 251–268. doi.org/10.1177%2F2516602620936028.

3. Chowdhury, R., Heng, K., Shawon, M. S. R., Goh, G., Okonofua, D., Ochoa-Rosales, C., & Shahzad, S., (2020). Dynamic interventions to control COVID-19 pandemic: A multivariate prediction modeling study comparing 16 worldwide countries. *European Journal of Epidemiology, 35*(5), 389–399. doi.org/10.1007/s10654-020-00649-w.

4. Bodrud-Doza, M., Shammi, M., Bahlman, L., Islam, A. R. M., & Rahman, M., (2020). Psychosocial and socio-economic crisis in Bangladesh due to COVID-19 pandemic: A perception-based assessment. *Frontiers in Public Health, 8*(3), 1–19. doi.org/10.3389/fpubh.2020.00341.

5. Khambule, I., (2020). The effects of COVID-19 on the South African informal economy: Limits and pitfalls of government's response. *Loyola Journal of Social Sciences, 34*(1), 91–109.

6. Wells, C. R., Stearns, J. K., Lutumba, P., & Galvani, A. P., (2020). COVID-19 on the African continent. *The Lancet; Infectious Diseases.* S1473-3099(20)30374-1. doi.org/10.1016/S1473-3099(20)30374-1.

7. Sekyere, E., Muller, N. B., Hongoro, C., & Makoae, M., (2020). *The Impact of COVID-19 in South Africa.* Africa Program Occasional Paper, Wilson Center. https://reliefweb.int/report/south-africa/impact-covid-19-south-africa (accessed on 26 June 2021).

8. BusinessTech., (2020). *Flood of Complaints Around Coronavirus Corruption in South Africa.* https://businesstech.co.za/news/government/422148/flood-of-complaints-around-coronavirus-corruption-in-south-africa/ (accessed on 26 June 2021).

9. Staunton, C., Swanepoel, C., & Labuschagine, M., (2020). Between a rock and a hard place: COVID-19 and South Africa's response. *Journal of Law and the Biosciences, 3*(2), 1–7. Lsaa052, doi.org/10.1093/jlb/lsaa052.

10. Byaro, M., (2020). *Comment: Africa Lockdowns Due to COVID-19 and Its Effects on Household's Socioeconomic Livelihood, 12*(1), 73–83.

11. Melzer, I., & Rust, K., (2020). *COVID-19 and Housing - Strategies for Resilience in South Africa.* http://housingfinanceafrica.org/documents/covid-and-housing-strategies-for-resilience-in-south-africa/ (accessed on 26 June 2021).

12. Department of Health South Africa, (2020). *Update on COVID-19.* Media Statement. https://sacoronavirus.co.za/2020/09/14/update-on-covid-19-14th-september-2020/ (accessed on 26 June 2021).

13. Wegerif, M. C., (2020). "Informal" food traders and food security: Experiences from the COVID-19 response in South Africa. *Food Security,* 1–4.

14. Ellis, C., (2020). Knowledge, attitudes, and practices towards COVID-19 among Chinese residents during the rapid rise period of the COVID-19 outbreak: A quick online cross-sectional survey. *International Journal of Biological Science, 16*(10), 1745–1752.

15. Parliamentary Monitoring Group, (2020). *COVID-19 State of Disaster and Lockdown Regulations: Update.* https://pmg.org.za/blog/COVID-19%20State%20of%20Disaster%20and%20Lockdown%20Regulations:%20Update%20(3%20August%202020) (accessed on 26 June 2021).

16. Wadvalla, B. A., (2020). *COVID-19: Decisive Action is the Hallmark of South Africa's Early Success Against Coronavirus.* PMID: 32332021. doi: 10.1136/bmj.m1623.

17. Reimann, N., (2020). *South Africa Readies 1.5 Million Graves For Coronavirus Mass Burials.* https://www.forbes.com/sites/nicholasreimann/2020/07/08/south-africa-readies-

15-million-graves-for-coronavirus-mass-burials/#73da78c745a6 (accessed on 26 June 2021).

18. Parliamentary Monitoring Group (PMG) (2020). Update on healthcare services in relation to COVID-19: Eastern & Western Cape Provincial Departments of Health briefings. https://pmg.org.za/page/Update%20on%20healthcare%20services%20 in%20relation%20to%20COVID-19:%20Eastern%20&%20Western%20Cape%20 Provincial%20Departments%20of%20Health%20briefings (accessed on 10 July 2021).

19. Basia, D., Khotso, T., & Eden, K. G., (2017). Evaluation capacity assessment of the transport sector in South Africa: An innovative approach research. *African Evaluation Journal, 5*(1), 1–8.

20. Polity, (2020). *COVID-19: Municipal Update.* https://www.polity.org.za/article/covid-19-municipal-update-2020-04-08 (accessed on 26 June 2021).

21. Arndt, C., Davies, R., Gabriel, S., Harris, L., Makrelov, K., Robinson, S., & Anderson, L., (2020). COVID-19 lockdowns, income distribution, and food security: An analysis for South Africa. *Global Food Security.* Elsevier B.V. doi.org/10.1016/ j.gfs.2020.100410.

22. TamFum, J. M., Kallay, M. S., & Nachega, J. B., (2020). Limiting the spread of COVID-19 in Africa: One size mitigation strategy does not fit all countries. *The Lancet Global Health, 8*(7), 24–39.

23. Corburn, J., Vlahov, D., Mberu, B., Riley, L., Caiaffa, W. T., Rashid, S. F., Ko, A., et al., (2020). Slum health: Arresting COVID-19 and improving well-being in urban informal settlements. *Journal of Urban Health: Bulletin of the New York Academy of Medicine, 97*(3), 348–357. doi.org/10.1007/s11524-020-00438-6.

24. Mehtar, S., Preiser, W., Lakhe, N. A., Bousso, A., TamFum, J. J. M., Kallay, O., & Nachega, J. B., (2020). Limiting the spread of COVID-19 in Africa: One size mitigation strategies do not fit all countries. *The Lancet Global Health, 8*(7), 24–39. doi.org/10.1016/ S2214-109X(20)30212-6.

25. Huck, K. A., & Shmis, T. (2020). Managing the impact of COVID-19 on education systems around the world: How countries are preparing, coping, and planning for recovery. https://blogs.worldbank.org/education/managing-impact-covid-19-education-systems-around-world-how-countries-are-preparing (accessed on 10 July 2021).

26. Gilbert, M., Pullano, G., Pinotti, F., Valdano, E., Poletto, C., Boëlle, P. Y., & Gutierrez, B., (2020). Preparedness and vulnerability of African countries against importations of COVID-19: A modeling study. *The Lancet, 395*(10227), 871–877. doi: 10.1016/ S0140-6736(20)30411-6.

27. Stiegler, N., & Bouchard, J. P., (2020). South-Africa: Challenges and successes of the COVID-19 lockdown. In: *Annales Médico-Psychologiques, Revue Psychiatrique.* Elsevier Masson.

28. Raaÿ, E. M., (2014). Opportunism and honest incompetence in public procurement. *Journal of Public Administration Research and Theory, 25*, 953–979.

29. Ross, S. A., (1973). The economic theory of agency: The principal's problem. *The American Journal of Economics, 10*(4), 23–39.

30. Mitnick, B., (1973). Fiduciary rationality and public policy: The theory of agency and some consequences. *Paper Presented at the Annual Meeting of the American Political Science Association.* New Orleans, L.A.

31. Gauld, R., (2007). Principal-agent theory and organizational change: Lessons from New Zealand health information management. *Policy Studies, 28*, 17–34. doi. org/10.1080/01442870601121395.

32. Simonsen, B., & Hill, L., (1998). Municipal bond issuance: Is there evidence of a principal-agent problem? *Public Budgeting and Finance, 18*(4), 71–100. doi.org/10.1046/j.0275-1100.1998.01150.x.

33. Devereux, S., (2016). Social protection for enhanced food security in sub-Saharan Africa. *Food Policy, 60,* 52–62. doi: 10.1016/j.foodpol.2015.03.009.

34. Jha, P., & Acharya, N., (2016). Public provisioning for social protection and its implications for food security. *Economic & Political Weekly, 51*(18), 99.

35. Moor, I., Spallek, J., & Richter, M., (2017). Explaining socioeconomic inequalities in self-rated health: A systematic review of the relative contribution of material, psychosocial and behavioral factors. *Journal of Epidemiology Community Health, 71*(6), 565–575. doi: 10.1136/jech-2016-207589.

36. Olivier, J., Kruger, A., & Johnson, S., (2020). Avoiding potential retrenchments flowing from COVID-19: Employment law/COVID-19. *Without Prejudice, 20*(4), 6–8.

37. Chagunda, C., (2019). The South African Social Grant System: A positive effect on poverty alleviation and unforeseen socio-cultural consequences. *Gender and Behavior, 17*(4), 14237–14250.

38. Shore, J., & Shore, & Plant, (2019). *Welfare State and the Democratic Citizen.* Springer International Publishing.

39. Loopstra, R., Reeves, A., McKee, M., & Stuckler, D., (2016). Food insecurity and social protection in Europe: Quasi-natural experiment of Europe's great recessions 2004–2012. *Preventive Medicine, 89,* 44–50. doi.org/10.1016/j.ypmed.2016.05.010.

40. George, R., & George, A., (2020). Compensation for occupationally acquired COVID-19. *SAMJ: South African Medical Journal, 110*(5), 1. doi.org/10.7196%2FSAMJ.2020.v110i5.14743.

41. Persson, T., Parker, C. F., & Widmalm, S., (2017). Social trust, impartial administration and public confidence in EU crisis management institutions. *Public Administration, 95*(1), 97–114. doi.org/10.1111/padm.12295.

42. Transparency International, (2020). *In South Africa COVID 19 Has Exposed Greedy and Spurred Long Needed Action Against Corruption.* https://www.transparency.org/en/blog/in-south-africa-covid-19-has-exposed-greed-and-spurred-long-needed-action-against-corruption (accessed on 26 June 2021).

43. Republic of South Africa, (1998). *White Paper on Local Government-1998 Pretoria.* Government Printer.

44. Seepamore, B., (2018). Indigenous social security systems: A South African perspective. *Indigenous Social Security Systems in Southern and West Africa,* 71–87.

45. Bhorat, H., Oosthuizen, M., & Stanwix, B., (2020). *Social Assistance Amidst the COVID-19 Epidemic in South Africa: An Impact Assessment.* Development policy research unit working paper 202006. DPRU, University of Cape Town.

46. Mukumbang, F. C., Ambe, A. N., & Adebiyi, B. O., (2020). Unspoken inequality: How COVID-19 has exacerbated existing vulnerabilities of asylum-seekers, refugees, and undocumented migrants in South Africa. *International Journal of Equity Health, 19,* 141 doi.org/10.1186/s12939-020-01259-4.

47. Yanow, S. K., & Good, M. F., (2020). Nonessential research in the new normal: The impact of COVID-19. *The American Journal of Tropical Medicine and Hygiene, 102*(6), 1164.

CHAPTER 2

The Responsibility of State in Combating COVID-19: The Experience of India, Pakistan, Afghanistan, and Maldives

DEBASISH NANDY

Kazi Nazrul University, West Bengal, India,
E-mail: debasishnandy.kc@gmail.com

ABSTRACT

The question of state responsibility has been raised in the wake of the pandemic COVID-19. The nature and profile of the South Asian states are different. The South Asian states have often been criticized for not performing their responsibilities. COVID-19 has changed this myth. The private-public debate has posed in a new manner. Despite constraints, the role of the states has been positively manifested in the South Asian context, but at the same time, there are so many critics raised against the state. In the era of globalization, a debate is raised about the existence of state welfares. This pandemic has proved the essentiality of the state. The new managerial perception of the state has come forward due to COVID-19. There are three objectives of this study: (i) to search the responsibility of the selected South Asian states in combatting COVID-19. (ii) To make a comparative study among the selected states to identify the managerial perspective in combatting the situation. (iii) To explore the new policies of the states to handle the pandemic. This study based on a mixed-method: (a) content analysis method; and (b) observation method. The current study offers a new dimension of state responsibility and how civil society does matter.

2.1 INTRODUCTION

The COVID-19 has posed a tremendous threat to human civilization. It appears to be the most dangerous threat to human security in the post-II World War scenario. The viral pandemic then started quickly in December 2019, spread worldwide, and shook the whole world. There is no doubt that fundamentally the pandemic will change the socio-ecological fabric of human communities and societies in the longer run [1]. Most of the countries have been highly affected due to coronavirus which originated from Wuhan city of China and later on, spread across the globe. The question of the responsibility of the state has been raised as a core question in the contemporary world order. The role of China in handling coronavirus and humanitarian treatment to the citizens of China by the Chinese government has been vehemently criticized by the global community. However, the present study will deal with the experience of selected South Asian states. How India, Pakistan, Afghanistan, and the Maldives have handled the COVID-19 that will be critically analyzed in this study. I have chosen four different types of countries in terms of the nature of the state and economy. I would make a comparative study on the responsibility of these four different states critically. Among the three South Asian states, Afghanistan is a war-torn and terrorism-affected state which has been struggling to get a bailout from restless terrorism. The Maldives is the smallest vulnerable island states of South Asia. The over-dependent state system has been facing financial and health care problems due to COVID-19. Both India and Pakistan achieved their independence at the same time based on two different nature of state systems. The post-colonial South Asian societies are suffering from social unrest, ethnic conflicts, religious riots, political violence, terrorism, and civil wars. It is also found that the state itself is responsible for the spreading and lingering of violence for the sake of certain groups. However, the pandemic COVID-19 posed a new challenge to the South Asian states which compelled to rethinking about Human Security through a new outlook. However, the concept of Human Security is a post-Cold War development [2]. The pandemic COVID-19 is considered non-traditional security that affected the entire world.

2.2 RESEARCH QUESTIONS

There are three research questions of this study:

1. Are all South Asian states duly fulfilling their responsibility equally in dealing with all sections of the society to combat COVID-19?

2. Is the state the only actor for rescuing its people in a pandemic? and
3. Are the financial and infrastructural factors crux of the COVID-19 challenges?

2.3   EXPERIMENTAL METHODS AND MATERIALS

The present study is based on two research methodologies:

- Content analysis; and
- Observation method.

The present study is based on both primary and secondary sources. I have used the reports, books, journals, newspapers, and various websites to conduct the study.

2.4   CONCEPTUALIZING THE STATE RESPONSIBILITY

In the era of globalization, the question of the responsibility of the states has revolved around the intellectuals. The common perception about the state now is less responsible state due to the interference of MNCs, and other private agencies in most of the sectors. The idea of global governance is an outcome of globalization, and the concept of the welfare state has been challenged. For, the third world states, whether the very concept of world government would be useful or not that has been questioned by eminent scholar of International Relations, Professor Jayantanuja Bandyopadhyaya. He said, "the inadequacy of their domestic power base makes it imperative for them to seek the assistance and protection of a democratic world government for ensuring development and welfare of their people" [3]. However, the South Asian states are not immune from the effect of globalization. The overwhelming involvement in state affairs by the non-governmental agencies raised several questions. Most of the debt-laden and vulnerable South Asian states are often reluctant to fulfilling their due responsibilities for their inability or do not care attitudes.

The nature of the state often does matter. For a military state or puppet state or terrorist state or a vulnerable state, the issue of state responsibility is a utopian idea. The nature of the social fabric and vibrancy of civil society is very important in this regard. The governments of some South Asian states often make them delinked with the people intentionally. It is also true that in a crisis period, it is very difficult to overcome the crisis without citizens' response. The social security emphasis on voluntary citizen involvement rather than on top-down governmental solutions [4]. Participation in civil society and voluntary organizations have made a positive change in many western societies. The will to engage in prosocial efforts to assist the fellow member of the society very much needs to overcome the crisis [5]. The citizens of a country are primarily responsible for protecting their own lives and property, and then they will try to assist others abiding the advisories given by the government. The pandemic situation cannot be overcome by the government alone without the equal response and cooperation of the citizens. The backward societies like Pakistan and Afghanistan and some parts of India are unconsciously disappearing in fighting with the pandemic COVID-19. We cannot avoid the corporate social responsibility (CSR). Often it has been found that the corporate houses are intentionally avoiding their committed social responsibility. The national and transnational companies often forget CSR to confronted with economic and social challenges [6]. It has been proven in the pandemic COVID-19 that the state is still the prime responsible institution to bail out its citizens from the crisis. Although there are lot of criticism about the state's responsibility, yet there is no alternative of the state. Technically speaking, it is necessary to establish coordination among different levels of the government to overcome the crisis. This study attempts to make a comparative study of the selected South Asian states regarding their responsibility in combatting COVID-19.

2.5 INDIAN EXPERIENCE

The post-colonial Indian state failed to meet the aspirations of either of the contending groups and antagonized both in process. The pandemic COVID-19 has brought about a new global order. Due to coronavirus, the entire global economy and international trade, services, and diplomatic relations have been rapidly changing. COVID-19 originated from Wuhan of China (November 2019) and rapidly spread across the globe. Indian economy and foreign policy badly effected due to COVID-19 and India's relational equations with other countries have been changed rapidly changed. The future direction of the Indian economy and Indian foreign policy is struck for further development of global order. The global economy has been in recession from December 2019 to July 2020. The global economic shutdown has raised concerns in the Ministry of Finance. The Central government of India has announced a lockdown for the country from 22nd March 2020. The Union cabinet had approved an ordinance on 6 April 2020 to reduce salaries of the Prime Minister, other ministers, and Members of Parliament. The Central government has given directions to the private sector to continue salary payment to their employees. Due to pandemic COVID-19, thousands of people have lost their jobs. India's response to COVID-19 is quite different than other South Asian states due to its capacity, size, global image, regional responsibility. Despite having internal challenges, India extended assistance to South Asian neighbors, South East Asian, and Middle-eastern countries to fight with COVID-19. The state responsibility of India being the largest democracies in the world made its own identity.

2.5.1   *FINANCIAL CRISIS*

Pandemic COVID-19 had posed a negative impact on the Banking system. Due to long-time lockdown, the domestic and international business and trading were suspended, and the transport system was also stopped, which made a negative impact on the Banking system. From March 2020 to July 2020, the Reserve Bank of India has reduced the rate of interest. Many people have lost their jobs. The remittance has been almost stopped due to COVID-19. The foreign currency reserve has also been reduced due to COVID-19. India is suffering from acute financial hardship and the descending curve of economic development has posed a low economic profile before the global economic order. Regional trade volume has been affected due to COVID-19. The land borders and airlines services are closed, except emergency services, which resulted in a negative impact on India's regional trade. Except for Pakistan, India is the key supplier of the South Asian states. Due to COVID-19, India's overseas business got a setback up to September 2020. Over 20% of export orders have been canceled due to pandemic COVID-19 has resulted in a huge deficit in India's overseas business. Export Promotion Council has warned of an additional $2.7 billion impact in 2019–2020. Similar things happened in the carpet export sector [27].

2.5.2   MARGINALIZED CLASS AND INTERNAL LABOR MIGRATION

Prime Minister Narendra Modi declared lockdown on 24 March 2020 evening without any prior intimation, which resulted in huge problems in socio-economic strata. People were not preparing to stock foods, necessary goods, collecting money, and complete their necessary work. The most problematic issue which has been strongly criticized is the migration laborer. Many migrant laborers were stuck-up stuck in different states and different parts of the globe. Due to lockdown, they had lost their jobs and could not return to their home states. Most of the laborers had to suffer an acute financial crisis. The government of the host states was reluctant to take care of migrant laborers. Due to the food crisis, and health security issues, the migrant laborers wished to return to their homes. Thousands of inhuman incidents took place during the lockdown period. After huge pressure, and criticism raised by the opposition and state government, the central government was agreed to arrange some special train for returning to the laborers to their places. The government is trying to bring back them all, and regarding the issue, political debate and narrow politics are being played by different regional political parties. Primarily, the central government and state governments have to bear the expenses of the fares, and later on, the migrants had to pay their fare. Some states had initiated to bring the laborers by road transport. On 22nd April 2020, a 12-year-old girl had died after walking 150 km from the Telangana to Chhattisgarh. This was not an exceptional incident. Thousands of cases came forward where the death incidents got highlighted by the media. The real economic scenario of the Indian rural economy has been negatively exposed. It was also proven that in handling the crisis in a pandemic situation, the governmental agencies cannot claim the credit. The governmental management system and accountability are unexpectedly dissatisfactory in handling the COVID situation.

There are more than 40 million migrant laborers across the country makes it difficult to provide relief to everyone [7]. Several fatal road accidents were found when the labor force started to move to their hometowns or villages. On 16th May 2020, a fatal road accident in Uttar Pradesh between two trucks carrying 104 migrant workers killed 25 laborers. In some cases, it also noticed that some laborers tried to reach their homes by walking on the train line whether they had been smashed by train engines. Many people have died due to hunger and dehydration. The Indian question is difficult due to overpopulation, poverty, and center-state complicated relations. The situation might not be that serious if the government was given more time to return the migrant laborers in their places or secure food and proper medical facilities. Both the central government and the state government had tried to arrange foods, and other necessities to the migrant laborers after returning home. Some state governments, like the government of West Bengal, had declared for distributing foods to the marginalized people up to June 2021. It was unexpected that, in the pandemic situation, narrow political exercises have been found at the state level, as well as the national level. The Centre-state tug of war regarding the migrant workers posed in a bad manner. The political consideration and voting politics got priority in some cases.

2.5.3 FINANCIAL ASSISTANCE AND FOOD SECURITY FOR THE COMMON PEOPLE

Due to lockdown, around 33 crore poor people had lost their jobs. As the welfare state, how the central government has assisted the marginalized class? The central government has announced a generous relief package for the 33 crore economically vulnerable people. On March 26, the Union Finance Minister, Mrs. Nirmala Sitaraman, announced the "Pradhan Mantri Garib Kalyan Package" of worth Rs. 31,235 crores [8]. The financial package was announced to protect poor people, including women and senior citizens, and health workers from lockdown impact due to COVID-19. Under this package, food grains, and liquid cash were distributed to the poor people. The government has arranged 40.3 metric tons of food grains and also distributed subsidized gas cylinders. The government has also arranged 100 days' work for those people who belonged below the poverty line under the MGNREGA project. Payment has been ensured for the 8.69 crore farmers under the Prime Minister-KISAN project. The state governments have also taken some assis-tance projects for the jobless and poor people providing food grains. During the lockdown period, the state government-run schools have distributed food grains, potato, pulse, sanitizers to the family members of the needy students. Around 20 crore women have received an extra amount of Rs. 500.00 per month as the part of Jan Dhan project. It has been declared by the Union Finance Minister that the government will provide medical insurance to the frontline fighters of COVID-19 which will cover of Rs. 50,00,000 per person.

2.5.4 MANAGING THE PUBLIC HEALTH

Due to the outbreak of COVID-19, the public health sector of India has been severely challenged. The infected cases have been rapidly increased across the country, and in mid-August, it crossed 17,00,000. The government of India had focused on surveillance and screening of all incoming passengers from China. The government of India arranged a thermal checking system in all international airports. Primarily, lacing was found on surveillance. The declaration of suspension of international flights has been delayed. The domestic flight operations and passenger trains were lately stopped. During the ample time-space, coronavirus rapidly spread in the country. The central government has primarily tried to send the medical teams to the states. The number of government hospitals was not adequate in taking admission to COVID patients. The testing kits were not available for the people as per requirement. All state governments have not been able to handle the situation. The country office of WHO has taken several initiatives in association with the government of India in combatting coronavirus. The government of India and WHO collectively set up preparedness and response measures for COVID-19, including surveillance, tracking of COVID-19 affected areas, testing, prevention measures from central to state, and district. At the national level, the country office of India has provided technical support to the Ministry of Health and Family Welfare through the Joint Monitoring Group. It is jointly working with NCDC, ICMR, Disaster Management Authority, and other prime medical and health institutions of India.

The role of all states in combating coronavirus is not satisfactory. Due to lack of medical infrastructure, testing kits, number of doctors, nurses, and ambulance, most of the states have not been able to manage the pandemic situation properly. The center-state debate and political rivalry were shown in many cases regarding the procedure of treatment. There was a strong allegation against some states for hiding the actual figures of infected people. However, the role of the Kerala government in handling the pandemic situation can claim praise. The first Novel Coronavirus Dieses was detected in Kerala. Since the beginning, the government had taken the issue seriously. Kerala has 35 million populations which had been experienced devastating floods in 2018. The presence of governance in Kerala was manifested innovatively. The disaster management was applied in facing the pandemic situation. The government has deployed the management team in infected areas, and surveillance was done from the central control room. Adequate training was given to frontline workers and health personnel. The appreciable thing is that the State Emergency Operations Centre and the office of the Kerala State Disaster Management Authority had jointly provided support to the health sector. The state government has followed the guidance of WHO by tracing, testing, and isolating as many as possible. The lockdown, social distancing, and sanitization process were strictly maintained by the people under the surveillance of the state authority. The Community Kitchen initiative was taken by the local self-government department (LSGD).

2.5.5 IMPACT ON EDUCATION

After the declaration of the lockdown by the central government, the schools, colleges, and universities across the country got closedown. From the last week of March to mid of August 2020, all educational institutions remained close. No decisions have been taken by the central government and state governments regarding the opening of the educational institutions and conducting the examinations. All entrance tests and interviews are suspended. As per the constitution of India, the higher education is in the concurrent list, that is why no unanimous decision cannot be taken by the central government.

In July, the UGC has given directives regarding the conduct of the university examinations in a physical mode in September, but most of the states have opposed this decision looking at the uncontrolled pandemic situation. However, during the lockdown period, online classes have been conducted by educational institutions. The irony of online education is that most of the students who reside in remote areas having economic vulnerability have not been able to take benefit from the online platform. The government of India has encouraged universities and other educational institutions to commence online classes through a digital device. The underprivileged students could not be benefited by online mode of classes due to lack of capacity to access the internet. The Prime Ministers' e-VIDYA scheme has been introduced by the central government amid the lockdown period to encourage technology-based education.

2.5.6 THE VANDE BHARAT MISSION

I have visited Australia via Hong Kong on 10th February 2020. I had stayed there and noticed the effect of coronavirus within the airport and Hong Kong city. In Australia, the effect of the corona was comparatively less. The government of India has taken a very active role in the evacuation of Indian citizens from abroad. The responsibility of the government once has been praised by a section of people, but the opposition parties are very critical about this policy because of demanding a high rate of air ticket from the passengers. However, the government of India can expect credit. Passengers traveling to or through the USA, UK, or Singapore, where foreign nationals are being permitted to travel or transit, are required to show a visa with at least six-month validity. Indians flew in and foreigners flew out on these first-time direct routes like Auckland, Christchurch, Wellington, and Brisbane in Australia, Dublin in Ireland, Lubumbashi in Congo, and Minsk in Belarus. However, other private airlines also started their charter flights operation from Delhi to various destinations of the globe. The 5th phase of the Vande Bharat Mission started on 1st August 2020 for bringing passengers from 52 countries home.

2.5.7   INDIA'S ROLE IN SAARC TO COMBAT COVID-19

Being the second-highest populated country in the world, India has been one of the worst-hit areas by coronavirus that crossed 700,000 by July 2020. Bangladesh and Pakistan together have a larger population than the United States. The two countries combined have more than 200,000 COVID cases in July 2020. Both countries have relaxed their lockdown restrictions. However, India has initiated to ensure treatment for the citizens of SAARC countries through raising funds by the SAARC countries. India started to evacuate her citizens from different countries then citizens of other SAARC member countries were also evacuated by Indian national air careers. India also supplied medical equipment and essential medicines to the SAARC countries like Maldives, Sri Lanka, Bangladesh, Afghanistan, and Bhutan. India initiated a virtual meeting with SAARC countries in March 2020 to raise emergency funds for COVID-19. Except for Pakistan, all countries have contributed as per their capacity. India was the highest contributor and India's paid amount was 10 million USD.

2.5.8   COVID-19 AND INDIA'S RESPONSE TO SOUTH-EAST ASIA

India has extended its cooperation towards selected South-East Asian countries to combat COVID-19. The Indian government has agreed to help some southeast Asian countries like Vietnam, Singapore, and Indonesia to combat COVID-19. India has assisted the South-East Asian countries to overcome the healthcare and economic challenges caused by a coronavirus. India has also agreed to supply HCQ tablets and COVID-19 testing kits to Malaysia. The Indian embassy of Manila has initiated to distribute masks, sanitizers, and medicines to Philippine government officials, university students, and regular citizens. Over the last few years, the Indian healthcare industry has made a commendable contribution to the South-East Asian region. As per the agreement of India-Cambodia bilateral trade, India is playing a very active role in Cambodia also. The EXIM-BANK has decided to assist Myanmar in healthcare in the post-COVID-19 period.

2.5.9   INDIA AND MIDDLE-EAST IN RESPONSE TO COVID-19

In the wake of pandemic COVID-19, India has provided medical assistance to Middle-east countries for strengthening its cooperation in the post-CAA period through 'extended neighborhood policy.' India has provided medical equipment and medicines to the Middle-eastern countries to fight with COVID-19. Iran's President Hassan Rouhani requested to Narendra Modi to provide necessary supports to fight against COVID-19 in Mid of March 2020. The Indian medical team in Iran helped a lot to fight against COVID-19. There is a need to have a comprehensive understanding of the security challenges COVID-19 between India and the Middle-eastern countries.

2.5.10   NEW MANAGERIAL PERSPECTIVE: FROM CHINESE DEPENDENCY TO SELF-RELIANCE

During the crisis, what has been raised in the academic discourse that the importance of the state actors would remain the same or not. It has been proven across the globe the state has taken a major role in rescuing the people from the crisis as per their capacity. New Public Management has taken the public sector as a key sector and has become the principal paradigm since the late 1970s [9]. This paradigm has been challenged due to the globalization since 1991. In the era of globalization, through open market and private sectors-led business, the government wanted to introduce a new managerial system to improve their activeness and realize their goal [10]. Corporate responsibility has not been significantly shown. Although a few corporate houses have taken generous policies for helping the people and the government as well, those were not adequate as per the required demands. However, the new managerial challenges came before the Indian government in handling the situation. In the globalized world, all states are interdependent to each other, and relationally engaged with reciprocal. India is not exceptional in this regard. Due to the outbreak of COVID-19, the supply chain has been broken down. India's overdependence on medical equipment and medicines in China has created a crisis. Due to COVID-19, medicine, and other medical equipment imports have been interrupted. The testing kits of coronavirus were imported from China. In addition to that the Indo-China border stand-off at Galwan valley of Ladakh in on June 15, 2020, the governmental managerial strategy got changed. The government of India has emphasized on self-made products and encouraging self-reliance. Anti-Chinese sentiment has been started to grow in India in the post-Galwan period [11]. China is India's biggest source of imports. India imports more than 3,000 products from China. In the long run, Indian's self-reliance policy will not resolve its medicinal crisis, but also help to generate new revenue from its own-made products. The pandemic COVID-19 has given a new lesson to India for adopting a new managerial strategy.

2.6   PAKISTAN

Pakistan is a state without nationalism. Despite being an Islamic state, it has failed to secure human rights for all. Political violence is a language of Pakistani politics [12]. Pakistan is considered as a failed state for restless ethnic conflicts, intra-religious clashes, terrorism, religious orthodoxy, and military intervention. Being a democratic country with a federal structure, Pakistan has not been yet to fundamental rights and human rights for the citizens nor able to ensure equal opportunity to all ethnic groups. Over the years, the federal government of Pakistan has witnessed several ethnic conflicts for pro-Panjabi policy and pampering of the Sunni community. The process of Islamization in every sector of society collapsed its democratic structure. Pakistan has gone through military regimes after several intervals. The economy of Pakistan is very vulnerable due to many reasons. The developmental activities are immensely hampered for many reasons. The internal conflict is the major reason. The extremist policies are imposed on Shia and Ahamedia community. According to T. Paul, "Pakistan's ongoing war-making efforts have deeply affected its prospects for emerging as a tolerant, prosperous, and unified nation-state. This has major implications not only for Pakistan but also for global and regional security orders" [13].

Pakistan has been highly affected by a deadly coronavirus. Thousands of people have highly infected, and the economy of Pakistan has been slow-downed. The Pakistan government announced a lockdown in March 2020, when the situation went out of control. All educational institutions were closed down. The domestic and international flights were grounded. Primarily, the attitude of the government was so much reluctant. The negligence of the government has been manifested when it denied evacuating the citizens from abroad. The inhuman attitudes of the government with COVID-19 patients were highly neglected by the global community. If we talk about the human rights and human security of Pakistan, then it can be easily stated that Pakistan is the worst example of human exploitation and human rights violations. However, due to domestic compulsion, the Pak government had lifted the lockdown on May 9, 2020. After lifting the lockdown, the COVID-cases have rapidly increased due to the least 'caring attitude of the common masses. The entire healthcare system was broken down due to the overwhelming pressure of COVID patients. Testing kits were not available in Pakistan. Due to the infection of countless health workers from the very beginning, the failure of health management of the Pakistan government was reflected. When the Pakistan government decided to lift the lockdown, then Prime Minister Imran Khan addressed to the Pakistani people in saying that they must live with the virus. The voice of the Supreme Court of Pakistan was very surprising.

The apex court of Pakistan ruled that COVID-19 is 'not a pandemic' and ordered the stakeholders for reopening of shopping malls. The role of religious master, like ulema, was very orthodox. They urged the faithful to fill up mosques for Eid prayers. I am mentioning the role of these institutions and states pillars to understand the nature of Pakistan's state. The people of Pakistan, could not be secured by the government economically, socially, religiously, and medically also. The government of Pakistan never gives priority to human security before the military, ISI, and religious factors. Many people of Pakistan relied on the words of leaders and experts to make critical health decisions. This outbreak is not only a public health crisis but also a public communication crisis.

2.6.1 IMPACT ON HEALTHCARE AND THE ROLE OF THE GOVERNMENT

The COVID-19 has immensely affected the public healthcare system of Pakistan. The healthcare system in Pakistan is very weak. Some standard hospitals and medical centers are situated in big cities. The health security issue is closely related to social security. The Pakistan government spends only 2% of its GDP, which is much lower than the global average of 11%.

Social security and public health are notably weak in Pakistan. The World Health Organization (WHO) recommends and encourages the member states to spend at least 5% of their GDP on public health. The developed member countries are spending more than the suggested percentage of their GDP. But, for the least developing countries, Like Pakistan, it is far from the suggested percentage. In the case of Pakistan, it spends the lowest amount in developing public health and education. In FY 2006–2007, the governmental expenditure on healthcare was 0.5% of the GDP [14]. The inadequacy in health sector budgeting compelled the citizens to be more dependent upon the private heal care system.

The indigenous medical equipment is unavailable in Pakistan. Due to the overwhelming pressure of coronavirus infected patients, government hospitals cannot accommodate more patients due to a shortage of beds and ventilators. In Karachi, there are 15 hospitals (including private and government) that are dealing with COVID patients. The total number of ventilators in all of these hospitals is 136. In Lahore, there are 539 beds and 200 ventilators are available for patients infected by COVID-19 [28]. The Pakistan government has spent $298.94 million to purchase medical equipment. The government of Pakistan has taken some initiative to make awareness among the people for healthcare to combat the pandemic situation. The local governmental agencies have announced that maintaining social distancing and using masks as mandatory. The government had also enforced some directives to the local government for sanitizing. To promote public awareness, the government has taken several programs on sensitization. The particular governmental agencies have regularly sent a message to the people for making awareness. The health department has tried to identify the coronavirus affected areas to conduct rapid tests.

2.6.2   IMPACT ON THE ECONOMY

To sustain, Pakistan will have to overcome the current economic hardship. They have assumed that Pakistan's economic growth will be reached around 1–2% in the next year, and the government's revenue will be hugely reduced. Due to negative economic growth, the State Bank of Pakistan has decided to reduce interest rates by 2%. The government has decided to cut down the expenses of selected sectors. To rejuvenate some selected sectors, the government has taken some generous steps by declaring some relaxation on taxes and providing subsidies. The State Bank of Pakistan has declared a temporary economic refinance facility to encourage the new investments. The government has also announced a special package for the small entrepreneurs. The government of Pakistan has offered them to establish new hospitals and medical centers by offering low-interest loans for 5 years. As Pakistan is a federal state, that is why the provincial government has some special provisions to deal with the deadliest situations in their ways. The coordination between the federal and provincial have found to combat the coronavirus. The economic status of Baluchistan, NWFP, and FATA is not at par with Sindh and Punjab. So, all provinces have not been able to ensure subsidies to their needy provincial people. Sindh is the first state which announced curfew and lockdown in major cities to stop the spreading infections. The Northwest Frontier Province has also declared a partial lockdown to stop social interaction. The provincial governments have also announced some special packages for the economically backward classes.

2.6.3   DISCRIMINATORY ATTITUDES TOWARDS RELIGIOUS MINORITIES IN FOOD DISTRIBUTION

Constitutionally Pakistan is an Islamic Republic, but practically, it is a multi-religious country with Islamic factionalism. When the entire world has been fighting with COVID-19 unitedly, then in Pakistan, governmental discriminations have been found in treating with religious minorities. Religious intolerance has been manifested in Sunni Muslim dominated Pakistan. The coronavirus has been referring to as the 'Shia viruses to make more social pressure on the socially cornered minority Shia community. During the pandemic, an allegation has been raised against the Sunni-owned ration shop for pressurizing Christians to recite the kalma for getting ration. The same attitudes were shown towards Hindu. Some government distribution centers had denied giving ration to the Hindu despite showing the national identity card. This is the hard fact of Pakistan, where the state agencies or allied agencies often do discriminatory acts towards the religious minority. The governmental policy of exclusion has been implied in society also. In many places, relief was distributed by private foundations and trusts. These organizations often deny assisting the non-Muslim people to provide aid [15].

During the pandemic situation, the Hazara Shias were victimized due to the government. The government has tagged them as non-Muslim, that is why they are socially isolated. In a democratic country, is it expected that any public notice can be issued for a particular community in a discriminatory manner? As far as public health is concerned, no public notice can be issued to isolate any particular community by the government. The police authority of Baluchistan has made an announcement for the Hazara Shia community for confining themselves within the home. On another notice, issued by the Water and Sanitization Authority of Baluch Government on March 13, it was said that the two Shia-majority inhabited towns namely Marriabad, and Hazara will be treated isolated. The Shia people of these two cities were restricted to go outside of their homes during the amid of pandemic. Interestingly, other communities were remained free to go outside. However, to establish itself as a self-dependent county, the Pakistan government should abandon the policy of exclusion and ethnoreligious division policy within the state. It should be more aware of its economic development and self-reliance.

2.7 AFGHANISTAN

Afghanistan has failed to maintain human security. For Afghanistan, human security always exists in a volatile situation. The war-torn Afghan society is suffering from the inadequacy of human rights. There are several reasons behind the fragile human security in Afghanistan: (i) lawlessness, unstable government, absence of governability, restless political and social unrest; (ii) Taliban militancy; (iii) violence against women; (iv) ethnic conflicts and civil wars; (v) bombing and firing by external forces [16]. The relative autonomy of Afghanistan has been immensely questionable. Afghanistan got underway following the Soviet pull-out in February 1989, the forces which the CIA and ISI had gathered for the jihad begun realizing their importance for jihad elsewhere [17]. What Afghanistan today, the responsibility of superpowers is highly questionable for that. The concept of peace has been a utopian dream for Afghan people. The government has no role in peacebuilding in Afghanistan. Since the Soviet invasion in 1979, thousands of Afghan people had left the country for saving their lives and took shelter neighboring Pakistan, Iran, and some central Asian countries, like Tajikistan, Uzbekistan, etc. Due to economic vulnerability and non-stop civil wars, and external wars, Afghan people use to take shelter in developed countries also. The inability and irresponsibility of the state are found in the case of Afghanistan in protecting human security. Since the invasion of the USSR in 1979, Afghanistan has been a place of restless conflicts, and pawn of global cheeseboard for exercising of power of global powers.

In 2001, a United States-led military coalition invaded Afghanistan to fight against the al-Qaida and Taliban groups. Afghanistan consisting of 38 million people, out of this figure, 1.11 million has already been internally displaced, and 1.7 million people had taken shelter in Pakistan, Iran, Tajikistan, and other countries due to civil wars, terrorism, food crisis, unemployment. The Taliban group is brutally attacking not only government offices, foreign diplomatic missions, but also educational institutions, and hospitals. The BBC News has reported that in May 2020, a deadly terrorist attack was conducted at Ataturk Children's Hospital, and another attack was done on a maternity hospital in Kabul. These incidents are not exceptional which probes the challenge of human security of Afghanistan [18]. The healthcare system of Afghanistan is very much fragmented and weakened. The capacity of the government is spending money on public health is minimal. The government of Afghanistan spends a little amount on health care due to insufficient budgetary allocation. However, in recent times, the government has initiated to develop the health system with external financial assistance. Now, for per 10,000 people, 1.9% of physicians and 9.4% of skilled health-care professionals have been allocated. Indian doctors and nurses are working in Afghanistan for providing advanced health care. The major challenge to President Hamid Karzai was to stop civil wars and decade-long terrorism.

2.7.1 COMBATTING COVID-19: FEW OBSERVATIONS

As human security immensely questionable in Afghanistan, that is why human assistance is immediately needed for 14 million people. The state authority is unable to arrange humanitarian assistance to all of them, that is why external assistance has pleaded by the government. During the last couple of years, the international community has been worried about the peace and development of Afghanistan [19]. The development and peace of a country cannot be ensured or installed from the outside. The response of the society and aspirations of the countrymen are essentially needed for that. Despite receiving external assistance, a humanitarian vulnerability has not been removed in Afghanistan. The most vulnerable among the vulnerable like rural poor, minority groups, internally displaced people, and returned refugees from the neighboring countries. The COVID-19 has been introduced as an additional hazard with internal conflict, poverty, and repeated natural disasters [20]. For an economically challenged, orthodox, and unconscious state, it is quite a difficult task to combat the COVID-19.

Since February 2020, the COVID-19 crisis has fueled due to the returning of thousands of Afghan refugees, and migrants from Iran, Pakistan, and Turkey. These reversed people had carried the coronavirus and reached different provinces by public transport without maintaining the minimum directives of WHO. The government agencies of Afghanistan are usually very casual about public hygiene, sensitization, and health care. In the case of COVID-19, the same attitudes of the government were found. Lawlessness has been an integral part of Afghan society, which caused the spread of COVID-19. Afghanistan is an uncertain country in true sense. The inhuman and barbaric actions of the Taliban have been restarted in the pandemic situation which violated its earlier promises the government in maintaining the ceasefire. The Taliban had conducted several terrorist attacks during the pandemic situation. At least 55 attacked were conducted by the Taliban from March 2020 to August 2020. Taliban had also promised to help the governmental initiatives with international organizations to fight against the COVID-19, but ultimately the Taliban chose its old way of violence. This is a problem for a war-torn, and terrorist affected country to take any step towards the welfare project despite huge challenges. Due to the escalation of violence, the Afghan government has to face double jeopardy in the pandemic situation.

The World Bank has approved $400 million to the Afghan government to fight against COVID-19. The Afghan government has received assistance for handling the COVID-19 from the Abu Dhabi, Germany, and other countries had assisted Afghanistan to combat with COVID-19, but mismanagement of funds at different levels of the government have been found. Another alarming concern is a low social hygienic sense among the people, and due to health illiteracy, the infections have rapidly increased across the country. The shortage of food is not a new phenomenon for Afghanistan. As I have mentioned that the Taliban is always a problem for Afghanistan, which has been more complicated during the pandemic due to the release of 933 Taliban prisoners from different prisons of Afghanistan.

2.7.2   THE TAKEN MEASURES

The Afghan government has taken some measures to control the pandemic situation. (i) The government has tried to make awareness among the people to use masks, sanitization, and social distancing. (ii) The government has initiated for testing the suspected COVID patents in government hospitals with its limitations. (iii) Some quarantine centers and isolated wards have been made by the government. The Kabul-centric health-care system could not mitigate the required public health demand for all provinces. (iv) The working hours in the government health centers have been increased, and shifting duty charts were made for the doctors and health staff. (v) The government advisory was given to the people. The aged employees and pregnant women were advised to do work from home (WFH). (vi) The government offices were asked to avoid the gathering of more people. (vii) New budget allocation was made for fighting with coronavirus offices [21].

For fighting with coronavirus, Afghanistan is not in a position to arrange isolation centers for the majority of infected people. The country has only 991 beds for COVID patients. Kabul has a capacity of 50 tests for COVID-19 per day. It is quite difficult to afford foreign testing kits for the common people. The situation of provincial governments is very worst. Afghanistan has a total of 172 hospitals. The well-trained doctors, healthcare staffs, and nurses are inadequate in Afghanistan. There are only 9·4 skilled health professionals and 1·9 physicians per 10,000 citizens in Afghanistan. The physicians are disproportionately distributed across the country [22]. The overdependence on foreign countries in health care and other infrastructural developments are to be reduced by the government. The state management strategies are to be introduced by the Afghan government. In the post-COVID-19 world order, it would very difficult to receive foreign assistance by any economically vulnerable states, as most of the donor countries already cut up their budgetary allocation for the aid due to the acute financial crisis. The Afghan government should move to explore its sources in handling the further crisis.

2.8   THE MALDIVIAN EXPERIENCE

The Islamic Republic of Maldives is a vulnerable state in every sense. The tourism-dependent economy has to face an acute financial crisis. It is the least developed country, as it depends on tourism, and fishery being as its main sources of income [23]. As the state economy is overly dependent on tourism that is why it has immensely weakened the economy. The international assistance has been received by the Maldivian government from various sources. The Maldivian president Ibrahim Mohamed Solih has been democratically elected with a lot of promises in 2018. The state government led the economy of Maldives has a stronghold in the society. The role of private sectors in the Maldivian economy is not significant due to the lack of indigenous industries. The influence of the Chinese government and companies have been drastically changed the economic autonomy of the country since 2012. A huge amount of Chinese liquid assistance has been received by the Maldives over the last few years. The complex financial conditions have been imposed on the Maldivian government, but when the question of social responsibility comes, the Chinese government is used to keep mute itself. Maldives has pleaded for getting financial assistance from the different international agencies and countries as well to procure personal protective equipment (PPE) and medical supplies. The World Bank has approved a fast-track aid package of $7.3 million to strengthen the preparedness of the country.

2.8.1   HEALTH CARE FACILITIES

The health care system of Maldives is very vulnerable. The Indira Gandhi Memorial Hospital in Male is the biggest in the country. Due to a shortage of money, doctors, nurses, and backwardness in medical research, Maldives is struggling with the health care system. The population of Maldives is sacredly leaving in different islands. Most of the islands have no medical facility, and the transportation system merely depends upon waterways. It is a less populated country. As per the record of 2018, the total population of Maldives is 516,000. Less population has given an extraordinary facility to the Maldives. Several islands and the resorts are uninhabited, which are providing space for isolation or quarantine facilities. However, facilities for test and treatment of COVID-19 patients are available only in the capital city. A limited number of ambulances are available in the country. The total number of ventilators in the Maldives is 97. After observing the situation, the National Health Emergency was declared in the country [8]. According to the report of the health emergency operations plan (HEOP), the primary objective of this plan to strengthen the health sector and to take emergency preparedness to handle epidemics and pandemics; and other types of emergencies which has a substantial impact on people 's health and society [24]. To tackle the COVID-19, from the very beginning, the thermal screening facilities were set up at all international airports and seaports to identify passengers with possible symptoms, who would require isolation. Subsequently, a temporary ban was imposed on travelers and flights from the most affected countries in March. The issuance of visas for foreigners was suspended from March 27, 2020 [8].

The Maldivian government has decided to produce food grains and vegetable uninhabited islands to reduce dependency on other countries. Due to the acute financial crisis for the pandemic, the government of Maldives has decided to cut the salary of the government employees. With a limited capacity, the government has also announced some generous financial assistance for the fishermen, farmers, small and medium scale businessmen. The Maldivian government declared a special financial package of 2.5 billion MVR. Through the experience of the pandemic situation and acute financial crisis and shortage of foods, the Maldivian government decided to reduce its imports of staple foods, and over-dependence on tourism. The tourism-based economy struck at the lowest point, so alternative sources of revenue generation will be to find out by the Maldivian government. The government has decided to vacant land for those people who are interested in cultivation. To continue unimpeded imports during the crisis, the government has decided to establish state shipping lines in March 2020. The pandemic COVID-19 has given an unfolded experience to all states, which compelled those state authorities to explore new managerial perspectives of the state. The Maldivian government has also learned new things and tried to manage the crisis in a new manner. The Maldivian government has fallen in double jeopardy in the pandemic situation due to the overwhelming pressure imposed by China. The Maldives had taken a huge amount of loans during the regime of Abdulla Yameen.

The debt-burden economy of Maldives has been newly challenged by China by asking to repay the loan. In this unexpected crisis, it is very difficult for the Maldives to repay the Chinese loan. The Maldivian new government has started to re-establish friendly relations with India, making the country under the pressure from China. The Maldivian government has been received enormous assistance during the COVID-19 crisis in the form of foods, goods, and medical equipment. Now it is a great challenge to the Maldives to manage India and China in a balanced manner. The new managerial strategies are to be formulated by the government, which will be an additional lesson of COVID-19 for the Maldives. The Maldivian Government has been quite proactive in fighting against COVID-19. The government has started to explore new alternatives to be self-dependent. However, being a vulnerable state, the Maldives has been dealing with COVID-19 very well in comparison with other South Asian states.

2.9 CONCLUSION AND FUTURE SCOPE

The responsibility of selected South Asian states is different in their performance. The experience of India is widely different from the other states. Being the regional power and core state of South Asia, the responsibility goes beyond the state boundary. Despite having loopholes, India has tried to combat with COVID-19 internally. At the same time, India has extended its helping hand to a large number of countries across the globe, including the USA by supplying hydroxychloroquine. For a vibrant democratic country, the responsibility of the state is the key concern due to voting politics. The nature of the civil society, rate of literacy, social awareness, and corporate social responsibilities are interrelated and essential in combatting major crises, like COVID-19. The state managerial skill is not the same for all countries. The issue of corporate social responsibilities does not apply to the non-globalized states, like Afghanistan. One of the major outcomes of the study for India is the adoption of a policy of 'self-reliance.' The countries like Maldives and Afghanistan which are over-dependent on external supports and supply will have to rethink about indigenous production and the medical system. For Afghanistan, there are so many challenges that are difficult to overcome. The war-torn, economically vulnerable, and socially fragmented Afghanistan will have to develop its civil society and its resources. Pakistan stands for a military state which concentrates on the war-making process with an outlook of social exclusion. The shortcomings of the government's distributive policy are recognizable. The attitudes of the governmental agencies towards COVID-19 patients were not only reluctant but also inhuman in many cases. The responsibility of the state is not a mechanical thing; humanitarian outlook is very much needed for it. The new managerial perceptions have been fixed by the states of South Asian as per their capabilities.

The responsibility of South Asian states in combatting coronavirus is extensively different. Based on the entire study and observation, a few recommendations can be done: (i) the capacity of all states in the health care system is to be increased; (ii) self-dependency in health care, economy, and foods are to be ensured by Afghanistan, Pakistan, and the Maldives; (iii) the new managerial perspective is to be developed by each country as per their capacity for handling such type of pandemic situation; (iv) the attitude of the government towards a particular religious community in Pakistan is very discriminatory. The humanitarian and impartial governmental policies are to be implemented in Pakistan; and (v) The role of corporate houses should be more responsible. The state governments will compel the big corporate houses to perform cooperate social responsibility.

KEYWORDS

- **COVID-19**
- **globalization**
- **local self-government department**
- **managerial perception**
- **personal protective equipment**
- **South Asia**

REFERENCES

1. Mooney, J., Timo, H., & Dominelli, L., (2020). COVID-19: A new challenge for social work. In: Lena, D., Timo, et al., (eds.), *COVID-19 and Social Work: A Collection of Country Reports* (pp. 34, 35). COVID-19 Social Work Research Forum.
2. Chatterjee, A., (2017). Rethinking human security from a theoretical perspective. In: Madhuparna, G., (ed.), *Non-Traditional Security: Problems and Prospects* (pp. 25, 26). Avenel Press.
3. Bandayopadhyaya, J., (2002). *World Government: For International Democracy and Justice* (pp. 131, 132). Howrah: Manuscript India.
4. Linnell, M., (2014). Citizens response in crisis: Individual and collective efforts to enhance community resilience. *An Interdisciplinary Journal on Humans ICT Environment, 10*(2), 68–94. doi: 10.17011/ht/urn.201411203311.
5. Rodríguez, H., Trainor, J., & Quarantelli, E. L., (2006). Rising to the challenges of a catastrophe: The emergent and prosocial behavior following Hurricane Katrina. *The Annals of the American Academy of Political and Social Science, 604*, 82–101.
6. Idowu, S. O., Vertigans, S., & Burlea, S. A., (2017). *Corporate Social Responsibility in Times of Crisis* (pp. 1, 2). Springer International.
7. Mondal, K., & Mou, M. D., (2020). *Socio-Economic and Political Impact of Coronavirus on India: Challenges and Prospects* (pp. 15–20). Independently Published.
8. Sultana, G., (2020). *Maldivian Response to COVID-19*. Manohar Parrikar Institute for Defense Studies and Analysis, New Delhi. The Economic Times.
9. Diefenbach, T., (2009). New public management in public sector organizations: Dark sides of managerialistic 'engagement. *Public Administration, 87*(4), 892–909. doi: 10.1111/j.1467- 9299.2009.01766.x.
10. Goldfinch, S., & Joe, W., (2010). Two myths of convergence in public management reform. *Public Administration, 88*(4), 1099–1115. Doi.org/10.1111/j.1467-9299.2010.01848.x.
11. Dhar, V., (2020). *COVID-19 Effect: Time for Made-in-India Tag to Go Global*. Financial Express.

12. Ullah, H., (2014). *Vying for Allah's Vole: Understanding Islamic Parties, Political Violence, and Extremism in Pakistan.* Cambridge University Press.

13. Paul, T. V., (2014). *The Warrior State: Pakistan in the Contemporary World* (pp. 84, 85). Random House Publishers India Private Limited.

14. Ahmed, J., & Shaikh, B. T., (2008). An all time low budget for healthcare in Pakistan. *Journal of the College of Physicians and Surgeons Pakistan, 18*(6), 389, 390.

15. Mirza, J. A., (2020). *COVID-19 Fans Religious Discrimination in Pakistan.* Diplomat.

16. Nandy, D., (2019). Democracy, civil society, and human security in a war-torn state: A case study of Afghanistan. In: Pal, P., (ed.) *India in South Asia: Challenges and Opportunities* (pp. 50–67). Kunal Books.

17. Gul, I., (2009). *The Al Qaeda Connection: The Taliban and Terror in Pakistan's Tribal Areas* (pp. 120–125). Penguin Books.

18. https://www.bbc.com/news/world-asia-52631071 (accessed on 26 June 2021).

19. Sarkar, S., (2012). *In Search of a New Afghanistan.* Niyogi Books.

20. United Nations Office for the Coordination of Humanitarian Affairs (OCHA), (2020). *Humanitarian Response Plan Afghanistan 2018–2021.*

21. UNDP, (2020). *Afghanistan COVID-19 Impact: Short Term Disruptions and Policy Consideration.* https://www.undp.org/content/dam/undp/library/covid19/Afghanistan%20-%20Covid19%20Impact%20Note%20-%20Final%20%20April%2015%202020.pdf (accessed on 26 June 2021).

22. Shah, J., Karimzadeh, S., Al-Ahdal, T. M. A., Mousavi, S. H., Zahid, S. U., & Huy, N. T., (2020). COVID-19: The current situation in Afghanistan. *The Lancet Global Health, 8*(6), p.771. doi: 10.106/S2214-109.

23. Bussa, L., (2017). *India-Maldives Relations* (p. 62). Avni Publications.

24. Ministry of Health, Republic of Maldives, (2018). *Health Emergency Operations Plan* (HEOP). http://health.gov.mv/Uploads/Downloads//Informations/Informations(124).pdf (accessed on 26 June 2021).

25. Bhandari, A., & Jindal, C., (2018). *The Maldives: Investments Undermine Democracy.* Indian Council on Global Relations. https://www.gatewayhouse.in/chinese-investments-in-the-maldives/ (accessed on 9 July 2021).

26. https://reliefweb.int/report/afghanistan/afghanistan-humanitarian-response-plan-2018-2021-2020-revision-december-2019 (accessed on 26 June 2021).

27. The Times of India (April 7, 2020), https://timesofindia.indiatimes.com/defaultinterstitial.cms (accessed on July 9, 2021).

28.. The Times of India (June 12 2020), https://timesofindia.indiatimes.com/world/pakistan/pakistani-hospitals-running-out-of-space-with-a-spike-in-covid-19-patien, (accessed on 9 July 2021).

CHAPTER 3

COVID-19 and the Discourse on Human Rights

SUDAITA GHOSH

Department of Political Science, Raiganj University, Raiganj – 733134, West Bengal, India, E-mail: sudaitaghosh@gmail.com

ABSTRACT

The novel coronavirus infection, generally familiar as COVID-19 has first reported on December 2019 in the two provinces of China, Wuhan, and Hubei has now reached at the level of intercontinental epidemic. Absence of appropriate medicine to stop the alarming level of spread and severity of the virus resulted in the rising number of deaths of the human population worldwide. Though efforts are being made to develop vaccines to combat the COVID-19 virus, however, it is most threatening, particularly to the life of the underprivileged people, children, and old age of developing nations where health infrastructure is relatively inadequate than the developed nation. The World Health Organization's (WHO) COVID-19 protocols that involve social distancing, proper sanitization and complete lockdown of cities and towns resulted in breaking down the rapid infection rate. However, the scale and severity of COVID-19 pandemic pose a serious threat to the public health management system in India. In addition to this, imposition of nationwide lockdown, quarantine, and isolation also restricted certain human rights. Imposition of lockdown alone cannot be a viable option in India, where a large section of people are daily-based wage earners, including the migrant laborers. A humble treatment to human rights, including equal opportunity, transparency, and respect for humanity, and more importantly, establishment of the provisions within Three Generation of Human Rights are some delicate and critical issues whose solutions will come through judiciously. The study gives an overview of the present status and trend of COVID-19 pandemic in India call attention to human rights, which is under threat and disturbed because of a pandemic. Finally, a set of recommendations has proposed to successfully deal with the issues of principle rights and liberties in addition, the protection of civil liberties of individuals, which are thoroughly affected after the COVID-19 disruption.

3.1   INTRODUCTION

Human Rights are those basic rights, which confirm human dignity. The origin of Human Rights has been tracing back in the period of the Post-Cold War period. The Universal Declaration of Human Rights (UDHR) starts functioning since 10 December 1948 which has structured with 30 articles. Every article in the Universal Declaration is expressing the dignity and safeguard of the basic rights of the individual. The Preamble of the Declaration holds, the acknowledgment of intrinsic nobility along with the inseparable rights for entire civilized clan are the basis of liberties, rights, equity, and the security of the universe [3].[1] Human family is suffering from slavery, oppression, discrimination, refusing freedom and even genocide since the establishment of civil society, and the journey of negating and fading rights either from society as well as family or from authority is continuing. Struggling for rights are common even after the establishment of a democratic form of government. The goal of the establishment of UDHR to confiscate all the difficulties in the way of development consummated human dignity and respect. UDHR became new and refined behind the inauguration of Three Generation of Human Rights by Karel Vasak in 1977 [24]. First Generation of Rights established after the French revolution and guaranteed the Civil and Political Rights. Second Generation Rights had confirmed its importance after the Russian Revolution and initiated to established the economic, cultural, and social rights. Third Generation of Rights found the de-colonization with the inception of Developing countries and established the rights of peace, rights of environment, rights about common heritage, etc. International initiative to protect the rights of the people can be considered as the victory of humanity. Globally each nation is duty-bound to uphold the fundamental rights of their citizens. A nation can preserve the human of the people through the Constitution of the State. Statute literature must constitute the basic rights to sustain an individual's dignity and respect. However, rejection of human rights is now a very common phenomenon. Despite the Constitutional assurance of the Rule of Law, legal punishments and penalty, human rights are still struggling to prevail. Worldwide people are abiding by the torture of terrorism, war, discrimination on race, color, and

---

[1] UDHR, (1948) (UNGA).

gender, poverty, hunger, poor health, illiteracy, and are grieving for conserve their rights. State as a protector also acts as a violator of the rights in some cases. People scuffling by State made terror. An absence of moral respect for rights also a reason for not implementation of protection of rights.

3.2 HUMAN RIGHTS IN INDIA

India since its inception as an independent country, was very much aware of the prerequisite of autonomy and sovereignty of the citizens. The Constitution of India incorporated the Civil Liberties for the citizen of India in Section III has demonstrated within the Statute Book of the country. Section III of the Constitution incorporated the Chapters 14–18 for prohibition of the legal inequalities for the citizens of India, Chapters 19–22 confirms Freedom of Speech, expression assembly-associations, movement, settlement within the territory and selecting the profession, Freedom from Exploitation explains within Chapters 23 and 24, rights for free religious activities by Chapters 25–28, freedom in maintaining language, Cultural, and establishment of Educational institution described in Chapters 29 and 30 and Right to Constitutional Remedies in Chapter 32 [5][2], are the replica of UDHR. A growing number of violations of rights, dearth of awareness, and ignorance about protection of rights created the background for the formation of the National Human Rights Commission (NHC). Finally, on 12th October 1993 NHC began its functioning. Journey of the Human Rights Commission was not all about a smooth one [7]. Larger population, parochial nature of the society, economic insufficiency, and paucity of literacy all has created the hindrances in the way of success of the Commission. Human Rights Commission, with all these challenges, has functioned well in the cases of human trafficking, child prostitution, child labor, rights for the displaced people, domestic violence, old age problems, violence against women, problems of mental health, and so many. However, infringement of law, crimes, violence, and other activities are disallowing the enjoyment of basic rights. And most vulnerable sections who are enduring most women, children, old age people and underprivileged sections of the society [8].

Present COVID-19 affected India badly and jeopardized the life of the people. World Health Organization (WHO) Secretary recently comments for COVID-19 emphasized, that all nations should draw equilibrium between protecting health together with minimizing social and economic disruption,

---

[2] The Constitution of India.

with expecting human rights [24].[3] Violation of Human Rights is increasing regularly in India. At present COVID-19 preponderance the violation of rights in general worldwide [2]. Going by the WHO, the initial case of COVID-19 in humans, caused by the novel coronavirus, which has, latterly named SARS-CoV-2, had initially appeared in Hubei Province of China, in December 2019. Careful inspection by the health administration of China had able to traced patient with all sign of the Corona disease as early as December 2019 [21].[4] Majority of the World believed that it is a bioweapon, a manmade virus prepared to kill people. However, the WHO claimed that this virus has not manipulated and constructed. The first case was identifying in Wuhan province in China. Controversy is that initially it was hiding that the coronavirus is an infectious disease, misinformation leads towards misguiding and mishandling of the most delicate issue, which has already claimed million lives. This is a respiratory disease and contagious.

The majority of the population affected by the coronavirus may meet the problem of breathing troubles and demand total medical intervention for proper healing. Aged and those who are suffering from co-morbidities like cardiac unrest disease, diabetes, asthma, distress from kidney disease and carcinoma are more prone to build medical complications.

The Corona infection escalates from human to human generally via aerosol of dribble or discharge of saliva [23][5].

The WHO has issued instruction referring to Human Rights as crucial part after the Corona disease reaction. WHO accentuates the significance of human rights-based perspective in this pandemic situation and focuses on considerations regarding offense and injustice, interruption of brutality facing by the female, maintenance for helpless people, social segregation and limited medical facilities, scarcity of other facilities [21].[6]

3.3   CORONAVIRUS INFLUENCE ON HUMAN RIGHTS ON INDIAN SUBCONTINENT

3.3.1   HUMAN RIGHTS OF MIGRATORY LABORERS

Coronavirus outbreak is intensifying the incidents of human rights violation in India. Civil liberties in India like Equality before Law, freedom against

---

[3] Media Briefing, by WHO Director-General on 11 March 2020.
[4] Novel coronavirus (2019-nCoV) situation report 1, 21 January 2020.
[5] www.who.int. Health Topics.
[6] www.who.int/defoult-source/coronavirus/situation-reports/20200423.

Exploitation and Writs under statute book are infringing mostly. In India, the first case related with coronavirus infection has reported in January 2020 from Kerala. Next, the confirmed cases were coming from other cities as Bengaluru, Delhi, Hyderabad, Mumbai, and Patna. Initially maximum cases had travel history. To control the community spread Government of India had decided to shut down the nation, imposed lockdown since March 2020.

Suspension of economic activities due to lockdown has created a major impact on the life of migratory laborers. As per the World Bank Report, the figure of inland refuges in India is near about 450 million, according to the 2011 census, which has expanded up to 45% in comparison with the 2001 census which was 309 million. This exceeded the population growth rate of 18% during 2001–2011. Percentage of internal migrants increased from 30% in 2001 to 37% in 2011 [22]. Another report of the World Bank expressed that, more than 40 million internal migrations have been in troublesome condition because of COVID-19 and about 50,000 to 60,000 individuals revert cities to their own locality from their workplaces within a span of few days. People are shifting places for several reasons. Better opportunities, good education, and discrimination in distribution of wealth, environmental exploitation can be identified as the major reasons for the internal migration.

Lockdown notification announced the partial adjournment of economic productivities. Created panic among the workers and remigration has started without any planning. Post phonation of the public transportation system enlarges the difficulties. Social segregation after the out-break of COVID-19 in India has influenced thousands of internal migratory workers. Dearth of food and essential facilities, insecurity of job, fear of the unfamiliar situation and absence of collective help in complicated situation were actual grounds behind the fight of that population.[7] These all issues are expecting the imbalance of mental health at present and near future, which also an issue of concern [15, 19].

Gross Human Rights abrogation has recorded during this phase. All human rights definition was failed when these marginalized migrated laborers died on the road, crying for food, water, and medicine [20]. Millions question, are arising about the importance of Fundamental Rights. The National Human Rights office (NHRC) received more than 2000 cases related with legal rights violation during strict lockdown period by the NHC.

People specifically who migrated from rural to urban and belong to unorganized sectors were under miserable conditions. These unskilled laborers alone or with their families shifted to different corners of the country for

---

[7] Papers.ssm.com.

their livelihood. And experiencing physical exploitation, socio-economic exploitation viz. unpaid or low payment, denied from good shelter, nutritious food, safety, and secure life, rejected from educational opportunity for their children, physical harassment, rape specially among the female in their daily life, showing a clear picture of negligence by the authority and these are the cases of serious violation of human rights. Their states failed to insulate their livelihood, the government pledged it to protect their basic rights of food, shelter, and education. In consequence, people migrated from their own places and took shelter in another place. Their human rights violation has expected as natural by society and by the state also.

After debate, discussion, and criticism, the Government of India has initi- ated to take major steps on the way to the safeguard of the basic rights of this marginalized segment. The government released funds for providing food and shelter. The National Migrant Information Centre has formed to collect and record all information. Government-issued an order about the payment of wages without any deduction. Relief fund has developed and 1.7 lakh crore allocated for the poor including cash transfer. Allotted 11.092 crore to the states. Announcement of free rationing is also ensuring to the poor. State Governments and Central also initiated transportation for the traveling of the workers.

The Commission for protection of Citizen rights (NHRC) has registered the maximum number of cases about violation of fundamental rights during the time of lockdown. It is affected *"Right to Equality, Right to Freedom, Right to Education,"*[8] including socio-economic rights. Expelling from the job sector due to lockdown is a real violation of economic rights of the migrated workers. Workers of unorganized sectors predominantly marginalize and this section of the people faced major violation of basic liberties confirmed in the Constitution of India. Individual dignity, respect is hampering into every step because of an unplanned lockdown. Starvation, poor health, ignorance with some other problems migrated workers suffered during this pandemic period critically.

Government authority is also under pressure for preserving the natural rights to the individual in COVID situation. During that shutdown mob, violence against the police officer is another example of violation of rights. Multiple cases also came where people's rights have been interrupting because of over activism of Police personnel. Public harassment, arbitrary harassment in the name of lockdown order also disturbed human rights

---

[8] The Constitution of India.

several times. Harassment of the migratory laborers during the vigilance by the police authority also annihilates the dignity of the individual.

The UN High Commissioner for Human Rights Michelle Bachelet, on April 2, 2020, too showed deep worry at the circumstances of India's in land migrants and opined that more needs to be done as the human calamity continues to unfold before the world.

Further Committee of Economic, Social, and Cultural Rights in UN has address to every States to executed selected programs to protect the remuneration of the workers and benefits of all job seekers and take actions to secure the remarkable mobilization of resources to tackle the COVID-19 pandemic [4].[9]

3.3.2   RIGHT TO HEALTH

Chapter 25 (one) of UDRH declared, about individual's right of respectful life, health right, right of take care and welfare measures of a person and his family, included fooding, shelter, and pharmaceutical care and requisite community welfare matters, and the guarantee of safety, in the case of jobless, disease or illness, physical disorder, dowager, elderliness or related difficulties like loss of earning the recourse for living within the unrecognized situation [3][10]. Rights related with Health is disturbed because of coronavirus drastically. India's public health system is well and sophisticated. India can claim good healthcare facilities from rural to urban sectors. Notwithstanding all better health care, the majority of the citizens cannot avail the amenity of a good healthcare system. In the interior rural area, people are incompetent to get minimum health care system. Maternity death, infant mortality, and death for critical illness are the major problems of the rural poor. For any better health care system, they have to spend more money. During any crisis, the disorganized picture of the healthcare system can be visualized.

Urban India also envisages the challenges of medical facilities. Government Hospitals and Primary Health Care organizations with private health care facilities collectively are insufficient for providing the good service facilities. Unplanned development, rapid increase in population, neo-migrants, shortage of medical staff creating conditions imposing critical pressure on the urban health system. Urban slams belong in the most vulnerable section [6]. The middle income and low-income groups in the cities are enduring

---

[9] www.icj.org-india-the authorities-must-act-immediately.
[10] www.un.org-udhr.

more for good medical facilities. Better medical systems are provided by private medical care centers with huge expenses. In this way, the health care system in India is predominant by the private sector. Therefore, the general health system is not for all, which triggers the clear violation of Health-related rights that sanctioned the health as right for All, has pronounced in the Article 25 of UDHR. The Central Government as well as State Governments are concerned and arranged several schemes and health care facilities. However, these are not adequate in this large populated country.

At present by virtue of COVID-19 disease the world has experienced the worst healthcare problem specially countries of the Global South. Now India is in the highest position of COVID patients. Due to infectious viruses, patients are facing social stigma. A number of patients is increasing every day with a new record created pressures on medical care systems along with increasing the probability towards the collapsed health facilities. India is already suffering from a deficiency of medical staff, doctors, and emergency facilities; in that case, the present situation creates more complications. As a result, many emergencies medical treatments are not available for the non-COVID patients like Cancer, HIV, Kidney, Cardiac patients are hurting for medical help [13].

Coronavirus has brought massive disarray in the public health sector worldwide. Medicine or vaccine is under trial. Until today, no good news reached about laboratory success on discovering the medicine [9]. In India, initially, it was under control, but at present India is in the highest position in the number of infected people. Limited health staff and limited health care institutions are creating obstacles for treatment for COVID and non-COVID in both the cases. Right to Health has denied without any arguments. Additionally, Government shelter houses for COVID patients are administered in a ruthless manner. Unhealthy food, non-purified drinking water and improper sanitation have generated conditions more critical. COVID patients' lives and rights are excessively disturbed. Social stigma for COVID-19 is also responsible for the inhuman treatment of the patients.

3.3.3   RIGHTS OF OLD AGE PEOPLE

Old-age people are facing critical health challenges, and their human rights have been grossly affecting after the outbreak of COVID-19. Nowadays, safety security is an important issue, especially in the urban and suburban cities regarding the old age people. Maximum of them is living alone at their own residences or in old age homes, are finding difficulties in accessing good medical facilities and other necessary things in daily life, even nutritious food, safety-security is also a matter of concern for the elderly people. Since before the emergence of COVID-19 disease rights had been neglecting and were not secure. Crimes against old age people in metro cities are very common due to lacking proper security. Old age group of people who are living in some deprived socio-economic conditions, now in more adverse situations. Many of them survive because of their resilience [11]. COVID-19 situation creates conditions more critical and envisages more challenges. Now their human rights are violating rapidly. Character of the disease guaranteed that probabilities of infections are high for the old people. Protections through mask, glove, PPE are not easily available for the old age people, mainly those who are poor and this is a clear prove of discrimination from health facilities. Consequently, normal life came under criticality. It is now the question of livelihood maintenance for the underprivileged old age section. The old age group is also not confident about technology in their daily life. Therefore, COVID-19 can be treated as a direct threat to human rights violations of the people who belong to the old age group.

3.3.4   RIGHT TO EDUCATION

COVID-19 snatched the right to education of the children. It has a tremendous impact on their education and mental health just because of the closing of educational institutions [12]. Many students are going to schools for nutrition. Feeding in school has started with the goal of ensuring nutrition, preventing hunger, improving school enrollment, and reducing the dropout problem. But in this COVID situation food distribution is not possible in many remote rural areas. In many schools, students are coming for food and secure shelter because their parents both are working. Presently the whole education system is haphazard in the country. Discontinuity of education of the mass population would have hamper for producing human capital in the near future. Current educational circumstances strongly violate the Article 26 of UDHR connected to secure the Right to Education [3], in India Article 21 of the Constitution also guaranteed education for all (EFA) without any discrimination, COVID situation is forcing for non-implementation of Article 21. The Government has initiated online EFA students, primary to higher to make it continue.

Government aided educational institutions are facing the challenges after this decision. Teachers of Government education institutions are not well educated about technology-related with education. After understanding the impossibility of returning to normalcy, many private educational institutions have started the initiative to resume the teaching-learning procedure online. Normal chalkboards are transforming into online. However, Governments schools are not able to implement this. Now debate is not about quality education but ensuring the education for every child. Post-COVID situation would have escalated the dropout number. The quality difference between the government and private education system is degreasing the prosperity of the education system. Moreover, maximum of the students in the country have failed to avail the online education. Instead of classroom teaching-phones, the internet, social media has been selected for delivering knowledge. Poor, marginalized students are most vulnerable in this new method of teaching. The private education system is also disrupting to some extent because of problematic economic conditions. A vast number of Private educational institutions are in favor of continuing fees hike, which has been interrupted by the parents due to the poor economy in this pandemic. The new model of education is creating trouble for teachers as well. Many rural and backward area's schoolteachers are not fully trained for online teaching. Several rural and sub-urban schoolteachers are surviving for their livelihood due to lack of proper technical knowledge about online teaching and inaccessibility of the internet connection, especially teachers who are employees of private schools.

3.3.5 RIGHTS OF THE WOMEN

COVID-19 situation has immense social impact. Even domestic violence is increasing after the COVID outbreak. Laws against domestic Violence has introduced in India in 2002. Domestic violence is a global problem for women. Mental, physical, sexual harassment, abusive behavior are the parts of Domestic Violence and instantaneously hampered Human Rights. According to the data published by the Women Commission of the country (NCW) in April 2020 reported that violence against female have increased and 100% raised in cases associated to brutality against female after and during the countrywide lockdown was forced on March 2020 [17]. Being patriarchal society, women are dominating by male. COVID brought income disparity among the male and female members in a family, lockdown was the cause of unemployment of either male or female members in a family, unusual distribution of householding works, increase of alcohol consumption intensified domestic violence during this COVID period [1, 17].

Victims are unable to complain in the majority of cases because of lockdown. Victims of Domestic Violence are not only the female member but male and lesbian also. Some social stigmas are dominating in Indian society and that problems are not accept them to come forward and complain. This is not only the problem of India; reports show that the number of increasing violence is a worldwide problem. As observed globally, including India, the lockdown has resulted in a remarkably steep increase in domestic violence cases. According to a present report by UN Women, 243 million women and girls in the past 12 months globally have envisages sexual and/or physical violence by their intimate partner within the age group of 15–49. Further, National Commission for Women (NCW), which has observed the increasing number of complaints related to gender-based violence during the national coronavirus lockdown period. This can be imputed to family violence exhibiting as a form of release by rude partners who are currently obligated to stay at home [18][11].

In India, the Domestic Violence Act (2005) is subsisting for the protection, but in these pandemic situations, it looks difficult for the spreading awareness about the act [25]. Presently Judiciary is also in paralyzed mode and law protectors are busy with the activities to control the community spreading of the disease within the society. All are giving a boost in favor of growth about domestic violence. After filing of large number of cases, the Government is proceeding with some initiatives through spreading awareness. At the same time, the Government is utilizing social media also. What's App, Twitter, and Facebook are the important platform for spreading the legal helping hand. Recently States by their own are taking several initiatives in this matter. Chuppi Tod is a famous campaign among this, which has been initiating by the UP-State Government. Delhi Government has introduced a helpline number for taking calls from the victims and for counseling.

3.4 CONCLUSION

Absence of exact medicine COVID is dominating. This unknown dominance disturbed largely the social life. Especially developing countries are more sufferers of this unusual situation. People of these countries are struggling for their minimum rights, and this struggle is perpetuating for COVID. Moreover, Post COVID conditions might bring more complications.

---

[11] www.indianexpress.com.

Economy would be more influence by other consequences. Job loss will inevitable, collapsing of small farms, Government is unprepared for this. Increasing number of infected people bound the government to take some strict decisions. To tackle this complication, the government has to be more active and stronger about welfare measures. Existing legal support is not sufficient available, but the present situation demands more. These new normal needs exceptional support from administrative and legal authority. Some extra initiatives are crucial in this juncture for fighting with the disease and restoring fundamental human rights.

Right about Health facilities and right about food for all are the predominant issue at present. The Government of India has been initiating to guarantee these rights by announcing a single Card for Public Distribution system along with other schemes. Ayushman Bharat for Health. Pradhan Mantri Garib Kalyan Package now ensures Health Insurances Schemes for COVID workers. Cabinet of Indian Parliament has approved memorandum of understanding (MoU) between India and Zimbabwe on the area of coop- eration regarding the Traditional System of Medicine and Homeopathy also introduce guidance for general medical and specialist mental health care system, Niti Aayog Lounge Behavioral Change Campaign-Navigating the New Normal. Arogya Path, a web-based solution for real-time availability of critical health supplies has launched. Core treatments provided under Ayusman Bharat Pradhan Mantri Jano Arogyo Yojona.[12] However, these are not abundant support unless the launch of a free health scheme for every citizen including free test and medicine for the marginalized. Senior citizens should get medical insurance, free treatment in hospitals. For elderly people it is very important to arrange some caregiver with a helpline number. In this COVID-19 situation for social distancing and other reasons, old age community is denying even from routine health checkup.

To make it easy and available, every state government should arrange at least one or two hospitals only for non-COVID elderly people. It is necessary for the Government to increase the surveillance, spreading right and proper information to the community and prepared guidelines to combat the disease and Arogya Setu App. is a government initiative, fulfilling the purposes [10].

Article 32 of the Constitution of India also declined during this period. Normal Judiciary works have also postponed. Justice is delaying for those who are under trial. It feels positive to experience that the administration is well informed and aware about the breach of Human Rights. In response, the Administration is trying to take necessary measures. To ensure the food and

---

[12] nhp.gov.in/whatsnew.

shelter for the marginalized section Central and respective State Government declared some policies including direct transfer of money. The significant obstacle about the imparting of income support for the metropolitan unwaged people is the absence of a proper data archive as an information resource. For quicker dispatching of welfare, employer's help could be sort out. State government should take the initiative to register their ID and details in case of DBT.[13] It is expected that not fully but partially it will provide the relief. At this moment, more steps are necessary for universal preservation of Human Rights.

Based on the present status of the COVID-19 pandemic and its effect on the Human Rights, a set of recommendations can be propose.

- Firstly, because of this coronavirus people are under the profound economic crisis. Rate of unemployment is higher gradually. Free Credit cannot be effective to solve the long-term economic problems. Government ensures about monitory support but they must secure the maximum employment as soon as possible.
- Secondly, special attention is requisite for the marginalized section. Government already has promised to work in favor of them, but strict vigilance is necessary for the implementation of support schemes. Regular intimating and knowledge campaigning about the disease including the free of cost sanitizer and masks supply particularly in the over crowed slams locality should be consider as an urgent. Supply of drinking water should not be interrupt.
- Thirdly, for the old age people, free home delivery of food and medical help is require. Government must confirm this. To reduce the psychological problem of this group of people State should initiative some entertainment through telephonic and television. Special shows for grannies and grandpas possibly organize along with their active participation, so they can feel that they are still in life.
- Fourthly, Judiciary must arrange the procedure of speedy trial. Many are unnecessarily suffering in cell for non-trialing of their cases. Video conference should allow in every case in this pandemic situation. It is also important to curving the digit of prisoners. Simultaneously the Prison Administration must consider every day health checkup for every prisoner as the routine task.
- Fifthly, for ensuring Right to education needs free digital equipment and uninterrupted internet, facilities are prerequisite. The Education Department of India has promoted an E-Learning Platform that covers

---

[13] www.thehindubussinessline.com.

School and Higher Education.[14] Diksha, E-Pathshala, Swayam, Swayam Prava are also available for Higher Education [14]. This system of education is unsuitable for socio-economic backward children. Government can take the initiative to distribute free Laptop or Smartphone and free internet service for the underprivileged section of the students in both primary and higher education. Education for food is not possible in the New Normal condition for that government can transfer money to the students' bank account, so they can arrange nutritious food for themselves. Employers who are very less paying and working as daily wages in government offices need special care and monitory protection for their livelihood.

- Finally, in order to defensing and protecting of women rights in the COVID circumstances every police station across the nation must open a Centre especially for the women. This Centre will receive online and offline complaints about domestic violence and other brutalities against men, women, and LGBT into 24×7 during this period.

It is very unfortunate that during this crisis period, Indian states are engaging in narrow politics as a corollary of Vote-Politics. The Central-State issue again came into debate, blame game, controversial comments continued to keep good place in news headlines and most detrimental is corruption even in public distribution during this pandemic. The system made the criticality for human rights protection [16]. Judiciary interference is an urgent task to protect Human Rights when the executive to some extent failed to protect the basic human rights of the citizens. Human civilization is accountable for protecting, spreading, and demonstrating humanity through the preservation of Human Rights.

KEYWORDS

- **COVID-19**
- **human rights**
- **lockdown**
- **National Commission for Women**
- **National Human Rights Office**
- **Universal Declaration of Human Rights**

---

[14] Government.economictimes.indiatimes.com.

REFERENCES

1. Acharya, S. S., & Dutta, C. (2020). The Shadow Pandemic in India: 'Staying Home' and The Safety of Women During Lockdown. *Gender In Crisis. COVID-19 and Its Impact*, 46.
2. Amon, J. J., & Wurth, M., (2020). A virtual roundtable on COVID-19 and human rights with human rights watch researchers. *Health and Human Rights, 22*(1), 399.
3. Assembly, U. G., (1948). Universal declaration of human rights. *UN General Assembly, 302*(2).
4. Bachelet, M., (2020). Lecture: Challenges to the protection of human rights today. *American University International Law Review, 35*(2), 5.
5. Chandrakanthi, L., (2016). Human rights and fundamental rights in Indian constitution: An assessment. *International Journal in Management & Social Science, 4*(6), 754–763.
6. Corburn, J., Vlahov, D., Mberu, B., Riley, L., Caiaffa, W. T., Rashid, S. F., & Jayasinghe, S., (2020). Slum health: Arresting COVID-19 and improving well-being in urban informal settlements. *Journal of Urban Health*, 1–10.
7. Das, A. K., & Mohanty, P. K., (2007). *Human rights in India*. Sarup & Sons.
8. Desai, A. R., (1986). *Violation of democratic rights in India*. Popular Prakashan.
9. Awasthi, A., Vishwas, S., Corrie, L., Kumar, R., Khursheed, R., Kaur, J., & Kumar, A. (2020). Outbreak of novel coronavirus disease (COVID-19): Antecedence and aftermath. *European Journal of Pharmacology, 884*, 173381.
10. Garg, S., Basu, S., Rustagi, R., & Borle, A., (2020). Primary health care facility preparedness for outpatient service provision during the COVID-19 pandemic in India: Cross-sectional study. *JMIR Public Health and Surveillance, 6*(2), e19927.
11. Golechha, M., (2020). India should ramp up its emergency medicine and critical care infrastructure to combat COVID-19. *Postgraduate Medical Journal*.
12. Gupta, A., & Goplani, M., (2020). Impact of COVID-19 on educational institution in India. *Purakala Journal U (CARE Listed), 31*(21).
13. Hebbar, P. B., Sudha, A. N. G. E. L., Dsouza, V. I. V. E. K., Chilgod, L., & Amin, A. D. H. I. P., (2020). Healthcare delivery in India amid the COVID-19 pandemic: Challenges and opportunities. *Indian J. Med. Ethics*, 1–4.
14. Jena, P. K. (2020). Impact of pandemic COVID-19 on education in India. *International journal of current research (IJCR), 12*.
15. Kochhar, A. S., Bhasin, R., Kochhar, G. K., Dadlani, H., Mehta, V. V., Kaur, R., & Bhasin, C. K., (2020). Lockdown of 1.3 billion people in India during COVID-19 pandemic: A survey of its impact on mental health. *Asian Journal of Psychiatry*.
16. Kumar, C. R., (2011). *Corruption and Human Rights in India: Comparative Perspectives on Transparency and Good Governance*. Oxford University Press.
17. Malathesh, B. C., Das, S., &Chatterjee, S. S., (2020). COVID-19 and domestic violence against women. *Asian Journal of Psychiatry*.
18. Mittal, S., & Singh, T., (2020). Gender-based violence during COVID-19 pandemic: A mini-review. *Frontiers in Global Women's Health, 1*, 4.
19. Mukhra, R., Krishan, K., & Kanchan, T., (2020). COVID-19 Sets off Mass Migration in India. *Archives of Medical Research*.
20. Negi, A. C., (2020). *Human Rights Violations of Migrants Workers in India During COVID-19 Pandemic*. Available at SSRN 3629773.

21. Patil, P. K., (2020). COVID-19 Pandemic & Its Impact on the Mental Health of Youth. *Research Analysis and Evaluation*.

22. Sharma, A., & Jose, A. M. Internal Migration: Issues Prevailing in the NCT (National Capital Territory) of Delhi.

23. World Health Organization. (2020). Infection prevention and control during health care when novel coronavirus (nCoV) infection is suspected: interim guidance, 25 January 2020 (No. WHO/2019-nCoV/IPC/2020.2). World Health Organization.

24. Domaradzki, S., Khvostova, M., & Pupovac, D. (2019). Karel Vasak's Generations of Rights and the Contemporary Human Rights Discourse. *Human Rights Review*, *20*(4), 423–443.

25. Sharma, I. (2015). Violence against women: Where are the solutions?. *Indian journal of psychiatry*, *57*(2), 131.

CHAPTER 4

The Pandemic of COVID-19 and Inhuman Wrongs

SUBIR KUMAR ROY

Registrar (Addl. Charge) and Associate Professor, Department of Law,
Bankura University, Bankura, West Bengal, India,
E-mail: dr.roysubir@gmail.com

ABSTRACT

The COVID-19 pandemic has posed the greatest challenge to the very survival and existence of humankind since the Second World War. The pandemic with its ugly face is tormenting the daily life pattern of human beings throughout the world. Already it has stormed with social, political, economical, and cultural changes. The world is facing the acute humanitarian crisis occurring from a virus about which our knowledge is visibly poor and still now we are incapable to accept the challenges thrown by the above microscopic creature and as a consequence, we are observing a global public health emergency across the globe. The whole world is stunned with the devastative impact of this novel coronavirus. The outbreak of COVID-19 exposed the vulnerability of the poorer sections of the society, their sufferings and inhuman wrongs being perpetrated on them. The aim of this chapter is not to discuss about the scientific and technical matters related with COVID-19 or to discuss about its physiological impact or the scientific ways to arrest the above but to discuss the issues from the prism of human right, beckoning for a changing social order based on the principles of interdependence, coordination, and solidarity. This chapter is based on the analytical study of the existing literature and information.

4.1   INTRODUCTION

It is needless to mention that the whole world is witnessing an unprecedented calamity caused by COVID-19. The devastating impact of novel coronavirus endangers the life of many and completely disrupts the daily activities of life. It is severity of contagiousness breaks the record of all previous pestilence, and almost all the nations of the world are trembling with its lethalness. It has decimated lives, crumbled down the economic structure, displaced millions, smashed, and speared the hopes of life and mental peace, derailed the health system, and engulfed the whole humanity in its destructive mechanism. Day by day, the above menace is assuming a gigantic shape worldwide, thereby causing a deadly impact on the life of the people, and with the pace of the above, the death toll is also rising. Keeping this horrid human crisis in mind, the World Health Organization (WHO) declared the situation caused by the novel coronavirus as Public Health Emergency across the globe on 30th January, 2020. International Health Regulation (2005) defines such situation as potential for international spread and requires a coordinated international step to combat the above situation [12]. This situation caused a grim global crisis which has affected both the advanced economies and emerging markets and developing economies and thereby the situation led the IMF to project growth in advanced economies at –6.1%.

We should not forget that shadows of cloud cannot hide the sun for long and after every dark night, a glorious morning comes. Pained with the casualty caused by World War II, the representatives of 50 nations met at San Francisco in the year, 1945 to draft the United Nations (UN) Charter and kept the UN under the obligation to promote and estimate for inalienable natural rights and for essential core freedoms for all without making any discrimination and ultimately which has been coined through Article 55 of the UN charter. Through Article 56 of the UN charter, the members pledged themselves to cooperate with the organization in order to achieve the noble ideals of Article 55. The San Francisco conference was followed by a number of covenants and conventions. Similarly, the COVID-19 fiasco brought all the countries more interdependent and interconnected in dire search of a healthy life supported by a strong economy to uphold the humanity. The pandemic of coronavirus and the massive health disorders that arise out of it will surely compel the world order to rethink about incorporation of inner-state bio-security and to take meaningful step for making this earth free from starvation or hunger, pollution, and diseases. This alarming situation demands to intensify the war against the bio-terror and bio-weapons,

weapons of mass destruction and terrorism. This pandemic has opened our eyes that still, how much we are helpless despite of our boasts of advancement of modern science and technologies and thereby claiming ourselves as the smartest human beings. The states should come together with all their strength, power, values, and interest to intensify the collaborative effort to arrest this pandemic situation and also to engage in finding the solution to save humanity from this disastrous and delirious situation. But in practice, we are finding completely a reverse picture in the world order where the nationalism is increasing and gradually the 'One World Theory' is becoming thinner and narrower. The tensions are growing in between China and the USA, and the impact of this equation perceives in the ongoing strenuous relationship of USA with WHO. The drastic deterioration of Indo-Sino relationship, the drastic erosion in the cohesion of the European Union, the adamant stand of USA regarding lifting of ban on Iran to make way for humanitarian aid, the displeasures of Baltic Nations about addressing their problems to tackle the pandemic situation by the European Union, the closure of boundaries, severance, stoppage of supply chain among the states and closure of international flights axing on the very root of globalization. However, the world polity is bound to adopt the concerted and coordinated approach to overcome this human crisis as this is a global and transboundary issue. The outbreak of COVID-19 exposed the vulnerability of the poorer sections of the society, their sufferings and inhuman wrongs being perpetrated on them, especially in developing countries, including India. During this period of human crisis, the third world countries have to reconsider and reassess its health system. COVID-19 with all its ugly face sending the message that the ill health of one may prove fatal for the health of a considerable size of population.

4.2 A CAGING LIFE: PSYCHOLOGICAL AND MENTAL DISORDER

We can imagine of a new world order with changed philosophy of life, inclining towards a more humanistic approach, in aftermath COVID-19 episode. The boring and distressful life in quarantine, isolation, and staying at home reminds us of the basic tenets of the human beings, i.e., being social creatures, we cannot survive outside the society. During this period of lockdown and social distancing, we are madly feeling the urge and need for the company of our family members, our relatives, neighbors, colleagues. People are longing for the company of others no matter known or unknown, to feel and trace their own existence and identity as a human being by sharing the warmth, ethos, pathos, and feeling of humanness with each other. People have learned about 'privacy' during the industrial revolution and felt the pain of isolated life in a pandemic period of COVID-19. The practicalities of caging life prompted us to revisit the prime philosophy of life, which teaches us that the aim of life cannot be the selfish survival but to sacrifice the same for the sake of others as nothing can be greater or important than humanity. The sociologists are claiming that we are entering into a world of new sufferings and pain arising due to the initiation of the steps for staying away from the people to breakdown or cut-off the route of transmission as it is reported to be transmitted from human to human. It is axiomatic, that to curb the transmission of the coronavirus social distancing, isolation, lockdown, quarantine, etc., are essential but at the same time evidently the method of withdrawing the people from their society and to confined them within the four walls of their house is causing the mental and physiological disorder to human beings in a devastating proportion. Beside the physiological illness it is seriously impairing the mental ability by inflicting the disorders like mental anxiety, depressions, mental stress, agony, fear psychosis, etc. There is a dearth of data available on how the current pandemic situation is affecting and impairing emotional, behavioral, and mental hygiene, but on the basis of different case histories, as appearing, it can be said that this pandemic will give birth to unparallel mental health issues and psychological distresses. Psychological disorders, mental trauma, behavioral health threats persist for a long time among the affected groups and multiplies with the loss of lives of the close and dearest relatives, change in socioeconomic status and by the change of the surroundings such as diminishing of the comfort of habitual zone, but the irony of the issue is that a large section of society pays little attention towards the mental illness to get rid over it[15]. Public health planning and policies should give priority to address the mental hygiene as it silently destroys the families and thereby ultimately weakens the whole race. The Corona pandemic has dumbfounded the global community; people accepted the life of isolation out of fear psychosis, advice of governmental agencies, and afterwards by legal enforcement, which astonishingly dented the freedom and liberty of the people. The emergency public health laws, besides the physiological disorders, should also take care of the psychological disorders by ensuring the instruments like counseling and an enabling environment, especially to children, aging, and other vulnerable groups.

---

[15] James, G. H. Jr., Lainie, R., & Aubrey, J. C., (2010). *Mental, and Behavioral Health Legal Preparedness in Major Emergencies*. Public Health Reports, Sage Publications. Accessed from: https://www.jstor.org/stable/41434834 (accessed on 3 July 2021).

4.3   ISSUES OF HEALTH AND ECONOMY: CONTESTED OR COMPLEMENTARY

The COVID-19 episode is also raising one another burning issue which has not yet been addressed seriously and almost a neglected issue, i.e., the cross issues or the contested questions in between health and economy. Which should be the matter of prime concern health or economy? This cross-issue gets emphatic from the policy decision of imposition of lockdown and social distancing to hammer the transmission of coronavirus from human to human because till the information, human beings are the sole carrier of this virus, which spread and transmitted through droplets. Since the outbreak of the respiratory disease caused by the COVID-19 at the end of 2019 in Wuhan, China yet, till writing of this chapter, our scientists have failed to understand the nature of this virus, its incubation period and about its different forms happening due to its rapid mutation. From the above; we can easily imagine the disastrous, devastating, notorious, and dangerous impact of this virus. As, still we have failed to develop any kind of protective shield like vaccinations and effective medicines globally, the nation-states are giving priority to lockdown, social distancing, etc., which is no doubt ruining the growth of the global economy. The above non-medicinal interventions have almost crushed down the economy, across the globe. No other remedial measures incorporated globally raised so many global, legal, ethical, moral, and political issues. The pandemic of COVID-19 and the worldwide lockdown as a remedial measure has caused the worst recession even worse than any other previously occurred global economic crisis and economical disaster[16]. It has challenged and crushed the global economy in such a magnitude that no other worldwide crisis had ever done. As per the Global Financial Stability Report, April, 2020 the social distancing measures are seriously impairing the global economy and caused 3% negative growth instead of the expected 3% positive growth in only three months which is even worse than the worldwide financial recession happened during 2008–2009[17]. It has devastatingly affected the trade, business, commerce, etc., and has completely disrupted the market mechanism. The COVID-19 pandemic is engulfing the vibration of life and is presenting itself as unprecedented disastrous to world

---

[16] Gita, G., (2020). *The Great Lockdown: Worst Economic Downturn Since the Great Depression.* Accessed from: https://blogs.imf.org/2020/04/14/the-great-lockdown-worst-economic-downturn-since-the-great-depression/ (accessed on 3 July 2021).
[17] International Monetary Fund, (2020). *Global Financial Stability Report: Markets in the Time of COVID-19.* Washington, DC, April. Accessed from: https://www.imf.org/en/Publications/GFSR/Issues/2020/04/14/global-financial-stability-report-april-2020 (accessed on 6 May 2020).

economy. According to the Creon Butler, Director of Global Economy and Finance Program at Chatham House, the world has never before witnessed such a 'global economic shock' resultant from the pandemic of COVID-19[18]. Many economists and the thinkers like James Meadway compared the economic debacles caused by this pandemic with the economic disaster happened due to Second World War and disagreed to compare it with either the recent economic recession happened during 2008 or the great depression of the 1930s[19]. Now, under the above backdrop, the whole world is very confused on the very proposition that which one will prevail over the other-life or economy. It is a great challenge before the policymakers and the whole system-the Government, Governance, and the Governed that whether they will drive for protection from sickness and death or pay attention to save the economy which is in a moribund condition. Protective measures, as already described, most of which are non-pharmaceutical in nature, from contamination as well as revival of economy from its ruining position, both are the urgent need of the hour to save life and livelihood. Life and livelihood both are the intrinsic part of each other. Life cannot exist without livelihood and the question of livelihood arises only where there exists life. This pandemic has raised a very important and crucial cross issue of health and economy. Many economists opine that if the world will remain in lockdown for some more months, then a large chunk of people from the developing country will die out of starvation. But at the same time, it is also true that the right to health is certainly more precious and valuable than any other rights as it is an intrinsic, integral, inalienable, and sacrosanct part of the human right to life. Article 25 of the UDHR[20] considered right to health as an inseparable and inherent part of the human rights. The states are under the obligation to ensure the right to life of the people threatened by any private individual[21]. The same analogy can be used in the matter of threat to life of the persons caused by other affected with the contagious disease caused by the novel coronavirus and States by the above dictum of Un Human Right Committee

---

[18] How to Survive the coronavirus? (2020), *The World Today*. April & May 2020, Royal Institute of International Affairs Accessed from: https://www.chathamhouse.org/publications/the-world-today/2020-04/how-survive-pandemic (accessed on 6 May 2020).

[19] James, M., (2020). *Capitalism's Gravest Challenge: How COVID-19 will Reshape the World?* New Statesman. Available at: http://iproxy.inflibnet.ac.in:2111/ehost/pdfviewer/pdfviewer?vid=11&sid=92558615-2d5c-4561-bfc4-87fd9ffc992a%40sdc-v-sessmgr02 (accessed on 3 July 2021).

[20] Accessed from: https://www.ohchr.org/EN/UDHR/Documents/UDHR_Translations/eng.pdf (accessed on 3 July 2021).

[21] General Comment No. 36, (2018). *On Art. 6 of the ICCPR on the Right to Life of UN Human Rights Committee*. UN Doc CCPR/C/GC/36, paras 7, 21.

are liable to protect the life of the people diligently[22]. The right to health is also recognized by Article 12 of the International Covenant on Economic, Social, and Cultural Rights (ICESCR) which states that everyone has the right to enjoy the highest attainable standard of physical and mental health and it is the cardinal obligation of the States to ensure the mechanism so that all can realize the above rights full and effectively and must include the provisions for improvement of child mortality, healthy environment and hygiene, curb, and treat epidemic, endemic, occupational, and other diseases and mechanism for healthcare[23]. This provision is very important as it bestows the legal right on everyone to protect themselves from the ongoing pandemic and also the COVID patients to get proper healthcare especially in the light of the commitment of the UN Committee on Economic, Social, and Cultural Rights which states that it is the obligation of the States to respect, protect, and fulfill the rights related to health. So right to health is an indispensable, inseparable, and integral part of the human right. WHO treats right to health as "the enjoyment of the highest attainable standard of health[24]." Health is a comprehensive term, requires all those ingredients and elements without which a person cannot attain the physical, mental, and spiritual growth. Right to health demands for its proper enjoyment and implementation, the basic necessities of life like food, clothing, shelter, security along with the medical and pharmaceutical care and of course in an enabling environment. It is an undebatable issue, that to ensure sound health, sound economy is sine qua non. The issue is how long the non-pharmaceutical intervention will create impediments into the way of economy to stop its growth and thus this virus has thrown a strong and unwelcoming challenge to the policymakers of the different nation-states to resolve and tackle the situation in an alternative way to ultimately uphold the humanity. As per the estimation of the World Bank, the global economy will decline by $4.2 trillion, between 2019 and 2020 which is much greater than the global economy of South Asia[25]. Millions of people may lose their jobs and to face the hunger, food insecurity, starvation, malnutrition in a horrified scale. As per the study of World Bank, four out of five people in the global workforce of 3.3 are facing the full or partial closures of their avocations[26]. As per a report,

---

[22] Ibid

[23] Art. 12 of the Covenant on Economic, Social, and Cultural Rights, opened for signature on December 1966 and came into force, 3rd January 1976.

[24] WHO, Our Guiding Principle. https://www.who.int/about/what-we-do/who-brochure (accessed on 3 July 2021).

[25] Axel, V. T., (2020). *Voices.* Accessed from: https://blogs.worldbank.org/voices/broad-fast-action-save-lives-and-help-countries-rebuild (accessed on 3 July 2021).

[26] Ibid.

updated as on May 1, 2020, of the Congressional Research Service, this pandemic will shrink the global economic growth by as much as 2.0% per month if the COVID episode will continue in its present form[27]. It further forecasts that the global trade could fall by 13% to 32%, depending upon the extent of spread of the contamination[28]. In the first quarter of 2020; 4.8% drop in US GDP has been indicated and this figure is 3.8% reduction in Euro-zone economy[29]. The rating agency Moody's forecasted that the in the current fiscal year, India's economic growth will be 0% due to the impact of the coronavirus[30]. On the other hand, the death toll as well as the number of the patients affected with the COVID-19 is rising day by day. It has already engulfed 190 countries and case counts are changing daily and of course with increasing rate which is very worrying. Now at the above juncture it is a billion-dollar question that whether the non-pharmaceutical measures will persist over the economic activity or something else. The situation has thrown tough challenges to the policymakers whereby all are bewildered, how to tackle a situation where the nature and whereabouts of the enemy is largely invisible. It is the high time that UN, WHO, and other International Organizations should come ahead to cooperate and compel the state parties, especially the developing countries to comply with the International legal mechanism to ensure the right to health of the people in this pandemic situation and should also ensure hygiene and biosecurity and to impose liability, if any state or states are liable behind the outbreak of the novel coronavirus otherwise the International Legal Mechanism concerning health will turn into ridiculous position.

4.4 COVID-19 AND CHANGING DIMENSIONS OF LIFE

The COVID-19 pandemic has posed the greatest challenge to the very survival and existence of the humankind since Second World War. The pandemic with its ugly face is tormenting the daily life pattern of the human beings throughout the world. Already it has stormed with social, political, economical, and cultural changes. Social distancing, masking, hand washing, sanitization, cleaning is going to be a part of our culture and handshaking,

[27] James K. J., Schwarzenberg, Weiss, & Nelson, (2020). *Global Economic Effects of COVID-19.* Accessed from: https://crsreports.congress.gov/product/pdf/R/R46270/20 (accessed on 9 May 2020).
[28] Ibid.
[29] Ibid.
[30] https://www.ndtv.com/business/coronavirus-news-moodys-sees-indias-economic-growth-at-zero-in-current-financial-year-amid-covid-19-2225381 (May 8, 2020 03:10 pm IST) (accessed on 3 July 2021).

hugging, kissing, etc., may take farewell from the public life, permanently, in the near future, if the danger of the contamination persists for long. The political scientists are confused in portraying the future shape of the world. We can observe the sharp differences and divergent opinions in forecasts of the experts on the issues of nationalism, globalization, democracy, inter-relationship of states, etc., in the aftermath COVID situation. However, all agree on this point that the composition of the inter-state and intra-state relation will change radically to address the issues of public health, hygiene, employment, trade-commerce, etc. Apart from the above, it will bring massive changes in the pattern of livelihood. Due to the apprehension of the spread of the contamination of coronavirus, the tendency of work from home (WFH) will grow more and more. This changing attitude will further boost to the development of computer science, information technology, and the artificial intelligence. To save the humankind from the disastrous impact of COVID-19 the human mind will compel to further explore the I.K.B.S., i.e., Intelligent Knowledge-Based System, Preparation of Robotics, Computational Metaphor, and more sophisticated, advance, and effective Communication System, however the present article does not intend to involve the legal, ethical or any moral issues associated with the above. The COVID-19 pandemic is also causing the behavioral changes among the human beings with its unwelcoming presence in the human habitat. Such as, no one should suppose to spit indiscriminately in public places. Many countries have already have initiated the legal measures to refrain people from causing such nuisance, since this virus spread through the droplets. People for their own survival will avoid the public gatherings so long we are not getting the triumph over this pandemic. Most of the countries have already imposed ban on any kind of social, political, or religious gatherings and till the date nobody can predict how long it will continue. Sometimes the over protectionism attitude may make a section of people maniac or crazy.

4.5   COVID-19 AND CHALLENGE TO LIFE AND LIVELIHOODS

The ugly face of COVID-19 blatantly exposed the distinction in between the have and have-nots. Though this virus itself does not discriminate the people on any ground like status, race, religion, caste, etc., while contami-nating people but it unveils the present human crisis-vulnerabilities of a large chunk of people, who are in a position of hand to mouth and is dying out of starvation, needs immediate humanitarian aid. When the migrant laborers cover mile after mile in India by walking with a dream in their eyes to return back to their own house-may be tiny, congested or in a ruinous condition-but after all their own house inhabited by their own family members-a thirst for getting a glimpse of their faces-exposes the hardest truth, a grim reality-at what level the poverty exists and how a considerable section of the society live even worse than the animal life. As per the report of Spokesperson of world food program (WFP), 40 million people across West Africa will encounter the shortage of food due to the preventive measures initiated to restrain the contaminations[31]. As per the estimation of the WFP 12 million children less than 5 years old in this region could face the malnutrition during the period of June to August compared to 8.2 million in the same period last year[32]. WFP forecasts the same situation for the West Africa too[33]. As per an independent UN human rights expert, Philip Alston, if USA will not take immediate preventive and welfare measures millions of middle-class Americans will be in acute poverty[34]. According to him if the beneficial measures will not be initiated on behalf of the Government of USA, precisely Congress then a considerable section of the Country will soon face destitution[35]. As per the Bureau of Labor Statistics (BLS) April Employment Situation Report nonfarm payroll employment fell by 20.5 million and unemployment rate reached from 10.3% points to 14.7%[36]. The report further said that the unemployment rate was 3.5% in America which is lowest in the past 50 years of history of the country[37]. The people with lower academic qualifications are experiencing the largest job losses which, rose from 14.4% to 21.2% in April, 2020[38]. Bureau of Economic Analysis (BEA) estimated 4.8% contraction at an annual rate in the first quarter of 2020 and the consumer behavior is showing that Americans are dramatically curtailing the expenditures due to the COVID tragedy[39]. The above statistics manifesting the unexplainable sufferings of the disadvantageous sections even inside the 'superpower country' like the USA. It is exposing how the deprivation and discrimination is deep-rooted even in the developed countries

---

[31] Available at: https://news.un.org/en/story/2020/05/1063232 (accessed on 3 July 2021).

[32] Ibid

[33] Ibid

[34] Available at: https://news.un.org/en/story/2020/04/1061982 (accessed on 3 July 2021).

[35] Ibid

[36] Available at: https://www.whitehouse.gov/articles/aprils-job-losses-show-many-workers-still-connected-employers/ (accessed on 3 July 2021).

[37] Ibid

[38] Ibid

[39] Available at: https://www.whitehouse.gov/articles/depth-look-covid-19s-early-effects-consumer-spending-gdp/ (accessed on 3 July 2021).

like USA where the people belonging from the lower strata of the society are in panic about the guarantee of their life and livelihood. The disastrous economic condition of the USA and the tragic conditions of a considerable number of masses, happened due to the COVID catastrophe unveils the truth that just by preparing atom bombs, deadly weapons for mass destructions, blind automation, Star Wars, creating material gains by ruthless exploitation of natural resources, a state cannot become a superpower. To become a real superpower the primary concern should be to focus on the protection of health, life, and livelihood of the people. Despite of its ugly face, COVID catastrophe gives us a clear lesson that we require to pay attention towards the sustainable development, pleasure, and peace instead of the development of the weapons of mass killing. The attack of coronavirus reveals the truth that our boasting about our knowledge and wisdom has no foundation at all and for the existence of our own race it is the need of the hour to strengthen our relationship with the nature more closely and to pay attention to develop the mechanism for the survival of mankind in a sound ecosystem.

The world itself is reeling under hunger, unemployment, gender discrimination, diseases, rising crimes against humanity, cultural estrangement, growing hardcore ideologies to accelerate the tendency of separatism and segregation, terrorism, poverty, drug addiction, etc., and thereafter the current explosion of COVID-19 expedite the human tragedy and human crisis. All our so-called development proved dwarf to face the challenges thrown by a microscopic creature. We innovate more for the destruction of mankind than its survival and development. We have spent most of our resources and precious time to respond for wars and interventions, involving in arm race, engaging in power struggle, and in ruthless exploitation of natural resources but never tried to make this planet a pleasure shelter for all human beings irrespective of any discrimination where no one will have to die out of starvation and no one will have to face the exploitation.

4.6 COVID-19 AND TALES OF UNDERPRIVILEGED

We are passing through a peculiar situation, where everyone is spending their days with an apprehension about their very survival, fear, and agony grasping the mind and anxiety is manifesting about our own lives and livelihoods. The outbreak of the ongoing pandemic in almost all part of the globe and its horrible impact into the lives and livelihoods of the people has exposed our helplessness to fight with a microscopic creature. The whole humanity is reeling under fear and susceptible to panic as the threat is posed directly to their existence. Practically we are hiding ourselves as much as possible within the four wall of our house and saving ourselves from mixing with our near and dear ones as still, we don't have any effective remedy against it. As the prime importance before the nation-states are to protect the precious lives of the people, they are compelled to adopt the policies of lockdown and social distancing as a natural course of action to slow down the transmission of the virus. These policies have far-reaching consequences which are affecting the economic, social, cultural, and political lives of the people globally. State authorities are waging war on different fronts with huge pressure and facing the one after other challenges appearing with new features and dimensions. The prime challenges before the policymakers are obviously to provide health care facilities, to make an arrangement at war footed for the treatments of the coronavirus affected patients and at the same time the separate arrangements for the patients affected with the other non-COVID diseases, to make arrangements for food, water, sanitation, education, emergency services, security, to take care of the economy which has almost slipped into moribund condition, to provide foods and shelters to marginal and vulnerable section of the society, to maintain law and order, to take steps for eliminating the risk factors to the lives of the doctors, health workers, workers involved in cleaning and sanitizing activities, police personnel. Armies, etc., this pandemic has not only changed our lifestyle and our perceptions about it rather it also changes the whole social system. The sea changes are approaching in all the sectors-be it is political, social, economical, and cultural or any other branches of life. This pandemic is no more confined only within the gamut of public health emergency rather it triggered serious crisis to lives and livelihoods of the mankind. The human civilization has witnessed the pandemics earlier too but not as contagious and disastrous as COVID-19. Almost all the countries in the world are being engulfed by this pandemic, thereby disrupting the normal lives of the people, which had never happened before. The affected people are striving hard to restore their health, and the unaffected persons are battling tough to protect their livelihoods. The protective measures incorporated to stop the transmission costs much as it slowed down the economy of the countries.

The whole world is stunned with the devastating impact of this novel coronavirus. It has triggered storm in social, economic, and political fronts and compelling the states to find the ways for restoring normalcy. This pandemic has forced us to consider our abilities and potentialities completely from a new perception, through a fresh outlook. Almost six months have elapsed, since the outbreak of this pandemic, reported in Wuhan, Hubei province, China in December, 2019 and yet, we have not been able to arrest it. This tragedy has shown the limitation of our knowledge, information, and our poor performance and preparation in struggle with the nature. In view of the above grim reality, it is the demand of the situation, that the states should not only work collaboratively to find the way out to tackle this grim situation but also come forward to work in a coordinated way with a spirit of solidarity to protect the lives and livelihoods of the people. Aftermath COVID-19 situation will be more horrible than the present COVID-19 affected situation where a large chunk of people will lose their jobs, the rate of economy will be sleuth, poverty, and hunger will increase and people will suffer the health disaster. Despite of its destructive nature this pandemic has given us the opportunity to reassess our strengths and weaknesses, our triumph, and tribulations and to take lessons from our failure happened due to our own faults so that we may take a positive and meaningful step to make our future, bright, and in no way can endanger the very survival of our future generation.

COVID-19 crisis has made the life of the underprivileged people miserable and worse. It has been proved more fatal for the older persons and persons having the poor immunity due to the morbidity like cancer, diabetics, heart ailments, kidney disorders, etc. As per UN, this pandemic has exacerbated the vulnerability of the least protected and highlighted the prevailing inequalities of the society[40]. The report of UN entitled, 'COVID-19 and Human Rights: We are all in this together' gives emphasis on the need of strengthening the public health and social support system[41]. The present pandemic situation has totally changed the long-accustomed lives and livelihoods of the people. Emergency situation has been imposed in many countries and many of them have extended their power to deal with this crisis. Though the people are also supporting their governments for extending such extraordinary power but needless to mention, in many matters, the people are forced to compromise with their civil liberties. To effectively deal with the COVID calamity, the policymakers have to formulate the policies to fight with the poverty, hunger, malnutrition, and the distorted health facility. In many countries, the life and liberty of the poorer section of the society are in an endangered state. Livelihoods of the considerable section of the society are in dwindling position. The people are facing discrimination on the basis of race, caste, religion,

---

[40] *COVID-19 and Human Rights: We are all in This Together*, (2020). Accessed from: https://www.un.org/sites/un2.un.org/files/un_policy_brief_on_human_rights_and_covid_23_april_2020.pdf (accessed on 3 July 2021).
[41] Ibid

etc., even in this pandemic situation. Crimes are being organized against the people on the ground of their religion, race by falsely implicating them for spreading the virus. People affected by the coronavirus as well as the corona warriors are witnessing a kind of stigmatization against them in many regions. Due to the lack of social support systems in many countries, the lives of the elders have become very insecure. In many regions, the prisoners, migrants, LGBTI community, disabled persons, and women are facing the acute violation of their human rights. The UN High Commissioner for Human Rights said that racial and ethnic minorities are the worst victim of the COVID-19 pandemic due to the discriminatory policies of the Governments of some countries[42]. The UN rights chief had given a statistic which shows that in Brazil's Sao Paulo state, the people of color are dying 62% more than the white-skinned people[43]. The report also says that higher mortality rates have been observed in Seine-Saint-Denis department in France which is being inhabited by many minorities[44]. Not only that, the available data from the UN establishes the very fact that COVID-19 death rate for African-Americans is more than double in comparison to other racial groups. Similarly, it has been appeared the mortality rate of black, Pakistani, and Bangladeshi people are double than white people in England and Wales[45]. Inequality, discriminations, and lack of distributive justice are the prime reasons for the occurrence of such disparities. The ninth Secretary-General of the UN Mr. Antonio Guterres said that the pandemic continues to spread hatred, xenophobia, scaremongering, blaming, and stigmatizing mainly against the vulnerable groups, minorities, migrants, refugees on them concocted, imaginary, and baseless ground disparaged that they are responsible for spreading the virus and denied from the medical facilities[46].

4.7   COVID-19 AND GENDER DISCRIMINATION

The sufferings of the women have increased beyond tolerance during this ongoing pandemic situation. Women across the globe are facing the economic crisis more acute than their male counterparts amid the grim reality that the

---

[42] Address of the UN rights chief on 'appalling impact of COVID-19 on minorities.' Accessed from: https://news.un.org/en/story/2020/06/1065272 (accessed on 3 July 2021).

[43] Ibid

[44] Ibid

[45] Ibid

[46] Antonio Guterres, (2020). *We Must Act Now to Strengthen the Immunity of Our Societies Against the Virus of Hate.* Accessed from: https://www.un.org/en/coronavirus/we-must-act-now-strengthen-immunity-our-societies-against-virus-hate (accessed on 3 July 2021).

lion sharer of them earn less, engaged in temporary and contractual jobs, and live in a hand to mouth position. Most women are engaged in informal economic sectors where the social security and assistance are generally not available. Due to the measures like lockdown and social distancing to curb the spread of the virus further, the informal employment sectors affected largely, which ultimately affected the life of the women. As per the report of UN over 80% of women in non-agricultural jobs are in informal employment, and this figure in sub-Saharan Africa and in Latin America and the Caribbean is respectively, 74% and 54%[47]. On the other hand, due to the lockdown, the workload of women at home increases to meet the growing care needs with children out of school, husband, and other relatives at home and for the elderly and ill members but with no pay. To meet this increasing demand for unpaid care work, many working women and girls fail to attend their scheduled job, which creates another hardship for them. As per the report entitled, 'Policy Brief: The Impact of COVID-19 on Women' the increased demand for care work is deepening the existing gender inequalities in the field of division of labor[48]. Due to the closures of schools, most of the girls and adolescent girls living in poverty, rural areas, or belonging to the family cares little for education are being engaged in household activities and are spending most of their time for the same instead of focusing on study. This situation may lead to the dropping out of millions of girls from schools which will negatively affect the development of the society. During this COVID-19 pandemic situation the gender-based violence and particularly domestic violence is increasing across the globe. Absence of social contact, confinement within home and lack of social and legal support due to this ongoing crisis, the women are experiencing the gender violence more than before. Most of the women are forced by the situation to share the dwelling place with their abusers. As per the information provided by UN in many countries with reporting system in place the upward of 25% has been recorded and in some countries said offense has been doubled[49]. In many countries, the victims are not getting the support from the law enforcement authorities and civil society as either they are constrained by the lockdown or the shifting of the priorities to control the situation. The reason, whatever may be, it is a gross violation of the dignity, integrity, privacy of the women which should be addressed and resolved with utmost priority by any society; if it is sufficiently civilized. Reports

---

[47] *Policy Brief: The Impact of COVID-19 on Women*, (2020). Accessed from: https://www.un.org/sites/un2.un.org/files/policy_brief_on_covid_impact_on_women_9_apr_2020_updated.pdf (accessed on 3 July 2021).

[48] Ibid

[49] Ibid

of domestic violence have increased by 30% since the lockdown imposed in France and similar report has been reported across Europe and North America. In China, their police reports show the domestic violence tripled during the outbreak of the pandemic[50]. As per the report of the UN Working Group on Discrimination against Women and Girls, many provinces within the United States arbitrarily interfering with the reproductive rights of the women by creating unnecessary hurdles in accessing abortion[51]. The states like Texas, Oklahoma, Alabama, Lowa, Ohio, Arkansas, Louisiana, and Tennessee are imposing the ban on abortion, which is very much discriminatory, gender insensitive approach and inhuman act. Access to abortion care is placing the health of the women at greater risk and thus infringing their right to life. It not only impairs the rights of the women to have sound health but also denial of the right to have control on their bodies and lives, which is inherently dangerous and barbaric attempt on the part of the state authorities. Gender Inequalities are compounding with the ongoing COVID-19 crisis and appearing in many forms to jeopardize their rights further. The non-pharmaceutical measures are imposing restrictions in accessing the necessary services from the entrusted authorities to enforce their rights as well as the necessary support, information, and medical assistance related to their sexual and reproductive health care. The women, mainly in rural areas, are not getting the required health services, medicines, and the reproductive health care. According to a study of UN Foundation in Latin America and the Caribbean, because of the coronavirus crisis, 18 million additional women will lose regular access to modern contraceptives[52]. This situation may cause increase maternal mortality, unwanted pregnancy mainly in adolescents and the sexually transmitted diseases (STDs) including HIV transmission[53]. The crisis of the above health care support is prevailing in other parts of the globe also. It had been found 70% increase in death of women at the time of delivery of child during the Ebola crisis in West Africa[54]. Across the globe, 70% of women are engaged with the health care services and actively participating to respond to health care during the ongoing pandemic situation. The women health workers who are the frontrunners in this battle are facing enormous difficulties and hardships including violent attacks from the communities and affected persons due to their unawareness and unnecessary

---

[50] See: https://unfoundation.org/blog/post/shadow-pandemic-how-covid19-crisis-exacerbating-gender-inequality/ (accessed on 3 July 2021).
[51] Accessed from: https://news.un.org/en/story/2020/05/1064902 (accessed on 3 July 2021).
[52] Ibid
[53] Ibid
[54] Ibid

phobia about the disease, dearth of protective equipment, lower-paid and lower status as their opinions never carry any importance to induct the same in policy decision.

The present crisis is a serious threat to the human rights of the people, and we can overcome the above situation through the collaborative governance, by practicing respect for the human rights guaranteed by the International Human Rights bill, covenants, and protocols and through the international treaties and judicial opinions. Complying with the sustainable development goals (SDGs), we can fight with this situation in a better way. The impact of the coronavirus is undoubtedly a greatest tragedy of the civilization but at the same time it is also teaching us the values of life and the need of incorporation of an egalitarian system. Till date, the concept of egalitarian system attains the academic value only and the policymakers always considered it as nothing more than a myth.

4.8 CONCLUSION

The COVID-19 pandemic has created a serious human rights problems to almost all the countries but of course with different degrees and challenges and largely dependent on the socio-economic situation of the countries. The prime focus on the part of the policymakers must be to save the lives and livelihoods. This is true that the above virus does not discriminate the people in making its victim but its impacts on different strata of the society are obviously different. The poorer sections of the society are the worst victim of the present crisis. The people working in the formal and informal sectors are losing their jobs due to the slowdown of the economy, and thereby they are compelled to survive with hunger, exploitation, malnutrition. Beside the threat to life, liberty, and livelihood the outbreak is also causing, serious problem to rule of law, impediments in getting justice, arbitrary imposition of decision by the governments violating the democratic norms so as to hide their incompetency to manage the affairs, peace, and security challenges, massive health crisis, threat to the life of the health workers, refugees, and other vulnerable groups. The international as well as the national mechanism must protect the right to life, right to livelihood, right to health, right to freedom, right to education, right to equality otherwise lots of precious lives will be at peril and will endanger the humanity. The international human rights bodies and the humanitarian agencies under the aegis of UN should come forward and assist the governmental and non-governmental actors so that they can provide good governance and incorporate the inclusive and equitable policies based on the principle pro-bono-publico. A nation alone cannot get triumph over this invisible and strong enemy. It is a battle needed to be fought jointly with joint effort. Developed states must provide the financial aids, medications, and other humanitarian assistance to third-world countries, especially the low-income states, so that they can also fight back to win the battle. The UN should more active in the creation of a public perception and opinion on a real issue that it is a fight in between the human being and a pathogen where human beings have to fight the battle united otherwise our existence will be in danger. Creation of a sustainable society should be our goal we must strive towards that end. The madness for nationalism should not deprive the states to share and access the latest technological developments and research on modern treatment, medications, and the potential ways to beat the crisis.

KEYWORDS

- **COVID-19**
- **gender discrimination**
- **human rights**
- **marginalized people**
- **public health**
- **World Food Program**
- **World Health Organization**

REFERENCES

1. James, G. H. Jr., Lainie, R., & Aubrey, J. C., (2010). *Mental and Behavioral Health Legal Preparedness in Major Emergencies*. Public Health Reports, Sage Publications.
2. Gita, G., (2020). *The Great Lockdown: Worst Economic Downturn Since the Great Depression.* https://blogs.imf.org/2020/04/14/the-great-lockdown-worst-economic-downturn-since-the-great-depression (accessed on 26 June 2021).
3. How to survive the coronavirus, (2020), The World Today, April & May 2020, Royal Institute of International Affairs Accessed from https://www.chathamhouse.org/publications/the-world-today/2020-04/how-survive-pandemic (accessed on 6 May 2020).
4. Han, R., & James, M., (2020). *Capitalism's Gravest Challenge: How COVID-19 will Reshape the World.* New Statesman.

5. Axel, V. T., (2020). *Voices*. Accessed from: https://blogs.worldbank.org/voices/broad-fast-action-save-lives-and-help-countries-rebuild (accessed on 26 June 2021).
6. James K. Jackson, Schwarzenberg, Weiss & Nelson, (2020). Global Economic Effects of COVID-19, CRS Report, Congressional Research Service, R 46270, Accessed from https://crsreports.congress.gov/product/pdf/R/R46270/20 (accessed on 9 May 2020).
7. COVID-19 and Human Rights: We are all in this together (2020); UN Policy brief on human rights and Covid Accessed from https://www.un.org/sites/un2.un.org/files/un_policy_brief_on_human_rights_and_covid_23_april_2020.pdf (accessed on 14 May 2020).
8. Address of the UN rights chief on 'appalling impact of COVID-19 on minorities,' UN News, Global Perspective Human Stories, Accessed from https://news.un.org/en/story/2020/06/1065272 (accessed on 2 June 2020).
9. Antonio Guterres, (2020). We must act now to strengthen the immunity of our societies against the virus of hate, United Nations COVID-19 Response, Accessed from https://www.un.org/en/coronavirus/we-must-act-now-strengthen-immunity-our-societies-against-virus-hate (accessed on 3 June 2020).
10. Policy Brief: The Impact of COVID-19 on Women, (2020), United Nations Accessed from https://www.un.org/sites/un2.un.org/files/policy_brief_on_covid_impact_on_women_9_apr_2020_updated.pdf, (accessed on 3 June 2020).
11. News Releases, Bureau of Labor Statistics, US Department of Labor Accessed from https://www.bls.gov/news.release/archives/empsit_05082020.pdf (accessed on 26 June 2021).
12. Robert L. Cubeta, Catherine E. Shuster, & Stuart Smith (2020). New Models for a New Disease: Simulating the 2019 Novel Coronavirus, Institute for Defense Analyses, Accessed from https://www.jstor.org/stable/resrep22747 (accessed on 10 April 2021).

PART II

Health Challenges and Consequences of COVID-19

CHAPTER 5

Maternal and Reproductive Health in the Midst of COVID-19: The Case of Africa

PINKY LALTHAPERSAD-PILLAY

Department of Economics, University of South Africa, South Africa,
E-mail: lalthp@unisa.ac.za

ABSTRACT

Sub-Saharan Africa has persistently steep maternal mortality rates (MMR), accounting for as much as 66% of the global share of maternal deaths. The region is also home to extremely high levels of adolescent pregnancy. However, between 2000 and 2017, there was a 40% reduction in the maternal mortality ratio. There is a danger that this gain could be wiped given the effect that the COVID-19 pandemic could unleash on health systems, especially on the delivery of an array of maternal and reproductive health care offerings. Health care service disruptions will deny women access to potentially life-saving healthcare services, negatively affect access to contraception as well as increase maternal mortality and morbidity. This will affect the globally endorsed endeavors to end the unmet need for family planning and bring down preventable maternal deaths. The objective of the chapter is to contextualize the effects arising from the disruptions in service delivery due to the COVID-19 pandemic on various aspects of maternal and reproductive health care provision. It is therefore imperative that the full package of care in respect of maternal health and reproductive rights be sustained throughout the pandemic to ensure maternal and reproductive health benefits and gains for women and girls.

5.1 INTRODUCTION

Maternal health care is inclusive of a number of healthcare offerings and interventions such as prenatal care, post or ante-natal care, delivery care, and emergency obstetric care [1]. Reproductive health care entails the extension of family planning measures to prevent unwanted pregnancies [1]. Both maternal and reproductive health are essential in lowering maternal mortality and morbidity. Maternal and reproductive health outcomes are less than ideal in many African countries due to inadequate healthcare provision. Sub-Saharan Africa faces dual trepidations relating to high maternal mortality and steep adolescent pregnancy rates, which are odious for the overall health standing of women and girls [2]. The strain that COVID-19 exerts on healthcare systems is likely to further weaken vulnerable health systems. Disruptions in the delivery of health services will also have catastrophic effects on women's and girl's ability to manage their reproductive and maternal health needs due to shortages in contraceptives, the closure of clinics, costs incurred in traveling to far off clinics, and a shortage of healthcare workers to provide services. This will push up the tally of maternal deaths and unwanted pregnancies. The chapter begins with a contextualization of maternal and reproductive health care interventions. This is followed by an overview of maternal mortality and adolescent pregnancy rates. The possible bearing COVID-19 will have on the provision of contraception, and delivery care is then considered. Lastly, some policy measures are put forth.

5.2 PROBLEM STATEMENT

Maternal and reproductive health outcomes are less than ideal in many Africa as evidenced by the high numbers of maternal deaths, a steep adolescent pregnancy rate and high unmet need for family planning. Sub-Saharan Africa has persistently steep maternal mortality rates (MMRs), accounting for as much as 66% of the global share of maternal deaths. It is also burdened by steep levels of adolescent pregnancy [2]. However, between 2000 and 2017, there was a 40% reduction in the maternal mortality ratio [3]. There is a danger that this gain could be wiped out given the effect that the COVID-19 pandemic could unleash on health systems, especially on the delivery of maternal and reproductive health. This will impede progress in achieving broader global goals such as ending the unmet need for family planning and preventable maternal deaths [2]. The objective of the chapter is to contextualize the effects arising from the disruptions in service delivery due to the COVID-19 pandemic on various aspects of maternal and reproductive health care provision.

5.3   BACKGROUND TO THE STUDY

5.3.1   THE MATERNAL AND REPRODUCTIVE HEALTH CARE AGENDA

The provision of both maternal and reproductive health care offerings is singularly important to the well-being and upliftment of women and girls [4]. Maternal and reproductive health care are crucial in lowering maternal mortality as they provide a continuous stream of care before, during, and after pregnancy and childbirth, as well as preventing unwanted pregnancies. "Maternal health refers to the health of women during pregnancy, childbirth, and the postnatal period" [1]. On the other hand, sexual and reproductive health, and rights (SRHR) "encompass efforts to eliminate preventable maternal neonatal mortality and morbidity, to ensure quality sexual and reproductive health services, including contraceptive services, and to address sexually transmitted infections (STI) and cervical cancer, violence against women and girls, and sexual and reproductive health needs of adolescents" [5]. The WHO [5] points out that the provision of SRHR is beneficial for development at large, aside from fulfilling the health needs of women and girls and acceding to the ambit of their human rights.

Globally, protocols have been put in place over the years to deal with maternal and reproductive health care provision. The Convention for Elimination of All Forms of Discrimination Against women require governments to extend to women the full range of pregnancy-related services before, during, and after childbirth [6]. The conferment of SRHR was endorsed at the International Conference on Population and Development in 1994 [7, 8].

From a regional perspective, the African Charter implored governments to assure every person the right to health. More expressly, Article 14 of the African Women's Protocol impels states "to promote women's right to health, specifically recognizing that this includes their sexual and reproductive health and stresses that this right calls for the provision of adequate, affordable, and accessible health services" [6, 9]. In Article 14(2b), it succinctly requires states to create and bolster existing health services pertaining to delivery, as well as pre- and post-natal care [6]. The Maputo platform of action (MPoA) that was adopted in 2006 provided guidelines on issues pertaining to SRHR, maternal, infant, and child mortality, sexually transmitted diseases (STDs), HIV, and adolescent health concerns [9, 10]. The Accelerated Campaign on Reduction of Maternal Mortality in Africa (CARMMA) put forth in 2008 by the African Union was primarily an attempt to impel African leaders to slash the maternal deaths tally in their respective countries. It also encouraged the delivery of SRHR services by 2015 [11].

Despite these protocols that have been enunciated over the years, maternal, and reproductive sexual health and rights have been overlooked by most African governments. In Sub-Saharan Africa, SRHR have not enjoyed the full support of governments resulting in skewed provision of health services. In Sub-Saharan Africa, maternal mortality is fueled by two factors, namely, poor provision of maternal healthcare targeting women and girls as well as the neglect of sexual and reproductive rights by governments [7, 10]. The abjuration of (SHRH) precludes women from obtaining essential information that empowers women to take control of their reproductive choices by preventing pregnancy or the ability to give birth safely [2].

The inclusion of the maternal health in the MDG reinvigorated interest in a hitherto very important public health issue. Likewise, the incorporation of different aspects of maternal health in the sustainable development goals (SDGs) as goal 3 subsumed under 'good health and well-being' reaffirms the import of this crucial public health issue and the delivery of timely health services to women [12]. Targets relating to maternal and reproductive health reside in Targets 3.1 and 3.7 of the SDGs [13]. Specifically, the targets are as follows:

- Target 3.1: "By 2030, reduce the global maternal mortality ratio to less than 70 per 100,000 live births" [13]. The MMR and the amount of births attended by skilled health personnel are the two indicators laid down.
- Target 3.7: "By 2030, ensure universal access to sexual and reproductive health care services, including for family planning, information, and education, and the integration of reproductive health into national strategies and programs" [13]. This target comprises two indicators. The first indicator pertains to the share of women of reproductive age (15–49 years) that are deemed to have their need for family planning satisfied by the use of modern methods. The second indicator addresses the adolescent birth rate (those aged 10–14 years and 15–19) gauged per 1000 women in the said age range [13].

5.3.2 OVERVIEW OF MATERNAL MORTALITY

A maternal death is deemed as "the death of a woman while pregnant or within 42 days of termination of pregnancy, irrespective of the duration and site of the pregnancy, from any cause related to or aggravated by the pregnancy or its management but not from accidental or incidental causes" [14] The extent of maternal deaths is captured by the MMR and is quantified as the number of maternal deaths per 100,000 live births [15]. Maternal deaths are termed preventable deaths as they can be prevented with timely medical intervention. The push to halt the maternal mortality remains a top priority on the global health agenda [16].

The number of maternal deaths has fallen sharply globally between 1990 and 2015 from 532,000 to 303,000 amounting to a 43% decrease. This decrease mostly occurred in developed countries whilst developing countries are still inundated with disproportionately high maternal mortality numbers [15]. Impressive progress attained in the past two decades did not halt the number of maternal deaths. WHO [3] adds that in 2017 close to 810 women died every day from complications stemming from pregnancy and childbirth.

The global MMR was estimated at 211 in 2017, falling by 38% between 2000 and 2017 [13, 16]. In 2017 close to 295,000 women (270,000–340,000) died due to pregnancy-related complications and childbirth. Most maternal mortality was in the main due to direct factors pertaining to severe blood loss, infection, conditions of high blood pressure, unsafe abortions, and obstructed labor. The indirect causes were sickness such as anemia, malaria, and heart disease [16]. Almost 94% of all maternal deaths take place in low and lower-middle income countries. The MMR in Sub-Saharan Africa was 542 in 2015, way above the global figure of 216. Approximately 86% or 254,000 maternal deaths of the estimated global deaths in 2017 took place in the Sub-Saharan African region and South Asia. In Sub-Saharan Africa, the number of maternal deaths is almost two-thirds the global figure or 196,000 in 2017. However, despite Sub-Saharan's steep MMR in 2017, the sub-region recorded a sizeable decline in MMR of nearly 40% since 2000 [3].

Maternal mortality is influenced by regional and income considerations. Whilst low-income countries in 2017 had an MMR of 462, high income countries had an MMR of just 11. In reality, the steep number of maternal deaths in some regions of the world mirror income inequalities and poor access to quality health care. Studies show that poor women in rural areas are bereft of good quality health care. Maternal deaths are calamitous events as they have far-reaching effects on immediate family members. Studies document higher mortality rates among children whose mothers succumbed to maternal mortality. Such families also suffer a loss of income and are likely to be subjected to cycles of intergenerational poverty [13].

Maternal and reproductive health indicators and COVID-19 infection numbers as at 5 August 2020 are listed per region:

1. Africa:
   - MMR: 542 [17];
   - Adolescent birth rate: 99 [17];
   - Contraceptive prevalence, any method: 56 [17];
   - COVID-19 infection numbers: 830, 456 [18].
2. Sub-Saharan Africa:
   - MMR: 549 [17];
   - Adolescent birth rate: 101.3 [17];
   - Contraceptive prevalence, any method: 30.5 [17];
   - Unmet need for family planning: 24.0 [17];
   - Proportion of births attended by skilled health professionals: 59.5 [17];
   - Antenatal care coverage: 81.4 [17].
3. World:
   - MMR: 216 [17];
   - Adolescent pregnancy rate: 44.0 [17];
   - Contraceptive prevalence, any method: 55.8 [17];
   - Unmet need for family planning: 14.4 [17];
   - Proportion of births attended by skilled health professionals: 86.5 (UNDP);
   - Antenatal care coverage, at least one visit: 87 [17];
   - COVID-19 infection numbers: 19.718.030 [18].

It is clear from the list above that Sub-Saharan Africa suffers from glaring drawbacks in all maternal and reproductive indicators compared to global estimates. The region has the highest maternal mortality and adolescent pregnancy rates, coupled with the lowest proportion of births attended by skilled health attendants and antenatal care coverage.

5.3.2.1   MEASURES TO REDUCE MATERNAL MORTALITY

Two measures to bring down the proportion of maternal mortality hinge on affording access to modern methods of contraception and secondly, providing high quality prenatal, post-natal, and delivery care. Studies show that MMR and contraception usage are inversely associated, that is, MMR are steepest when family planning needs (contraception needs met based on modern methods) is least met. Secondly, MMR and skilled birth attendance are inversely associated, that is, MMR is highest when the proportion of births delivered by a skilled birth attendant is lowest [2, 13].

Contraception has many benefits and has its utilization has surged rapidly over the decades. Fulfilling family planning needs allow for the spacing of births and ultimately lessens the maternal death count. Globally, the proportion of women whose family planning requirements were met with modern contraceptives saw a modest rise from 73.6% in 2000 to 76.8% in 2020. In Sub-Saharan Africa, coverage stood at just 55% in 2020 [16].

The second method to decrease maternal mortality is to make available good healthcare. The provision of skilled care before childbirth, during pregnancy and following childbirth are crucial in that both mothers and newborn lives can be saved [13]. At a global level, it is estimated that 81% of births between 2014 and 2018 had a skilled birth attendant present, which amounted to 64% an increment over the 2000–2006 period [7, 16]. However, the help of a skilled birth attendant is not uniform across all regions. Whilst the proportion of births attended by a skilled birth attendant stands at just 59% in the WHO African Region, the figure jumps to over 90% in the Region of America and in the European and Western Pacific Regions [13]. On the other hand, only 60% of births in Sub-Saharan Africa in the period 2014–2019 were assisted by skilled birth attendants [16]. Put another way, data shows that in excess 90% of all births in most high income and upper middle-income countries, have a skilled birth attendant (either a trained midwife, doctor, or nurse). However, less than half of the total number of births in low and lower-middle income countries have a skilled birth attendant present [3].

Health care provision is highly skewed with huge inequalities being evident. Research shows that poor women in far-off areas are most likely to be denied access to adequate health care [19]. This is particularly the case in regions that possess low levels of skilled health personnel, particularly Sub-Saharan Africa and South Asia [13, 20]. UNFPA [21] notes that 73% of the countries that have 96% of the global share of maternal deaths possess less than 42% of the world's complement of midwives, nurses, and doctors.

Pregnant women not seeking health care is another reason for poor maternal health outcomes. However, there are some genuine reasons why women do not opt for care during pregnancy and childbirth. This includes factors such as:

- Poverty influences;
- Distance to facilities and location;

- Limited or absence of information;
- Inadequate and poor-quality healthcare provision [3].

A key factor underlying elevated MMRs in Sub-Saharan Africa lies in the absence of basic maternal health interventions. Many African countries encounter challenges relating to the provision of proper health care services for women. Health systems are weak in most African countries, and funding of health is inadequate, which leaves glaring inequities in the delivery of healthcare services for women. In many African countries, health facilities are poorly equipped, do not have the skilled medical staff to undertake basic medical interventions and cannot provide emergency obstetric care [22]. Furthermore, high user fees exclude many women from accessing health services, as is the case in Nigeria, which has high out-of-pocket expenses. Even in some African countries where when free primary health care initiatives are in place, payment of fees are still expected which cause women to avoid them. This problem is markedly existent in Sierra Leone [23].

Other problems that plague maternal mortality is the shortage of skilled medical staff, stock-outs of medicines, no blood supplies to perform surgeries, poor infrastructure together with a lack of electricity and water. Health care worker density in SSA in most countries are below the WHO recommended numbers [24]. This is partly why so few cesareans or C-sections take place in African countries compared to developed countries. Estimates show that whilst the number of cesarean or C-sections stood at 44% in Latin America and the Caribbean in 2015, it was only 4% in West and Central Africa [25]. Another factor has to do with the low number of facility-based deliveries and a reliance on home births. For example, in Nigeria, which has extremely acute numbers of maternal deaths, only 36% of births occurred within the confines of a healthcare facility [26].

5.3.3   OVERVIEW OF ADOLESCENT PREGNANCY

Adolescent pregnancy is a growing concern in developing countries. Adolescent pregnancy is the pregnancy in girls aged between 10–19 years [27]. Estimates indicate that every year in developing countries, close to 21 million girls in the 15–19 age category fall pregnant, and almost 12 million of these adolescents give birth. This amounts to 44 births per 1,000 adolescent girls. Alarmingly in developing countries, approximately 777,000 girls below the age of 15 give birth each year. Whilst the adolescent-specific fertility rate fell by an amount of 11.6% in the last 20 years, stark differences across regions are apparent. The adolescent fertility rate is just 7.1 in East Asia but a staggering 129.5 in Central Africa. Adolescent birth rates are strongly influenced by income disparities. High-income countries have the lowest adolescent birth rates (12 births per 1000 adolescent girls) whilst low-income countries have the highest rates (97 births per 1000). There are also regional differences. The WHO Western Pacific Region boasts the lowest adolescent birth rate (14 per 1,000) compared to 99 per 1000 in the African Region. Despite reductions in the global fertility, the actual number of childbirths to adolescents has been on an upward trend. The biggest number of childbirths took place in Eastern Asia (95,195) and in Western Africa (70.423) [3]. Adolescent pregnancies are abundant in Sub-Saharan Africa due in part to the high number of child marriages that feed into it.

Pregnant adolescents face many adverse health consequences. Early childbearing is risky. Early childbearing has harmful effects not just on the health of newborn, but impacts on the health of the adolescent mother. Studies show that the risk of maternal death is greatest for adolescent girls below the age of 15. At the same time, adolescent girls aged 10–19 is more susceptible to many pregnancy and childbirth complications and difficulties than are women aged 20–24 [3]. Pregnant adolescents also risk endangering their lives by undergoing unsafe abortions. Estimates show that of the total 5.6 million abortions that take place each year among adolescent girls aged 15–19 years, close 3.9 million abortions can be deemed unsafe. Unsafe abortions push up the number of maternal deaths, causes morbidity and other health rigors [3]. Estimates show that in developing regions, as much 10 million unintended pregnancies take place each year among adolescent girls aged 15–19 [3].

There are many factors that give rise to adolescent pregnancies and births. In some societies, cultural, and religious influences encourage early marriage and early childbearing. However, many studies finger limited or no access to the full spectrum of contraceptive services as being a key factor. Such failure undermines the rights of those adolescents that do not want to get pregnant. It also likely adolescents may lack knowledge about the different contraception methods, how to use contraception and where to obtain them. At the country-level, obstacles in the guise of restrictive laws and policies along with stipulations on age and marital status tied to the provision of contraceptives may be obstacles holding back access. Importantly, the attitude of health workers also matters. Health workers may view adolescents that seek contraception negatively and be unwilling to dispense contraceptives. Adolescents may not have the transportation or finance to access contraception. Adolescents may also lack the know-how and freedom that allows them to choose the correct contraception and to make consistent use of it [13].

Studies underlie the importance of family planning and skilled birth attendance in respect of adolescent pregnancy and childbirth rates. It has been shown that firstly there is an inverse association between adolescent birth rates and meeting of contraceptive needs, that is, adolescent birth rates are highest where the need for family planning (or contraceptive needs) are not met or lowest. Secondly, there is an inverse association between adolescent birth rates and the proportion of births delivered by a skilled birth attendant, that is, adolescent birth rates are steepest when the number of births attended by a skilled birth attendant is lowest [13].

5.4   DISCUSSION

5.4.1   HEALTH AND GENDER CONCERNS OF THE PANDEMIC

The COVID-19 pandemic is a worldwide public health disaster not seen in recent times. It is causing unprecedented levels of mortality, morbidity, as well as taxing the economy and the health system [28]. Whilst there were close to 20 million cases worldwide as of August 2020, Africa had over 800,000 cases. South Africa with over 566,000 infections topped the list of African countries. The other nine African countries that the highest number of COVID-19 infections were as follows, namely, Nigeria (44,433), Ghana (37,812), Algeria (32,504), Kenya (23,202), Ethiopia (19,875), Cameroon (17,718) and Cote d'Ivoire (16,293) [18].

Given the absence of a vaccine to combat the virus, measures that limit the spread of the virus have been paramount. Social distancing measures practically mean that both large gatherings of people as well as avoiding close contact with people can stop transmission. As a means to slow down the spread of the virus, governments worldwide put their respective countries under lockdown, thereby forcing people to stay at home, with only emergency workers being allowed to operate as normal and with restrictions on the general movement of people.

The Beijing Platform for Action, which is being commemorated this year, underscored the notability of gender equality. However, the pandemic which is not gender-neutral is likely to rescind achievements made in the past, worsen inequalities, and undermine women's well-being economically, socially, and in terms of their health outcomes [29]. It possible that in under-resourced settings, the rerouting of scarce healthcare resources to dealing with the pandemic, could compromise the health needs of women and girls, including the extension of sexual and reproductive services [29, 30].

Acquiring treatment and health care services is arduous for women and girls during health pandemics. Women and girl's physiology means that they have unique health demands. But in reality, they are likely to be deprived of access to quality health care services, medicines, maternal, and reproductive health care, or health insurance coverage, especially in rural communities and low-income areas [29]. In low-income as well as humanitarian and fragile settings that already have weak economic and health systems, the pandemic is interrupting the delivery of reproductive health services. The pandemic is "also compounding existing gender and social inequalities" [28].

The fallout from COVID-19 is likely to be substantial for the health status and well-being of women and girls. During the 2014–2015 Ebola virus outbreak, the closure of health centers and the downscaling of routine health services, together with concerns about getting affected, caused women to stay away from health facilities that remained open [19]. The outbreak of Ebola in Liberia saw maternal health care service usage diminish rapidly, and the treatment of many basic obstetric problems fell by the wayside due to fear of being infected by the disease [15]. In Sierra Leone, the Ebola outbreak triggered many adverse reactions. Many health care workers simply left their jobs, there were closures of health care facilities, the number of facility-base deliveries fell by 25%, mistrust of health care workers and reversion to the use of traditional birth attendants. These factors caused maternal mortality to soar [31].

The pandemic will weaken already vulnerable health systems, such as in some African countries where the provision of proper reproductive and maternal health care is a major challenge. Two effects that will result from the pandemic, that is, one relates to everyday effects its terms of service disruptions that will felt at the country level. At a broader level, it will impact on overarching global goals. According to UNFPA [28], the 2030 Agenda aims "to ensure the health, rights, and dignity of all people, its achievement must not be derailed by the current global public health crisis." UNFPA [28] argues that the pandemic will have harmful consequences on the two 'trans-formative results' the organization would like to attain by 2030, namely, halting preventable deaths as well the unmet need for family planning. The pandemic will have negative repercussions on the goal of ending unmet need for family planning.

5.4.2 REPRODUCTIVE HEALTH CARE EFFECTS

It is widely accepted that extending voluntary family planning to all women is crucial given the wide-ranging benefits that family planning entails for women in general and the country at large. There has been significant headway in the past 25 years in terms of making family planning methods accessible to as many women as possible. Data indicates that the proportion of women utilizing modern contraceptive methods rose twofold from a level of 470 million in 1990 to top 840 million in 2018 [28]. A more recent estimate shows that as of March 2020, almost 450 million women spread across low-and-middle-income countries were using modern contraceptives [28].

The pandemic will have a bearing on the provision of sexual and reproductive health. The delivery of sexual and reproductive health services and maternal health care are crucial to the health, rights, and well-being of women and girls [4]. The redirecting of funding and health personnel away from maternal and reproductive health care could cause higher numbers of maternal deaths, maternal morbidity, push up the rate of adolescent pregnancies, HIV, and STDs [4]. In regions such as Latin American and the Caribbean, projected estimated that the pandemic will deprive an additional 18 million women of regular delivery of modern contraceptives [29].

Marie Stopes International, a global institution that has a presence in 37 countries and which caters for contraception and safe abortion services, has projected that the pandemic could mean that as many as 9.5 million women and girls around the world are being prevented from using their services in 2020 [32]. This interruption could instigate almost 2.7 million unsafe abortions as well as 11,000 pregnancy-related deaths [19]. The reality is that many countries governments have shut down sexual and reproductive health services as they were not deemed essential, in most instances the provision of abortion and contraception services [19]. The impact of this has been to deny women and girls access to timely and crucial life-saving services [19]. In East and Southern Africa, reports have already emerged of women being denied access to routine reproductive health offerings [29].

It is foreseeable that some of the restrictions on women's reproductive rights will extend to curtailing advice and support on abortion service and the delivery of maternal health care services. Measures such as social distancing, lockdowns, and other tactics to curb the spread of the virus will affect the ability of women to access ad to continue using modern contraception [28].

There will be severe aftershocks on family planning which will thwart efforts aimed at ending the unmet need for family planning. Moreover, it will disrupt and undermine efforts to meet family planning needs. These effects will be experienced as:

- The amount of services will be scaled down;
- There will be disruption of the routine delivery of maternal health services and contraceptives;
- Health care workers tasked with dealing with the pandemic may be too busy and not have time to provide the necessary services;
- Health care facilities are likely to reduce the expanse of the services by offering limited services or by closing down altogether;
- Worries about being infected or limits on the movement of people may force women to stop visiting health care centers;
- There could be supply chain interruptions that could affect the quantity and availability of contraceptives leading to stock-outs of certain types of contraceptives. UNFPA [28] adds that such a reality will occur in at least 12 of the lowest-income countries in the course of the next six months;
- Decreases in the manufacturing process will triggers shortages and stock-outs of contraceptive items invariable amounts to women not being able to continue with their current or routine method of contraception and may have to switch over to utilizing less effective short-term methods or stop contraceptive use altogether;
- Limited access to skilled health personnel will deny women and girls complete information on the most suitable and effective contraceptive method [28].

Estimates show that almost 47 million women living in low- and middle-income countries will be denied use of modern contraceptives methods if lockdown and scaling down of services continue for a period of six months [28, 33]. It further adds two alarming scenarios could play out. Firstly, where for every three months that the lockdown is in place and there are substantial levels of service interruptions, a further 2 million women may be not able to utilize modern contraception. Secondly, if the lockdown lasts for a period of six months and is accompanied by significant disruption of services, an additional 7 million pregnancies will take place. It is argued that the tally of unintended pregnancies will surge as lockdown and service interruptions endure.

A study by Avenir Health estimated that service interruptions could translate into between 13 and 51 million women that normally use modern contraception would be unable to acquire supplies. Furthermore, there would be more widespread disruptions of injectables than other short-term methods as they require the assistance of skilled health care providers. Secondly, the public sector will be more subjected to disruptions as they are likely to be swamped with COVID-19 cases. Thus, this decline in contraceptive use could have calamitous implications for women, with the likelihood of 325,000 unintended pregnancies should their disruptions of 3 months duration. As much as 15 million unintended pregnancies could result over a 12-month period of disruption [28].

5.4.3   MATERNAL HEALTH CARE EFFECTS

Measures to stop the spread of the virus will also impact on the offering of maternal health care services. Limited healthcare workers could also entail long waiting times, which may further deter pregnant women from accessing health services. As with case with the take-up of contraceptives, pregnant women may be reluctant to use visit health care facilities for fear of being infected and concern of how it may affect their unborn child. Limited health care workers at health care facilities could see women being turned away. The closure of facilities will entail higher costs for women as they are forced to travel to far off places to receive care. The diversion of resources and limited health workers could also impact on delivery care. UNFPA [28] and Cousins [19] predict that there could be in the region of 7 million unintended pregnancies, huge numbers of deaths arising from unsafe abortions and childbirth complications births that are untreated due to inadequate access to emergency care.

Service delivery disruptions, the diversion of resources to treat COVID-19 and the scaling down of health care offerings will have dire cost implications for women and girls, especially in low-income areas. The closure of health care facilities and traveling to far-off ones would mean higher travel costs. Also stock out of contraceptives at public health care facilities means that women may have meet the costs of purchasing needed items from private sector health providers.

5.4.4   EFFECTS ON ADOLESCENT PREGNANCY RATES

In March 2020, the United Nations Education and Cultural Organization (UNESCO) has estimated that the pandemic was keeping 1.52 billion children from attending school [32]. Being out of school put girls at risk of child marriage and will push up adolescent pregnancy rates as sex education and contraceptives will be unavailable. School closures will subject girls to many atrocities such as gender-based violence, early forced and child marriages, unwanted pregnancies, female genital mutilation, and HIV infections and STIs [29].

5.4.5   POLICY MEASURE

The gender dimensions of the pandemic must be acknowledged as its effects on the health of women and girls will be felt many years on. Governments need to ensure that their policy endeavors take cognizance of the health rights of women and girls [4]. Governments need to pay attention to the SHRH of women and girls [4]. Attempts must be made to ensure that student health services are catered for and adequately funded, especially for sexual and reproductive health care. Furthermore, the maternal healthcare services for women of reproductive age (15–49) must be accommodated or met, in respect of antenatal, post-natal, and delivery services, including emergency obstetric and newborn care [4]. Institutional support for and funding needs of existing gender and health policy needs must be met to ensure that the health and well-being goals of the SDGs are accommodated. This means that governments must ensure the reproductive health needs are catered for and the supply of modern contraception is not stalled [28].

5.5   CONCLUSION

Maternal and reproductive health are crucial in reducing the number of maternal deaths and morbidity and allowing women and girls both control over the number of children and as well as the spacing of births [22]. The COVID-19 pandemic and the strain that it puts on the healthcare system and resources is likely to rescind many of the gains made in the context of maternal and reproductive health. Efforts to contain and spread of the virus and restrictions of movement, additional patient burdens at health facilities, additional funding for medical supplies to treat COVID-19, a shortage of health care workers and personal protective equipment (PPE) will mean a diversion of resources away from maternal and reproductive health care.

It is therefore imperative that the full package of maternal and reproductive health care encompassing prenatal, post-natal, delivery care together with emergency obstetric care, as well as preventing unwanted pregnancy, be sustained during the pandemic to safeguard the health of women and girls. In Sub-Saharan Africa, the pandemic could undo gain made in reducing maternal mortality, whilst at a global level, it would endanger the achievement of goals in respect of ending the unmet need for family planning and preventing maternal deaths. The scope of future research stemming from the effects of the pandemic on maternal and reproductive care should include the ramifications for girl's education, women, and girls time allocation, household income levels, and women's labor market impacts.

KEYWORDS

- **adolescent pregnancy**
- **contraception**
- **COVID-19**
- **family planning**
- **maternal deaths**
- **maternal health**
- **maternal mortality**
- **reproductive health**

REFERENCES

1. WHO, (2020a). *Maternal health Fact Sheet.* Retrieved from: https://www.who.int/health-topics/maternal-health#tab=tab_1) (accessed on 26 June 2021).
2. UNFPA, (2017). *State of the World Population.* Retrieved from: https://www.unfpa.org/sites/default/files/sowp/downloads/UNFPA PUB 2017 EN SWOP.pdf (accessed on 26 June 2021).
3. WHO, (2019b). *Maternal Mortality Fact sheet.* Retrieved from: https://www.who.int/news-room/fact-sheets/detail/maternal-mortality (accessed on 26 June 2021).
4. UN, (2020). The 17 Goals. Retrieved from: https://sdgs.un.org/goals (accessed on 26 June 2021).
5. WHO, (2020b). *Sexual and Reproductive Health and Rights: A Global Development, Health, and Human Rights Priority.* Retrieved from: https://www.who.int/reproductivehealth/publications/gender_rights/srh-rights-comment/en/ (accessed on 26 June 2021).
6. Afulukwe-Eruchalu, O., (2014). *Accountability for Non-Fulfilment of Human Rights Obligations: A Key Strategy for Reducing Maternal Mortality and Disability in Sub-Saharan Africa.* Retrieved from: https://www.pulp.ac.za/edited-collections/

strengthening-the-protection-of-sexual-and-reproductive-health-and-rights-in-the-african-region-through-human-rights (accessed on 26 June 2021).

7. Lalthapersad-Pillay, P., (2019). Joyce Banda and Ellen Johnson Sirleaf - confronting the neglect of maternal health and women's rights in Malawi and Liberia. *Agenda.* doi: 10.1080/10130950.2019.1605679.

8. UNECA, AU, AFDB & UNDP, (2015). *MDG Report 2015: Lessons Learned in Implementing the MDGs.* Addis Ababa: UNECA.

9. PULP, (2014). *Strengthening the Protection of Sexual and Reproductive Rights in the African Region Through Human Rights.* Retrieved from: www.pulp.ac.za (accessed on 26 June 2021).

10. Munyati, B. M., (2018). African women's sexual and reproductive health and rights: The revised Maputo Plan of Action pushes for upscaled delivery. *Agenda.* doi.org/10.1080/10 130950.2018.1438962.

11. Department of Health, (2012). *South Africa's National Strategic Plan for a Campaign on Accelerated Reduction of Maternal and Child Mortality (CARMMA).* Pretoria: Department of Health.

12. UN Women & United Nations, (2019). *Progress on the Sustainable Development Goals: The Gender Snapshot 2019.* New York: UN.

13. WHO, (2019a). *World Health Statistics 2019 – Monitoring Health for the SDGs.* Geneva: WHO.

14. WHO, (1997). The World health report. Retrieved from: https://www.who.int.whr/1997/en/whr97 en.pdf (accessed on 26 June 2021).

15. WHO, UNICEF, World Bank & UN, (2015). *Trends in Maternal Mortality: 1990 to 2015.* Washington: World Bank.

16. WHO, (2020c). *World Health Statistics 2020 - Monitoring Health for the SDGs.* WHO.

17. UNDP, (2018). *2018 Statistical Update.* New York: UNDP.

18. WHO, (2020d). *COVID-19 Situation Update for the WHO African Region. External situation Report 23.* WHO Regional Office for Africa: WHO.

19. Cousins, S., (2020). COVID-19 has a devastating effect on women and girls. *The Lancet, 396*:310–302.

20. Egenberg, S., Masenga, G., Bru, L. E., Eggebo, T. M., Mushi, C., Massay, D., & Øian, P., (2017). Impact of multi-professional, scenario-based training on postpartum haemorrhage in Tanzania: A quasi experimental, pre-vs. post-intervention study. *BMC Pregnancy and Childbirth.* doi: 10.1186/s/12884-017-1478-2.

21. UNFPA, (2014). *State of the Worlds' Midwifery.* Retrieved from: https://www.unfpa.org/sites/default/files/pub-pdf/EN SoWMy2014 complete.pdf (accessed on 26 June 2021).

22. WHO, (2016). *World Health Statistics 2016 – Monitoring Health for the SDGs.* Geneva: WHO.

23. Edoka, I., (2016). Free healthcare for under-fives, expectant and recent mothers? Evaluating the impact of Sierra Leone's free health care initiative. *Health Economics Review, 6,* 19. doi: 10.1186/s13561-016-0096-4.

24. Ministry of Health and Sanitation, (2017). *Sierra Leone National Reproductive, Maternal, Newborn, Child and Adolescent Health Strategy 2017–2021.* Sierra Leone: Ministry of Health and Sanitation.

25. UNICEF, (2019). *Healthy Mothers, Healthy Babies: Taking Stock of Maternal Health.* Retrieved from: https://www.healthy-Mothers-Healthy-Babies-brochure(1).pdf (accessed on 26 June 2021).

26. Gage, A. J., Ilombu, O., & Akinyemi, A. I., (2016). Service readiness, health facility management practices, and delivery care utilization in five states of Nigeria: A cross-sectional analysis. *BMC Pregnancy and Childbirth, 16:29*7. doi: 1186/s12884-016-1097-3.
27. Loudermilk, B., (2017). *Countries with the Lowest Teen Pregnancy Rates.* Retrieved from: https://www.worldatlas.com/articles/countries-with-the-lowest-teen-pregnancy-rates.html (accessed on 26 June 2021).
28. UNFPA, (2020). *Interim Technical Note 27.* Retrieved from: http://www.unfpa.org/resources/impact-covid-19-pandemic-family-planning-and-ending-gender-based-violence-female-genital (accessed on 26 June 2021).
29. UN Women, (2020). Policy brief. *COVID-19 Ending Violence Against Women and Girls: Key Priorities and Interventions for Effective Response and Recovery.* UN Women East and Southern Africa: UN Women.
30. Care Emergency Fact Sheet, (2020). *Coronavirus Crisis. Emergency Fact Sheet.* Retrieved from: https://www.care.org/wp-content/uploads/2020/05/covid-19_two-pager_04.13.20.pdf (accessed on 26 June 2021).
31. Figueroa, C. A., Linhart, C. L., Beckley, W., & Pardosi, J. F., (2018). Maternal mortality in Sierra Leone: From civil war to Ebola and the sustainable development goals. *International Journal of Public Health, 63*, 431, 432. doi.org/10.1007/s00038-017-1061-7.
32. Burki, T., (2020). The indirect impact of COVID-19 on women. *The Lancet, 20*, 904, 905.
33. Dasgupta, A., Kantorova, V., & Ueffing, P., (2020). *The Impact of the COVID-19 Crisis n Meeting Needs for Family Planning: A Global Scenario by Contraceptive Methods Used* (Vol. 4, p. 102). Gates Open Res. doi: org/10.12688/gatesopenres.13148.1.

CHAPTER 6

Mental Health and the Psychological Effects of Isolation During COVID-19

WILLIAM B. BOWES

Department of Humanities and Social Sciences, University of Edinburgh, Edinburgh, United Kingdom, E-mail: W.Bowes@sms.ed.ac.uk

ABSTRACT

A significant aspect of the measures taken against the COVID-19 pandemic involves remaining physically distanced from others, and when necessary, remaining in isolation. While this is clearly an important measure for curbing the spread of the disease and its resulting physical consequences, this long-term, sustained isolation and social distance has its own costs and consequences for mental health. While building on the foundation of years of recent research showing the deep-rooted necessity for human beings to be socially connected and interpersonally close to others, this chapter will examine the mental health consequences associated with isolation and loneliness in the context of this pandemic. The purpose of this chapter is to highlight an otherwise overlooked aspect of the complex web of distress and need that COVID-19 has caused, and through doing this, various methods of addressing the problem and treating its consequences will be explored.

6.1 INTRODUCTION

A unique aspect of the COVID-19 pandemic is that it has created a sense of shared human experience. No one has been exempted from the measures and precautions taken against the disease, and therefore a sense of solidarity emerges and creates a commonality in the difficulty of the pandemic's attending circumstances. One clearly shared effect of the global situation has been the collective experience of isolation and social distance. During the early stages of the spread of the disease, when there is misinformation about the disease, confusion about the right course of action, and a lack of clarity about the future, one of the only consistent points of recourse to slow the spread of COVID-19 and to prevent exponential increases in the death rate has been to be distant or isolated from others. Even so, given the unpreparedness of many for this isolation and given the quickness, unprecedentedness, and overall inconvenience of the isolation itself, there are many costs and concerns associated with it. Perhaps the primary concern related to pandemic-necessitated isolation involves the mental health consequences of it, and how severe and long-lasting such consequences will be.

In the midst of many anxieties over what is still unknown about the virus, the deaths caused by it, the financial strain of it, and misinformation related to it, isolation, and separation from others is an immensely weighty burden. Some recent research has even shown that loneliness related to this pandemic-induced solation is the most common personal stressor that people identify in this context [1]. The effects of this mandated separation and distancing, many of which the world may be ill-prepared, will be the focus of this chapter. While physical protection from the disease is essential and physical safety is at the forefront of public discourse about the disease, there is a clear sense that the physical safety afforded by long-term isolation and social separation comes with a price to pay related to the mental health toll that such measures will take.

This chapter will thus seek to explore these negative effects, focusing on the human need for connection, community, and close interpersonal contact and how to understand the effects of the deprivation of these things. In it, the particularities of imposed isolation will be addressed, as will the mental health effects of perceived disconnections or separation from others. Finally, the chapter will explore forward avenues for addressing these problems and how this pandemic experience may shape approaches to both the treatment of mental health issues and the understanding of the human species as an incorrigibly social and communal being.

6.2   THE HUMAN NEED FOR INTERPERSONAL COMMUNICATION

Myriad studies have shown that humans have a need for connection, closeness, and intimacy [2–4]. The disruption of it, as imposed in the context of a pandemic, highlights the essential health-related effects of close contact with others and the problems related to the privation of this contact. Consistent, strong, interpersonal affiliations or relationships are good for mental health and well-being, as such ties provide a buffer against stress or anxiety, bolster self-esteem, and inhibit the symptoms of depressive disorders and anxiety disorders [3]. Without regular access to these supports or the opportunities to develop them, there is a greater risk of developing or lapsing into unhealthy behaviors such as addiction [5]. This is a particularly high-stress time for many because of a perceived lack of control over circumstances related to COVID-19 and a pervasive sense of uncertainty about the future, which makes it an especially risky time to be isolated from interpersonal connections, given their role as a buffer against stress [6].

The basic need for intimacy and affiliation among humans is part of what makes the abrupt, undefined nature of its deprivation during COVID-19 an uncharted area of concern for mental health professionals. As Coplan and Bowker put it, if sustained, a temporary failure to fulfill the human need for intimacy "can lead to significant physical and psychological distress…social neuroscientists now suggest that loneliness and social isolation can be bad not only for our psychological functioning and well-being but also for our physical health" [2]. This basic need pertains even to something as simple as being physically touched by another person. Researchers have found that not only do humans benefit from regular (even daily) touch, they need it. "When we are touched (in a positive way)," writes Megan McCluskey, "a cascade of events happens in the brain and one of the important ones is the release of a neurochemical called oxytocin" [7]. Oxytocin, research has repeatedly shown, reduces stress and improves immunity [7]. In times when social distancing is necessary to curb viral spread, this healthy, necessary touch is limited.

6.2.1   THE PROBLEM OF LONELINESS AND ISOLATION

Because there is a distinction between isolation as a state and loneliness as a related experience, it will be helpful to define these terms. Isolation here refers to an objective lack of social contacts in a quantitative measure, while loneliness is the perceived deficiency in one's social relationships as a subjective feeling [8]. As concepts, these two are related but independent of one another, in that one does not necessarily entail the other. Both, however, pose health risks. In the context of a pandemic, there is an experience of social isolation, but one that most people consider to be necessary and temporary. The more pronounced distressing element in this time is the experience of loneliness [9, 10].

Loneliness, as McGraw writes, "is principally the lack of intimacy" [11]. It is the unwanted absence of meaningful intimacy and intimate meaningfulness, drawing from the inherent need or desire of others, which manifests as a stress-oriented feeling of being alone [11]. The opposite of loneliness is belongingness or social embeddedness, which must indeed be the goal of those providing resources (however modified they may be) to the lonely in this time [12]. Loneliness and social isolation are both most significantly observed in older adult populations, and even before this present crisis, studies have shown that about 40% of older adults feel consistently lonely [13]. Older adults may also be the overall most affected now, because they are more at risk physically from COVID-19 infection than others, due to a generally weaker immune system from age [14]. Because of their susceptibility for infection (the average death rate in those above 80 is 15%, and the average age of death is 78), this population needs to self-isolation and distance more, which increases the likelihood of experiencing loneliness [15].

Interestingly, especially in western, individualistic cultures like that of the United States, the subjective phenomenon of loneliness can also be a source of shame. This is because a western, individualistic notion of the distress of loneliness sees it as being caused by personal shortcomings rather than circumstantial social inadequacies (like a lack of access to a broader network of connections) [11]. The evident problem with this cultural pressure to shame the lonely is that it makes it far more difficult for lonely individuals to talk about their experiences, which is the first step in adequately addressing their distress [12]. Those from communal cultures do not tend to stigmatize loneliness but do have a greater fear of isolation than those familiar with a more individualistic milieu [16]. In both cases, the isolation imposed as a necessity by the pandemic presents cross-cultural difficulties; in communal cultures there is anxiety and trepidation about the circumstances of social distance itself, and in individualistic cultures there are not only the subjective effects of social distance but a lack of familiarity, comfort or even ability to address them.

These observations about the need for intimacy and the effects of isolation offer a background for this topic and show why the solitary component of the COVID-19 pandemic is a mental health issue presently and will continue to be in the long term. The mental health effects of this sustained social distance do comprise an issue of global public health that transcends just the physical risks associated with the disease and is made more complex by the fact that this isolation (and its attending loneliness) is imposed and therefore much more difficult to remedy.

6.3   THE EXPERIENCE OF REQUIRED SOCIAL DISTANCING DURING COVID-19

According to the World Health Organization (WHO), because SARS-Cov-2 is a respiratory disease spread by human-to-human transmission and has no known treatment or cure, maintaining physical distance from others is essential [17]. Similarly, for those already infected, their guidelines require a 14-day quarantine in isolation from others, with a recommendation for more severe measures for the elderly or those with preexisting health conditions or immune system problems [18]. After employing these measures globally for several months, research has shown them to be effective as a prevention and control strategy in that they reduce the number of susceptible and infected people because of the resultant lack of proximity for the viral agent to find another host [34]. Social distancing reduces unknown spread, general isolation reduces potential spread, and absolute isolation in quarantine reduces known spread [19].

The primary issue with this approach is that while it is physically effective when followed, it is not sustainable from the standpoint of mental and emotional health. Specifically, while protected from possible infection, the vast majority of those isolated in homes do not have access to mental health care [20]. Thus, effective self-care and self-help methods, many of which the average person may not understand or practice, are basically the only available resource [20]. This is particularly true in the context of COVID-19 as distinct from other forms of isolation and loneliness because the present form has been acute and severe, leaving the average person with inadequate preparation and resources set in place to combat it [15]. An example of a problematic side effect from inadequate coping strategies for this isolation has been shown in the clearly observable double-digit increase in alcohol sales and consumption since the disease was declared a pandemic [20]. Increased alcohol consumption, of course, is an ineffective but widely practiced way of ameliorating anxiety and distress associated with circumstances outside of one's control [21].

6.3.1   GROUPS MOST AT RISK OF ISOLATION DURING COVID-19

The people most at risk during the isolation from this quarantine times are those with preexisting physical and mental health conditions, older people living in institutions like care homes and special needs facilities, disabled individuals, people with recent bereavement, hospitalization or illness, those subject to domestic violence or sexual abuse, people with drug and alcohol use disorders, individuals with caretaking responsibilities including childcare during school closures, the unemployed or those having lost income during COVID-19, people living with limited social capital or network, refugees, and immigrants [22]. For these groups of people, the normal mental health consequences of isolation and loneliness are augmented by other circum-stantial and situational factors which limit their ability to cope and adapt in a healthy way. While for many this temporary but sustained isolation and loneliness is difficult and inconvenient, for these groups, it can be devas-tating. If, for example, a person who is attempting to leave an abusive spouse or grieving from a loved one's recent death, isolation within the home can lead to worsening circumstances because of the difficulties associated with engaging in adaptive behaviors necessary to cope with such problems.

Since both the human need for contact and intimacy and the privation of those within the context of the pandemic have been explored, it will be necessary to understand what the precise possible consequences of long-term isolation can be. In knowing these dangers and possibilities, one can better prepare and develop more helpful interventions in the midst of the pandemic and as a safety measure once circumstances have changed in a post-COVID world.

6.4   SPECIFIC MENTAL HEALTH PROBLEMS ASSOCIATED WITH ISOLATION AND LONELINESS

That loneliness and isolation can have mental health effects is all but certain, as observed in recent research, but the significance of these effects varies. In general, researchers have noted that the longer a person is confined or isolated, the poorer the mental health outcomes [23, 24]. Both reported isolation and loneliness have been linked to depressive disorders, anxiety disorders, reduced executive functioning, reduced cognitive performance, and reduced immune functioning [8, 25]. As it relates to immune functioning, a 2005 study found that young adults who reported loneliness or had a small social network had a poorer antibody response to influenza immunization [8]. Long periods of time in isolation and quarantine have been connected to PTSD symptoms, avoidance behavior, and anger, indicating that "quarantine itself can be perceived and experienced as traumatic" [24]. In the context of previous pandemics (such as the SARS outbreak), suicides have been reported among those who have been quarantined [26]. Tragically, multiple suicides have been reported in different countries in the context of COVID-19 as well, both among the quarantined and among health professionals treating the sick [27].

Research has also indicated that among those who have been isolated in quarantine, their satisfaction with their treatment decreased and their anxiety increased based on whether or not they were uninformed about their health-care [28]. This is especially relevant in the midst of COVID-19, where there remains a significant public and private concern about both misinformation and a lack of information about the virus and effective measures to be taken against it [29]. A primary driving force behind the psychologically negative effects of isolation is uncertainty and loss of control, which is derived from various sources but ultimately stems from isolation itself [28].

While isolation and loneliness create depressive symptoms, the depressive symptoms within a pandemic may be more rightly associated with an adjustment disorder than with major depressive disorder, and thus time will tell whether such symptoms would necessarily necessitate pharmacological treatment [30]. However, beyond these depressive symptoms, loneliness also tends to increase problematic behaviors such as addictive patterns of technology or substance use [34]. Similarly, lonely people have a lower likelihood of performing healthy activities such as engaging in regular physical exercise, which is a necessary de-stressing activity [8].

Neurologically speaking, it is important to note that social behaviors go hand in hand with neural, hormonal, cellular, and genetic mechanisms or adaptation, and thus social isolation can be as strong a risk factor for morbidity as smoking, obesity, or high blood pressure [31]. Specifically, perceived isolation predicts "greater vascular resistance, elevated blood pressure, morning rise in cortisol, less salubrious sleep, and sedentary lifestyles" [31]. Given the reality of these varied consequences and dangers, there are a host of possible ways forward for those inside and outside the health professions in the context of this pandemic, and to an analysis of these positive avenues we now turn.

6.5 OPTIONS AND STRATEGIES FOR COMBATING THE EFFECTS OF LONELINESS AND ISOLATION

This chapter has shown the great importance of social connection for psychological and emotional well-being and what groups are most at risk in the context of this pandemic. Thus, the next step for mental health professionals and laypeople alike is to intervene among these groups to reduce their negative symptoms or risk factors for long-term consequences by creating methods of ameliorating the distress stemming from social deficits. In previous times of crisis, like during Hurricane Katrina in the United States, "social support and community ties played a crucial protective role in mental health recovery" [19]. Since that is not possible in the same way during this crisis, methodologies will have to become more creative.

The most obvious immediate approach, although limited, is to leverage technology to act as a buffer against loneliness and to raise awareness of the need for self-care, which is essential to reducing anxiety [19]. Many activities (whether for service or for leisure) have moved to online formats, but more needs to be offered for those for whom these activities have been limited or inconsistent. People must be encouraged to expend as much effort as necessary to maintain or create social interaction online, over the phone, or by letters, particularly when they are older and maybe experiencing increased isolation while also having a sense of unfamiliarity with new technology [32]. Especially for those who have never utilized mental health services before, there needs to be an easy, cost-effective way to receive telehealth services in a consistent manner. For mental health professionals providing telehealth services, supportive therapy, such as utilizing repeated reassurance and building skills to overcome helplessness by providing accurate information to correct cognitive distortions or persistent misconceptions, would be most helpful. As one psychiatrist puts it, during a pandemic, "empowering individuals to make decisions and by helpful them to restore or establish routines during the isolation, as well as directing them to utilize healthy defenses, including humor, may go a long way in maintaining mental health equilibrium" [30].

This task is not just one for mental health professionals, but primary care physicians also have a role to play in mental health support, as one in five patients has been shown to consult general practitioners for primarily social rather than medical problems [22]. Handling anxiety during isolation and quarantine necessitates a multi-pronged approach involving several different areas, which includes support and reassurance but also the provision of correct information and practical solutions to problems, and, when necessary, the utilization of medication [30]. Regardless of the type of provider, several studies have iterated that it is especially important in crisis contexts to prepare individuals emotionally beforehand as much as possible and to maintain consistent, regular communication with providers [28, 34].

In terms of practical interventions, psychologists recommend that isolated people attempt to structure out each and every day, maintain consistency in their activities, and vigilantly include relaxation-oriented, self-care activities like mindfulness, meditation, breathing exercises, taking walks outside, or practicing other relaxation techniques [2, 15]. Because of anxiety caused by an inundation of negative or frightening information through news sources, researchers generally suggest limiting the amount of information sources consulted and the duration for which they are consulted [33]. This is necessary to maintain a cognitive state that is able to focus on the positive and not only the negative aspects of isolation. Also important is for people to maintain regular diet patterns and to practice activities that engage them physically and mentally in order to ward off the risk of developing addictive behavior patterns. This could include activities such as physical exercise (such as cardiovascular training or weight training), reading, playing a musical instrument, engaging in games, or sporting activities, painting, sewing, or similar sorts of hobbies [33].

A practical series of interventions for mental health professionals is illustrated in Figure 6.1. This series is comprised of six steps, the first being to deliver positive virus-related information to optimize one's perception of risk, second to improve a person's isolation-related mental health symptoms by reducing one's various opportunities for negative or problematic behaviors, third to bring about or increase one's knowledge of stress management strategies and activities, 4th to alleviate any conflicts in one's family system or interpersonal network, 5th to practice the cultivation of more positive habits and behaviors to replace problematic ones, and 6th to adjust or modify one's expectations in preparing for the immediate future (where the virus is still an incurable threat) and for the far future (once there are safe and effective treatments).

Any intervening measures and techniques to fight against the loneliness and isolation of quarantine should keep in mind both preventative and remedial goals. That is, any intervention seeks to prevent the worsening of symptoms, but holistic interventions consider how a lonely or isolated person can prepare for life after the pandemic. Once this pandemic has run its course and effective treatment methods have been developed, all affected cultures and societies can hope that the broad-scale, shared experience of social distance can lead to a future where strong, meaningful interpersonal relationships are more celebrated and more actively pursued and recognized for their essential benefits, and also that long-term safeguards will have been put in place to serve as tools of transition for the chronically isolated or lonely. Even though various treatment methods are being developed at the time of this writing, even with widescale successes, the implementation of such treatments will take a significant amount of time. With this in mind, it is necessary not only to expend great effort to ameliorate the distresses of the lonely and isolated presently, but to prepare for a post-COVID world that will have many more resources for those that perennially struggle with these issues.

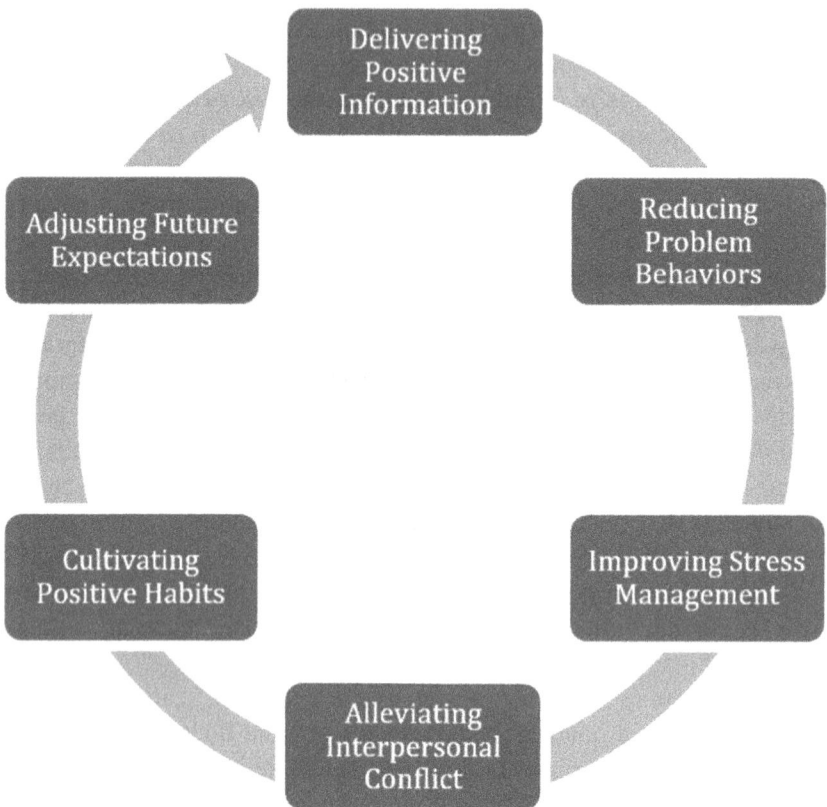

FIGURE 6.1   A series of cognitive-behavioral interventions.

6.6   CONCLUSION

This chapter has illustrated the need for close interpersonal contact among humans, the mental health effects of a sustained deprivation of this, and has explored forward avenues for treatment and alleviation of the negative effects that have come with this unique and difficult time. One can certainly hope that if there are positive outcomes from this crisis, one may be that the world becomes more aware of the importance of social connection, especially as loneliness and isolation has generally been on the rise [1]. This time may also help highlight to the world the usefulness but ultimate insufficiency of internet-based, social media relationships, which have their place, but do not actually fulfill the deep, human need for interpersonal connection that is required for people to flourish. Regardless of the various tools that have been and will continue to be used in this time to assist the isolated and lonely, it will continue to be necessary that those in the health professions emphasize the importance of mental health just as much as physical health during and beyond the context of a pandemic, and that societies as a whole move away from stigmatizing these mental health struggles and into viewing each and every person more holistically.

KEYWORDS

- **COVID-19**
- **isolation**
- **loneliness**
- **mental health**
- **pandemic**
- **quarantine**
- **social distancing**

REFERENCES

1. Smith, B. J., & Lim, M. H., (2020). How the COVID-19 pandemic is focusing attention on loneliness and social isolation. *Public Health Res. Pract., 30*(2), 1–4. doi: 10.17061/phrp3022008.
2. Coplan, R. J., & Julie, C. B., (2013). *The Handbook of Solitude: Psychological Perspectives on Social Isolation, Social Withdrawal, and Being Alone.* Wiley & Sons.
3. Rohde, N., D'Ambrosio, C., Tang, K. K., & Rao, P., (2016). Estimating the mental health effects of social isolation. *Applied Research in Quality of Life, 11*(3), 853–869. doi: 10.1007/s11482-015-9401-3.

4. Smith, K. J., & Victor, C., (2019). Typologies of loneliness, living alone and social isolation, and their associations with physical and mental health. *Ageing & Society, 39*(8), 1709–1730. doi: 10.1017/S0144686X18000132.

5. Dingle, G. A., Cruwys, T., & Frings, D., (2015). Social identities as pathways into and out of addiction. *Frontiers in Psychology, 6,* 1795–1817. doi: 10.3389/fpsyg.2015.01795.

6. Hostinar, C. E., & Gunnar, M. R., (2015). Social support can buffer against stress and shape brain activity. *AJOB Neuroscience, 6*(3), 34–42. doi: 10.1080/21507740.2015.1047054.

7. McCluskey, M., (2020). *Why Lack of Human Touch Can Be Difficult Amid Coronavirus.* Time Magazine. https://time.com/5817453/coronavirus-human-touch/ (accessed on 26 June 2021).

8. Beller, J., & Wagner, A., (2018). Loneliness, social isolation, their synergistic interaction, and mortality. *Health Psychology, 37*(9), 808–813. doi: 10.1037/hea0000605.

9. Killgore, W. D., Cloonen, S. A., Taylor, E. C., & Dailey, N. S., (2020). Loneliness: A signature mental health concern in the era of COVID-19. *Psychiatry Research, 113*–117. doi: 10.1016/j.psychres.2020.113117.

10. Rana, U., (2020). Elderly suicides in India: An emerging concern during COVID-19 pandemic. *International Psychogeriatrics, 1,* 2. doi: 10.1017/S1041610220001052.

11. McGraw, J. G., (2010). *Intimacy and Isolation.* Brill.

12. Gierveld, J., Van, T. T., & Dykstra, P. A., (2006). Loneliness and social isolation. *Cambridge Handbook of Personal Relationships,* 485–500. doi: 10.1017/CBO9780511606632.027.

13. Ring, L., Barry, B., Totzke, K., & Bickmore, T., (2013). Addressing loneliness and isolation in older adults: Proactive affective agents provide better support. In: *2013 Humaine Association Conference on Affective Computing and Intelligent Interaction* (pp. 61–66).

14. Nikolich-Zugich, J., Knox, K. S., Rios, C. T., Natt, B., Bhattacharya, D., & Fain, M. J., (2020). SARS-CoV-2 and COVID-19 in older adults: What we may expect regarding pathogenesis, immune responses, and outcomes. *Geroscience, 1*–10. doi: 10.1007/s11357-020-00186-0.

15. Cullen, W., Gulati, G., & Kelly, B. D., (2020). Mental health in the COVID-19 pandemic. *QJM: An International Journal of Medicine, 113*(5), 311–315. doi: 10.1093/qjmed/hcaa110.

16. Kim, K., & Markman, A. B., (2006). Differences in fear of isolation as an explanation of cultural differences: Evidence from memory and reasoning. *Journal of Experimental Social Psychology, 42*(3), 350–364. doi: 10.1016/j.esp.2005.06.005.

17. World Health Organization, (2020). *Advice for the Public on COVID-19.* https://www.who.int/emergencies/diseases/novel-coronavirus-2019/advice-for-public (accessed on 26 June 2021).

18. World Health Organization, (2020). *Considerations for Quarantine of Individuals in the Context of Containment for Coronavirus Disease (COVID-19).* https://www.who.int/publications-detail/considerations-for-quarantine-of-individuals-in-the-context-of-containment-for-coronavirus-disease-(covid-19) (accessed on 26 June 2021).

19. Saltzman, L. Y., Hansel, T. C., & Bordnick, P. S., (2020). Loneliness, isolation, and social support factors in post-COVID-19 mental health. *Psychological Trauma: Theory, Research, Practice, and Policy,* S55–S57. doi: 10.1037/tra0000703.

20. Matias, T., Dominski, F. H., & Marks, D. F., (2020). Human needs in COVID-19 isolation. *Journal of Health Psychology, 25*(7), 1–12. doi: 10.1177/1359105320925149.

21. Aldridge-Gerry, A. A., Roesch, S. C., Villodas, F., McCabe, C., Leung, Q. K., & Da Costa, M., (2011). Daily stress and alcohol consumption: Modeling between-person and within-person ethnic variation in coping behavior. *Journal of studies on alcohol and drugs, 72*(1), 125–134. doi: 10.15288/jsad.2011.72.125.

22. Razai, M. S., Oakeshott, P., Kankam, H., Galea, S., & Stokes-Lampard, H., (2020). Mitigating the psychological effects of social isolation during the COVID-19 pandemic. *BMJ*, 369–374. doi: 10.1136/bmj.m1904.

23. Cacioppo, J. T., Cacioppo, S., Capitanio, J. P., & Cole, S. W., (2015). The neuroendocrinology of social isolation. *Annual Review of Psychology, 66*, 733–767. doi: 10.1146/annurev-psych-010814-015240.

24. Usher, K., Bhullar, N., & Jackson, D., (2020). Life in the pandemic: Social isolation and mental health. *Journal of Clinical Nursing*, 2746–2757. doi: 10.1111/jocn.15290.

25. Cacioppo, J. T., & Hawkley, L. C., (2009). Perceived social isolation and cognition. *Trends in Cognitive Sciences, 13*(10), 447–454. doi: 10.1016/j.tics.2009.06.005.

26. Chatterjee, K., & Chauhan, V. S., (2020). Epidemics, quarantine and mental health. *Medical Journal, Armed Forces India, 76*(2), 125–127. doi: 10.1016/j.mjafi.2020.03.017.

27. Thakur, V., & Jain, A., (2020). COVID 2019-suicides: A global psychological pandemic. *Brain, Behavior, and Immunity*, 952, 953. doi: 10.1016/j.bbi.2020.04.062.

28. Abad, C., Fearday, A., & Safdar, N., (2010). Adverse effects of isolation in hospitalized patients: A systematic review. *Journal of Hospital Infection, 76*(2), 97–102. doi: 10.1016/j.jhin.2010.04.027.

29. Brennen, J. S., Simon, F., Howard, P. N., & Nielsen, R. K., (2020). *Types, Sources, and Claims of COVID-19 Misinformation* (pp. 1–13). Reuters Institute.

30. Huremović, D., (2019). *Psychiatry of Pandemics: A Mental Health Response to Infection Outbreak*. Springer.

31. Cacioppo, J. T., Hawkley, L. C., Norman, G. J., & Berntson, G. G., (2011). Social isolation. *Annals of the New York Academy of Sciences, 1231*(1), 17–23. doi: 10.1111/j.1749-6632.2011.06028.x.

32. Brooke, J., & Jackson, D., (2020). Older people and COVID-19: Isolation, risk and ageism. *Journal of Clinical Nursing*, 2044–2046. doi: 10.1111/jocn.15274.

33. Fiorillo, A., & Gorwood, P., (2020). The consequences of the COVID-19 pandemic on mental health and implications for clinical practice. *European Psychiatry, 63*(1), 1, 2. doi: 10.1192/j.eurpsy.2020.35.

34. Chen, B., Sun, J., & Feng, Y. (2020). How have COVID-19 isolation policies affected young people's mental health? Evidence from Chinese college students. *Frontiers in Psychology, 11*, 1–6.

CHAPTER 7

Health and Non-Health Care Challenges of COVID-19 Management

S. S. M. SADRUL HUDA[1] and SYEEDA RAISA MALIHA[2]

[1]Department of Management, School of Business, North South University, Dhaka, Bangladesh, E-mail: ssadrul@gmail.com

[2]Re-Think, Re-Search, Dhaka, Bangladesh

ABSTRACT

This chapter aims to collect insights regarding the medical sector of Bangladesh in the COVID-19 pandemic. The design/methodology/ approach of this chapter heavily relies on secondary research from different journals and newspapers. The findings of this research show some important dimensions of the country's health sector in the ongoing pandemic. This includes the sacrifice of the healthcare workers; initiatives taken to protect the healthcare professionals; faulty hospitals; unwilling healthcare professionals who denied providing proper treatment to the sufferers; uncooperative patients. Besides, healthcare management problems related to test kits and testing processes, short supply of medical equipment, personal protective equipment (PPE), corruption have been identified in this chapter. The role of citizen volunteers, social organizations, and corporate houses along with the government to combat COVID 19 also came up. Finally, the positive aspect among all-the perseverance of the scientists trying to discover a vaccine. The originality or the value of this chapter is that this is the first chapter that brings all the major challenges faced by the health care system of Bangladesh in managing the COVID 19 pandemic under a single framework. This identifies the nature of health service failure in public and private hospitals based on a review of newspaper reports. The challenges of delivering health care services at an adequate level have been identified. This chapter possesses the strengths of creating a theoretical ground for future studies as it covers not only the medical issues but also the social, cultural, and administrative issues of managing the COVID 19. Thus, this chapter may be the basis of developing future healthcare models of managing pandemic of this nature in a developing country. Policy/managerial implication of this chapter creates immense value for policymakers as it presents the challenges of healthcare management in different categories (e.g., social, hospital, patients), which help them to evaluate the gravity of the problem in different areas of healthcare management. The policymakers will get a direction to march forward to address the health care issues in a pandemic situation by focusing on the weaknesses of the system.

7.1   INTRODUCTION

In recent years, the health care system has improved a lot. The life expectancy at birth has turned from 44 years to 72 years from 1970 to 2014; rudimentary vaccination coverage of children by 12 months has risen to 78%, usage of contraceptive has improved from 8% to 62% and there has been a decrease of fertility rate from 6.3 per family to 2.3 [5]. All of this is good news. However, it is still not enough. The number of healthcare professionals is not adequate. We only have 0.5 doctors and 0.2 nurses per 1000 people, which is far from the standard, which is 2.28 per 1000 [1]. Their study also revealed that 76.2% of patients are satisfied with the treatment of private healthcare systems where 76.4% were dissatisfied with the service of public hospitals. Besides, there are numerous uncertified health advice workers such as homeopathic doctors, Hekim-Kabiraaj, even workers at the pharmacy that health tips to the patients. To make things worse, this year, a disease that has taken millions of lives all over the world has hit us, and the vaccine is yet to be discovered, which is known as COVID-19.

7.2   LITERATURE REVIEW

The recent outbreak of the COVID-19 has shown us how faulty our whole medical sector is, but then again, it also showed us how people will come forward to help others when it is needed, they will come up with something.

The government is taking initiatives here. They are ensuring that the infected are in fact in isolation and are not running around infecting others. So, importing or making N95 masks and PPEs should another major focus for the government. To make a better world, the study of Emanuel et al. [2] suggests four ideal values: saving as many lives as possible, treating patients equally, giving priority to the worst off, and promoting these ideals everywhere.

Boundary spanners are very important for every organization as they are the bridge between the company and the customers, and they are ones that conduct the exchange of information between these groups [3]. The outbreak of coronavirus has shown us the real-life version of such conflict. The doctors, nurses, police, and all frontline workers who are in direct touch with people are facing the person vs role conflict every single day.

This pandemic has also shown us a rise in voluntary activities to help people in need. The more the world is in crisis, the more the demand for social entrepreneurship, and that is why there has been a boom of social entrepreneurship in the past couple of years [4]. According to his study, such entrepreneurs can also bring a change by influencing society's behavior. In this pandemic, many dedicated individuals are coming up with low-cost necessary items for the low-income group of the country, many are working day and night to provide home delivery so that people can stay home in the lockdown, many are providing oxygen cylinders so on.

7.3   AN OVERVIEW OF THE HEALTHCARE SYSTEM OF BANGLADESH IN COVID-19

Bangladesh has not become proficient in this sector either. As a result, now we have almost 159,679 people infected in total with 1997 dead [6].

From our findings from the secondary research shows us some important dimensions of the health sector of Bangladesh. We can see praiseworthy initiatives taken by the government and other sectors to improve our healthcare system by providing gears and equipment. The sacrifice of healthcare workers is also another dimension that we have figured out. They sacrificed their lives, time with their families, and their mental health. Then we could see initiatives taken to protect the healthcare professionals as they are the frontline warriors in this battle and we cannot afford to lose any more of them. Also, we could see many ordinary citizens are trying to help the people suffering because of this pandemic.

However, some negative issues have come into discussion become known because of this pandemic. There are many hospitals and healthcare professionals, who denied providing proper treatment to the sufferers, many gave faulty treatment and were overall uncooperative. The test kits and the whole testing process had technical problems and were insufficient in number. Even many patients were uncooperative. Ordinary patients were misbehaving with COVID patients, while COVID patients were not complying with the rules; they were fleeing the hospitals, not staying in quarantine and things those sorts. Many evil-minded people started taking advantage of people's misfortune. They started selling fake certificates, sometimes with and sometimes without the patient's consent. In the end, there is a positive aspect to it. Scientists are constantly working on finding a vaccine for this life-threatening disease. They have already come up with some medicines that minimize the negative effects of COVID-19. Even Bangladesh has started trials for developing a vaccine for coronavirus and become the 11th country to start working on vaccines.

7.4   OBJECTIVES

The objective of this study is to gather insights into the medical sector of the country. This includes collecting and interpreting information regarding the sectors working directly to help corona patients, the impact of the pandemic on the boundary spanners of the medical sector, problems related to the health sector, and the efforts to bring solutions to this problem.

7.5   METHODOLOGY

Our hands are somewhat tied because of the pandemic. As a result, we could not outside to conduct surveys or take face-to-face interviews. Therefore, we had to rely on secondary data analysis.

We also went through the newspapers for the past six months and gathered more than 70 links that contain relevant information, and the reflection of it can be seen in the chapter. We specifically chose Prothom Alo as it is one of the most trustworthy newspapers in Bangladesh. Therefore, news gathered from there have proper details as well as credibility.

7.6 FINDINGS AND ANALYSIS

7.6.1 GOVERNMENT AND PRIVATE INITIATIVES (FIGURE 7.1)

Some of the initiatives from the government and private sides are setting up hospitals; providing ventilators; providing protective gear; tax benefit on manufacturing protective gear; healthcare service over the phone; and developing kits and medicine.

Government and private initiatives

→ Setting up hospitals
→ Providing ventilators
→ Providing protective gear
→ Tax benefit on manufacturing protective gear
→ Healthcare service over the phone
→ Developing kits and medicine

FIGURE 7.1   Government and private initiatives.

Navana Group has so far handed over 50 portable ventilators and other medical supplies from China across the country. Navana Group has introduced a DS-6 BIPAP ST30 ventilator manufactured in China. It is an easily portable ventilator, which is very easy to use. Also, Navana Group has distributed PPE (personal protective equipment) including N-95 masks, gloves, face shields, to various hospitals.

Health Minister Zahid Malek inaugurated the 2,013-bed temporary hospital set up for the treatment of COVID-19 at the International Convention City Bashundhara (ICCB) in the capital. The health minister said there are 2,013 state-of-the-art isolated beds. Of these, 61 have oxygen cylinders attached to them. Also, there are at least 400 more portable oxygen cylinders. With an intensive care unit (ICU) system, the hospital is no exception to the COVID temporary hospital in the developed world. This hospital has been started on the initiative of the Bashundhara Group. Within 10 days, 2,000 doctors and 5,054 nurses have been appointed. Work is underway to recruit at least 5,000 new medical technologists.

The government is working on importing more and more protective gear as well. A C-130J transport aircraft of the Bangladesh Air Force, directed by the government, has returned home from China with a variety of medical supplies, including glasses, 200 goggles, and 10,459 personal protection (PPE) items.

If any local organization produces these products, it will get a tax benefit, as taxes have been exempted from the manufacture and trade of protective gear. The department of VAT under the National Board of Revenue (NBR) issued a notification with this VAT exemption. This measure has been taken to encourage more people to start making and selling safety equipment so that we can meet the growing demand.

Officials say they now have the technology and manpower to handle 1,00,000 calls a day. The doctors of this organization have advised about 50,000 people about dengue treatment and services in the recent dengue outbreak. Consulting on health or medical care from 18,263 saves both time and money. Also, in the case of basic services, it is safe to seek treatment from a health window without taking the medicine yourself, following the advice of the drug store, or going to the quack. The government's Health Window 16,263-call center has advised on dengue to more than 60,000 people in the last four months. People have called this call center and asked 102 questions about dengue. The call center received 430,553 calls from June 1 to September 20. Of these, 233,398 phones were related to medical services. Among the medical services, 60,703 phones were related to dengue. Around 21 doctors from Jhenaidah are working to give medical advice to the patients sitting at home. They have reportedly provided digital healthcare to more than 1,000 patients using mobile phones and various social media. This service runs daily from 8 am to 10 pm. Physicians are all taking part in this activity on their initiative. Patients from different diseases are taking medication through this process.

Although COVID is a buzzing issue, which does not mean dengue is not there. That is why the government has started dengue tests free. The program started on May 11 in 5 urban maternity hospitals and 22 urban health centers in the DNCC area. Apart from this, in the case of a free dengue test, dengue tests can be done free of cost in urban maternity wards and urban health centers from 9 am to 2 pm every day except Friday. Adequate kits for dengue testing have already been provided at these centers. Dengue test results will be available immediately.

Doctors and researchers have been working on developing testing kits and medicine to fight the virus. VTM kit was developed at the Designated Reference Institute for Chemical Measurement (DRICM), a subsidiary of the Bangladesh Council of Science and Industry Research (BCSIR). The Department of Health wrote a letter to DRICM on May 18 stating that they had tested with the kit and got promising results. The department wants to use this kit for sample collection. Also, the public health center kit is 80% effective in detecting antibodies in people infected with COVID-19. The research team of Bangabandhu Sheikh Mujib Medical University (BSMMU) said this after evaluating the effectiveness of the kit at the public health center. This kit is not effective in diagnosing people with symptoms of COVID-19 disease. This means that the antigen cannot be identified with this kit. Plasma therapy is a type of corona treatment where the plasma of a person who has recovered is given to another patient assuming that it has antibodies. Whether or not there are, actually antibodies can be determined using a public health kit. The results can be known in five minutes by taking blood from the person's body.

7.6.2   CHALLENGES CONFRONTED BY THE BOUNDARY SPANNERS (FIGURE 7.2)

The problems faced by the boundary spanners are death of healthcare workers; getting detached from family; fear of getting infected; and suffering from depression, fear, and anxiety.

Problems Faced by the Boundary Spanners
- → Death of healthcare workers
- → Getting detached from family
- → Fear of getting infected
- → Suffering from depression, fear, and anxiety

FIGURE 7.2   Challenges confronted by the boundary spanners.

According to the Bangladesh Medical Association (BMA), 41 doctors died of coronavirus infection and corona symptoms as of June 18. Of these, 38 people died due to corona infection. Around 5 people died of corona symptoms. So far, 1,011 doctors across the country have been affected by corona. Around 1,331 people including technologists and other health workers have been affected. On the other hand, the Bangladesh Nurses Association says that 1,160 nurses have been infected across the country. Around 6,520 people have been infected in the country.

Not only the risk of being infected, has the pandemic separated them from their families as well. Take the story of Jhumu Das as an example. She is a Medical Technologist (Lab) at Satkania Upazila Health Complex, Chittagong. The in-laws told her to quit the job because her two children are very young, and one of them is a breast-feeding baby. Jhumu Das explained to them that if a soldier fled from the battlefield, she would be identified as a traitor, and in this time of the Corona epidemic, the opportunity to serve the people may not come later. As COVID-19 can spread easily, she has sent her children to her mother's house to maintain their safety. Another mother working in Rajshahi Medical College Hospital is working in the ICU on a daily wage basis. She is keeping the baby at home and she is staying in the hospital quarters with the responsibility of taking care of the COVID-19 patients. These women are not being able to spend time with their infants because they chose to save lives over their happiness.

Two technologists from Munsiganj general hospital, Shahidul Islam, and Abdus Salam have been working day and night to serve the ones in need. Sometimes they work in the hospital, sometimes they visit the patients' homes to collect samples without caring for their own lives and staying away from their family for two months. They have done the same last year when dengue started taking lives. So far, they have collected 2,691 samples, which constitutes almost half of the whole samples collected from that district.

7.6.3   INNOVATIONS TO PROTECT THE BOUNDARY SPANNERS (FIGURE 7.3)

Innovations to protect the boundary spanners are importing protective gear; implementing policies; and critical isolation chamber for doctors.

Innovations to Protect the Boundary Spanners

→ Importing protective gear
→ Implementing policies
→ Critical isolation chamber for doctors

FIGURE 7.3   Innovations to protect the boundary spanners.

Healthcare professionals providing direct patient care are at a very high risk of combating the current COVID-19 outbreak. Many have been tested positive by now, and several have died. Policy discussions that have taken place so far were mostly about the quality and quantity of the protective gear used by the healthcare professionals. However, they tend to forget that protective gears are not the only thing that they should be concerned about. Other measures like proper separation, ventilation, schedules also need to be employed. Hospitals must provide replacements for PPEs as well because they degrade over time, and using one that has been used multiple times can put the healthcare professionals at risk.

The statistical ratio of healthcare professionals to a patient is highly alarming. There is only one registered physician per 1,847 patients and 3.06 nurses per 10,000 patients. If these people start getting infected as well because of the negligence of the authority, the country will run out of healthcare professionals, causing distress for thousands of patients. That is why these people need to be under the utmost care and safety. They can take steps like-formulation of policy regarding the safety of the healthcare professionals; deploying surveillance systems for ill or injured employees; use the data collected from the surveillance system to create or modify policy; formulate and train special committee to look after the health and safety of the professionals, etc.

In this case, the specialty of this chamber is more than other chambers. In this chamber, doctors, and health workers will be able to provide services only after wearing special protective clothing or PPE. Even if the coronavirus is present in the patient's body, the doctor has no chance of being infected. On the advice of experts, the members of the Facebook group 'Team SOS' volunteered to design this isolation chamber, an architectural firm called 'Foundation Architects Limited.' With the help of these booths at the entrances of hospitals, factories, health centers, 'infection-free medical management' can be ensured through patient segregation.

7.6.4 SOCIAL ENTREPRENEURSHIP (FIGURE 7.4)

The social entrepreneurship providing oxygen cylinders; alerting the citizen; spraying disinfectants; and delivering groceries and necessities.

Social Entrepreneurship
→ Providing oxygen cylinders
→ Alerting the citizen
→ Spraying disinfectants
→ Delivering groceries and necessities

FIGURE 7.4   Social entrepreneurship.

The good news is that the pandemic has shown us a new rise of humanity.

Volunteers are appearing directly in front of the patient's home as soon as they call the hotline. So far, 26 patients have been given oxygen services and 13 patients have been rushed to the hospital.

Iqbal Tanjir, one of the employees of Pay It Forward, has already started service with 100 cylinders. Another organization called Nistha Foundation is also delivering oxygen cylinders to patients' homes.

Towards the beginning of the pandemic, Zakir Mandal alerted the locals about the coronavirus with a hand mic. Now he is spraying disinfectant water on various institutions, including mosques in the area. On May 10, Zakir started spraying disinfectant water. Earlier, on March 26, he campaigned against coronavirus with a hand mike. The locals used to make fun of him for doing such a thing. They used to call him 'crazy.' However, at one time the people of the area understood the importance of Zakir's work. Now no one in the area makes fun of Zakir. Rather, many help him in his work.

The first Bangladeshi patient infected with COVID-19 was identified on Women's Day. Hearing the news, Babli Akand who is a journalist, felt the urge to do something as a woman. With a group of volunteers, she started giving the message of maintaining social distance in the area, adhering to hygiene rules, adhering to lockdown. Many people in the area used to make fun of her for not taking the matter well in the beginning. However, after the situation changed, now everyone affectionately calls her 'Corona Apa.' She has 20 volunteers who are working with her.

Medium-term infected people also need to be supplied with oxygen. As a result, a kind of wailing has been created with oxygen at this time of COVID-19. The cause of this wailing is mainly the shortage of oxygen supply equipment. In this situation, a Facebook group called 'Connecting: Connecting People' is working with the slogan 'Give the cylinder, deliver oxygen.' If you want to know what will be the case for the patients in the house, it is known from "Shonjog" that if there is any COVID-19 patient in the house, he will be provided oxygen by showing the prescription of the doctor. In this case, a service charge will be levied considering the financial condition of the customer.

Very recently, Rajabajar has been declared a red zone, and a total of 145 volunteers (45 in day and 40 at night) have started working to help the people living in that area to buy their daily necessities. They are also monitoring the incoming and outgoing of the people from that area as well as taking their temperature before allowing anyone to enter or leave. Nevertheless, the sad part is, the people of that area are taking advantage of the situation and are making the volunteers do trivial work at inappropriate times, e.g., ordering ice cream at 2 AM, ordering pimple cream at 4 AM saying that it is an emergency medicine.

7.6.5 *PROBLEMS REGARDING HOSPITALS (FIGURE 7.5)*

The problems regarding hospitals are lack of infrastructure; denial to give treatment; and uncooperative doctors and staff.

Problems regarding Hospitals
→ Lack of infrastructure
→ Denial to give treatment
→ Uncooperative doctors and staff

FIGURE 7.5   Problems regarding hospitals.

Mishti Akhter went to Gaibandha Mother and Child Welfare Center with labor pain, but as she was not admitted, she gave birth in a battery-powered auto-rickshaw on the road. Her husband Abdur Rashid said that she had labor pains at home on Monday evening. She was then taken in a battery-powered auto rickshaw to the Gaibandha Mother and Child Welfare Center. Touhida Begum, the family welfare inspector in charge of the center at the time, asked him to take her to another hospital without any examination. Even then, he repeatedly requested the inspector to admit this to his wife, but she did not listen.

Many hospitals have only been set in paperwork, but the actual work is far from reality. In Chittagong, a 100-bed isolation ward has been set up at the General Hospital and a 50-bed isolation ward at BITID for corona treatment. Nevertheless, ICU services for critically ill patients have not been implemented yet. There are health centers in six unions of Badarganj Upazila of Rangpur. None of these health centers has any infrastructure. As a result, grassroots people are being deprived of access to healthcare. The number of beds and ICUs provided by the Department of Health for corona patients is much lower than it is. Additional Director General (Administration) Prof. Nasima Sultana told the Health Department's regular news bulletin that there are 13,984 beds for corona patients across the country. In reality, there are less than 5,000 beds. That being said, there are 216 ICUs. The number of ICUs that have not been introduced has also been added. There are less than 140 ICUs.

Some of the doctors and staff are very uncooperative as well. Chittagong City Corporation has sacked 10 doctors and a storekeeper for lack of training to treat COVID 19 patients. To treat COVID patients, 17 doctors and 20 more, including nurses and brothers were selected for the isolation center, 36 people were selected. The city corporation arranged for three days of training for them before launching the isolation center. Specialist doctors and government officials from the health department provide this training. However, 10 doctors and a storekeeper were absent from the three-day training, which began on Sunday. However, the remaining 19 people including 6 doctors and nurses took part in the training. The city mayor was upset due to their absence three days in a row. As a result, he fired them.

As coronavirus infections increase, more and more health care providers are becoming involved in tackling the crisis. At present, about 36 health care institutions in the country are directly engaged in corona coping. There is no treatment for anyone except for COVID-19 patients. Besides, out of about 50,000 beds in government hospitals, 6,000 beds have been prepared as isolation beds for COVID-19 suspected patients. The number of doctors or health care workers is not up to the mark. Overall, the treatment opportunities for non-COVID or general patients have been greatly narrowed; their health risks have increased a lot. There is no separate ambulance for patients suffering from corona at Dhamrai Upazila Health Complex. The same ambulance is being used to carry medicines, including corona and general patients. This increases the risk of spreading the virus in ordinary patients.

7.6.6   TEST KITS AND PROCESS-RELATED PROBLEMS (FIGURE 7.6)

The test kits and process-related problems are technical problems; and insufficient number of kits.

Test Kits and Process related Problems
→ Technical problems
→ Insufficient number of kits

FIGURE 7.6   Test kits and process related problems.

Only one-third of the institutions have six essential medicines for the treatment of children. Around 6% of organizations are not ready to provide family planning services. Around 70 institutions across the country tested the samples. Around 30 in Dhaka and 30 outsides. Samples of 326,942 people have been tested in Dhaka. Overall, testing coronavirus samples is now a difficult task. More than 200 samples are collected every day. However, the number of people who need to be tested for corona samples is much higher. To test the corona sample at BSMMU one has to register on the website of the institution. Here an average of 450 samples is tested every day. Besides, about 280 samples are collected.

Gajipur, Savar, Kaliyak, everywhere, people are struggling to be tested. The process of testing and calling for samples is very troublesome. As a result, many are forming lines on the footpath so that they can be tested fast. Very few of them are maintaining social distance and hygiene. People are worried that even if they were not infected before, they might get infected while waiting to get tested.

Many hospitals are now facing problems regarding faulty kits. The coronavirus detection test at the PCR laboratory of Sheikh Hasina Medical College in Jamalpur is closed due to a mechanical fault. According to the laboratory authorities, a mechanical problem was suddenly seen in the PCR lab yesterday morning. Since then, sample testing for coronavirus detection has stopped. Engineers from software and hardware supply and installation organizations are being contacted in the lab to solve internal problems.

Not only that, but also, the number of people being tested is nowhere near being adequate. In Bangladesh, an average of 6 coronaviruses (COVID-19) detection tests is being carried out for every 1 million people. Of the 8 South

Asian countries, fewer are being tested in Afghanistan alone. Although the laboratory in Bangladesh can test over 12,000 samples a day, so far, the highest number of tests has been 6,900 in a single day. This equation is only better than Afghanistan among the South Asian countries.

7.6.7 *CORRUPTION REGARDING CORONA CERTIFICATES (FIGURE 7.7)*

The corruption regarding corona certificates is maily selling fake COVID certificates.

Corruption regarding Corona Certificates
→ Selling fake COVID certificates

FIGURE 7.7   Corruption regarding corona certificates.

RAB has arrested four people for selling fake 'Corona Negative-Positive' certificates. The gang is collecting copies of positive and negative reports of corona patients from Magda Hospital, scanning them, and selling them by putting their names there. Originally, workers from private companies and ready-made garment factories were collecting these certificates. RAB says that whether the corona is positive or negative in Bangladesh, the report only mentions the name and age. There is no national identity card number or passport number. As a result, it is not known who the buyer of the fake certificate is.

Coronavirus samples were collected from houses if they were called. In exchange, a minimum of TK. 5,000 to a maximum of TK. 6,600 was taken. However, the test results were given one day later without any test of that sample. Such allegations have been made against Jobeda Khatun Public Health Services (JKG Healthcare). The Tejgaon area of Dhaka Metropolitan Police arrested five people, including JKG chief executive officer Ariful Chowdhury, on Tuesday. Police say they have initially confirmed that at least 36 people were given fake results.

Not only that, but hospitals are also now charging way more than usual to make a profit out of people's misery. Freedom fighter MD Mojammel Haque expresses his disappointment regarding the healthcare system of Bangladesh. He was infected with coronavirus, and while undergoing treatment at the hospital for coronary heart disease, he had to pay Tk 8,400 for only 30 minutes of oxygen use in two days. Not only that, no doctor except the duty doctor saw him in the hospital. However, the doctor's consultant fee was BDT 49000. Besides, no cleaner or anyone else went to his room. However, the service charge of the room has been fixed at BDT 45,400.

7.6.8 UNHELPFUL PATIENT ROLE (FIGURE 7.8)

Unhelpful patient role are COVID patients fleeing from hospitals; ordinary patients treating COVID patients poorly; and patients preferring homeo-pathic doctors, Hakim-Kabiraj over hospitals.

Unhelpful Patient Role

→ COVID patients fleeing from hospitals
→ Ordinary patients treating COVID patients poorly
→ Patients preferring homeopathic doctors, Hakim-Kabiraj over hospitals

---

FIGURE 7.8 Helpful patient role.

Many people nowadays try to go for self-medication or by using the internet or visiting homeopathic doctors, which can cause more harm than good. Most of the people in the country do not go to the doctor who has passed MBBS when they get the disease. Around 56% of the patients get treatment from drug dealers, homeopathic doctors, Hakim-Kabiraj, Ojha, Pir, Vaidya, and other people. Due to this, more than half of the patients do not get proper treatment. This information is from the Household Income and Expenditure Survey of the Bangladesh Bureau of Statistics (BBS). Not all people go to the doctor because of the disease. About 58% of people think the problem is not important. Another part does not take treatment due to high medical expenses. They are about 16%. Many refrains from seeking treatment due to the lack of doctors in their area. Many people think that going to the doctor can catch a big disease. Many do not go to the doctor because of this panic. It also happens that many people do not go to the doctor or hospital because there is no one to accompany them. According to the Bureau of Statistics, 23% of people seek treatment in private chambers for "incompetent physicians." Drug dealer employees and compounders treat 33% of people. Around 2.23% of patients go for homeopathy treatment. Around 0.76% goes to Hekim and Kabiraj. Also, people do not visit doctors right after feeling ill. They wait for an average of four days before going to the doctor.

7.6.9   INNOVATIONS TO BRING A SOLUTION (FIGURE 7.9)

Innovations to bring a solution are medicines like Remivir, Doxycycline; plasma therapy; and the first trial on a vaccine.

Innovations to Bring a Solution

→ Medicines like Remivir, Doxycycline

→ Plasma therapy

→ The first trial on a vaccine

FIGURE 7.9   Innovations to bring a solution.

SKF has completed the production of the drug in Bangladesh shortly after the United States approved the use of remedicative for corona patients. Doctors in the country got a weapon to fight against Corona. The sooner the drug is approved for marketing, the more the people of the country will benefit from it. SKF will market the drug under the name 'Remivir.'

A study is being conducted regarding the use of a parasitic drug named ivermectin, with subjects being the adult patients who have been admitted to the hospital. Beximco Pharmaceuticals Limited is providing financial support for their study. This study will be completed in two months. The purpose of the research is to reveal if Doxycycline with ivermectin or treatment with ivermectin alone can reduce the rate of infection and how long it takes to reduce fever and cough. The study also looked at changes in oxygen requirements, why patients cannot maintain more than 6% oxygen saturation despite being given oxygen, changes in the number of days oxygen is supplied to patients, and hospitalizations and attempts to determine the cause of death.

After being infected with COVID-19 or coronavirus, special antibodies are made in the human body that fight against the virus. Plasma is taken from the body of the recovered person and transmitted to the affected body for utilizing that antibody. It is hoped that the mature antibody will continue to fight the virus in the body of the newly infected recipient.

Although consuming those medicines without consulting a doctor can be harmful. Experts warn that dexamethasone, which scientists say is effective in treating critically ill patients with COVID-19, can lead to serious physical problems if taken without a doctor's advice. Using dexamethasone can reduce the risk of death in patients on ventilators by one-third, scientists say. Moreover, for those who are being treated with oxygen, the death rate can be reduced by one-fifth.

Globe Biotech Limited is one of the leading pharmaceutical companies in Bangladesh. They started inventing a vaccine to prevent the coronavirus. This time the organization in Bangladesh has claimed that they have made great progress in inventing the vaccine. They have been 100% successful with trials on animals. That is what the officials of that organization have demanded. And only one step left. If it succeeds, Bangladesh will be able to claim that it has invented the corona vaccine. The officials held a press conference at the company's head office in Tejgaon, Dhaka. There they reported great progress in the process of inventing the vaccine. The last step is still considered to be the real one in discovering the rest of the vaccine. That is the clinical trial in the human body. Animal models will also be tested in the second phase of vaccine discovery. According to the agency, after 6 to 8 weeks, the vaccine will ask the government for permission to go on a clinical trial. Only with permission will it go to the last stage of the trial. The company claimed that they had achieved a 100% success by conducting tests on the animal's body. The company hopes that the vaccine will work in the human body as well.

We do not know whether this will work or not, but it is good news. This will inspire more people to start working on vaccines. Moreover, if they become successful, it will be a huge milestone for Bangladesh.

7.7   CONCLUSIONS AND FUTURE RESEARCH

This chapter shows a reflection of how the healthcare systems of a third world country work during a pandemic. Thus, this chapter able to fulfill the basic objective of the research and contribute significantly to the health care literature related to pandemic management.

The biggest drawback of this chapter is its heavy reliance on secondary data. No primary data has been collected because of the current scenario. However, further research can be conducted based on primary data as well as its analysis and interpretation. Another flaw of this chapter is the point of view. In this research, the healthcare system has been observed from a neutral point of view. Future research can take place where the healthcare system is evaluated by a healthcare professional or even a patient. Finally, the chapter only highlights the medical care of Bangladesh. To get a comprehensive understanding of the healthcare system of third world countries in the pandemic, other countries in South East Asia should also be included. Future studies can look into that.

Coronavirus has taught us that you do not need wars or heavy machinery or guns to bring a collapse in any country's economy because one tiny invisible organism has enough power to press the pause button for giant countries like the US, UK, or China. Therefore, for a country like the one Bangladesh to survive in a world like this is going to be a very daunting task, and we can see the reflection of that fact in our findings. To make things worse, the number of infected and dead are increasing every single day. This chapter provides proper insights on why and how these incidents are taking place, which adds value to existing health care management literature.

KEYWORDS

- **COVID-19**
- **healthcare system**
- **healthcare workers**
- **hospitals**
- **pandemic**
- **patients**
- **social stigma**

REFERENCES

1. Dilshad, S., Akhtar, A., Huda, S. S., & Samad, N., (2020). Assessment of healthcare service quality: Tertiary care hospitals of Dhaka City. In: *Global Issues and Innovative Solutions in Healthcare, Culture, and the Environment* (pp. 271–291). IGI Global.
2. Emanuel, E. J., Persad, G., Upshur, R., Thome, B., Parker, M., Glickman, A., & Phillips, J. P., (2020). *Fair Allocation of Scarce Medical Resources in the Time of COVID-19.*
3. Friedman, R. A., & Podolny, J., (1992). Differentiation of boundary spanning roles: Labor negotiations and implications for role conflict. *Administrative Science Quarterly*, 28–47.

4.   Nicholls, A., (2008). *Social Entrepreneurship: New Models of Sustainable Social Change.* OUP Oxford.

5.   National Institute of Population Research and Training - NIPORT/Bangladesh, Mitra and Associates, and ICF International. 2016. Bangladesh Demographic and Health Survey 2014. Dhaka, Bangladesh: NIPORT, Mitra and Associates, and ICF International. Available at http://dhsprogram.com/pubs/pdf/FR311/FR311.pdf (accessed on 23 July 2021).

6.   Ministry of Health & Family Welfare. (2020). Bangladesh Preparedness and Response Plan for COVID-19. July 2020.

CHAPTER 8

The Impact of COVID-19 on Mental Health

TILOTTAMA RAYCHAUDHURI

Assistant Professor of Law, WBNUJS, Kolkata, West Bengal, India

ABSTRACT

The novel coronavirus or COVID-19 pandemic is unlike anything experienced by humanity in the recent past. To flatten the curve of the virus, countries across the world imposed lockdowns, resulting in the abrupt shutting down of economies and confinement of billions of persons to their homes. Along with the toll taken on economies and the human toll, the pandemic has created a plethora of psychological problems, the effects of which may be long term. Though the effect of the COVID-19 crisis is felt by everyone, there is not enough research to test its psychological impact on different sections of society. In this chapter, the author examines the impact of COVID-19 on the mental health of a section of people living in India's metropolitan cities, to assess the impact of the pandemic on the more privileged sections of society. It is largely felt that people belonging to urban, upper-middle-class backgrounds have been less affected by lockdowns and related measures. However, the survey reveals, in line with emerging global findings, that even amongst people who have access to resources, the psychological impact of the pandemic is of considerable concern. Hence, the situation is likely to be much worse with respect to the sections of society which have lesser access and privilege.

8.1 INTRODUCTION: PANDEMICS AND THEIR PSYCHOLOGICAL IMPACT

One of the biggest challenges faced by humanity today is the outbreak of COVID-19, caused by the severe acute respiratory syndrome coronavirus

2 (SARS-CoV-2). The name COVID-19 was given to the disease by the World Health Organization (WHO) on 11th February, 2020. The outbreak started in Wuhan, China, reportedly in December 2019 and then swiftly spread to almost all countries across the world. On 11th March, 2020, amidst widespread controversy, the WHO declared COVID-19 to be a pandemic. A pandemic, according to the WHO, is "*an epidemic occurring worldwide, or over a very wide area, crossing international boundaries and usually affecting a large number of people*" [1]. Throughout the course of history, there have been several pandemics which ravaged civilizations, from the Antonine Plague in 165 AD to the ongoing COVID-19 crisis. The first documented pandemic was the Spanish Flu of 1918 and COVID-19 is the 5th such documented pandemic [2]. Some of these pandemics, like the plagues and cholera were caused by bacteria which developed the ability to spread rapidly, while others like the Spanish flu, human immunodeficiency virus infection/acquired immune deficiency syndrome (HIV/AIDS), severe acute respiratory syndrome coronavirus (SARS-CoV), Ebola, and Swine Flu involved virus strains that could easily transmit between humans.

While the world is regularly emphasizing on the economic and social effects of the pandemic, and rightly so, one essential effect that needs to be focused upon is mental health. Emotional stressors such as isolation, confusion caused by misinformation, insecurity, stigma, economic loss due to depletion of resources, loss of job opportunities, work, and school closures, inadequate governmental and medical responses are causing unprecedented fear, stress, and anxiety on individual and community levels [3]. Researches on past pandemics reveal their profound impact on human psychology. For instance, a study conducted on the survivors of the Ebola outbreak reveals initial feelings of fear, denial, rage, social isolation, and increased risk of suicides [4]. The COVID-19 pandemic, its epidemiological features, transmission pattern and insufficient preparedness of health authorities, are similar to those of the 2003 outbreak of severe acute respiratory syndrome (SARS). In the absence of a precedent of the scale to understand the impacts on mental health due to COVID-19, a parallel could be drawn with the 2003 outbreak observations [5]. In China, there were 5327 reported cases and 349 deaths during the outbreak. In a 4 year follow up survey, 42.5% of survivors reported at least one diagnosable psychiatric disorder, most commonly PTSD, depression, and chronic fatigue [6]. Even health care workers reported a long-range of psychiatric morbidities in the aftermath of SARS. According to studies in other countries, mental health problems such as somatoform disorders and panic disorders, in addition to the psychiatric problems observed in China, were common amongst survivors [31]. Therefore, the experience of SARS is evidence of the high possibility of chronic mental health problems ensuing, well after the current outbreak is over.

8.2   EFFECT OF COVID-19 ON MENTAL HEALTH

COVID-19 is a highly infectious disease. According to the WHO, the spread of the virus occurs primarily through "droplets of saliva, or discharge from the nose when an infected person coughs or sneezes" [7]. To date, there is no vaccine or cure for this virus which has already claimed millions of lives across the world. Developing a cure or a vaccine for this virus has been a major challenge, as the virus has RNA as a genetic material and gets mutated frequently, as compared to DNA viruses like herpes, smallpox, and human papillomavirus [32]. To prevent the spread of the virus, the WHO recommends practicing respiratory etiquette like coughing/sneezing with the mouth covered, wearing of masks, hygiene/sanitization measures, maintaining social distancing and also self-isolation in case of symptoms such as cough, headache, mild fever [7]. There have been several studies conducted on the spread of the pandemic and the development of herd immunity, using mathematical models like the SIR model (susceptible-infectious-recovered) [8]. However, these studies are not conclusive and are used primarily for predicting the spread of the virus. In the absence of a vaccine or cure, countries globally have tried to minimize the spread of the virus through measures like travel restrictions, social distancing, and the imposition of periodic lockdowns.

Various initiatives have been taken globally to gauge the repercussions of the pandemic and its associated impact on mental health. A nationwide survey among Chinese people to understand the psychological distress due to COVID-19 was conducted in February, 2020 which reported that of the 52,730 responses recorded almost 35% reported psychological distress [9]. In Germany, the Hannover Medical School conducted a web-based cross-sectional survey and recorded that out of 3545 participants, 45.3% experienced worsened sleep, 50.9% reported being easily irritated, 29% reported more aggression and anger and 5% experienced inter-personal violence on a verbal, physical or sexual level. In the United Kingdom (UK), "population prevalence of clinically significant levels of mental distress rose from 18.9% in 2018–2019 to 27.3% in April, 2020" and in Iran, distress in the population rose to 60% during COVID-19. In April 2020, Ethiopia estimated a "33%

prevalence rate of symptoms consistent with depressive disorder" which was a three-fold increase from pre COVID-19 times [31]. Similar results were obtained from numerous other countries. The gamut of mental health problems enlisted in these reports ranged from insomnia, stress-induced anxiety, post-traumatic stress disorder (PTSD) to increased chances of suicide.

Though the pandemic has affected the lives of all-in-one way or the other, research reveals that some groups are more vulnerable than others, across nations:

- Healthcare workers being at the forefront are faced with extreme workload, unprecedented stress, risk of getting infected, spreading infection to families and communities, witnessing deaths on a relatively regular basis, stigma, and other stressors. Under these circumstances, there are significant adverse effects on their mental health [10–12].
- In addition to health care workers, infected victims and survivors of the novel coronavirus are at the center of the chain. Apart from isolation, lack of community and familial support, pressing physical issues and stigma also exacerbate the deterioration of their mental health.
- Next in line are the potential victims of the virus, the older adults, and people with pre-existing health conditions. Around 8 out of 10 COVID-19 deaths in the US have been amongst adults who are 65 years or older [13], whereas in Germany, 87% of all deaths were of persons aged 70 or older [2]. This group requires special care as they are more susceptible to life-threatening complications resulting from the virus.
- Women also constitute a category of substantial concern. Women are more vulnerable to stress and likely to develop PTSD [14]. This had been substantiated by previously discussed surveys in countries such as the UK and US, which revealed that women recorded more instances of clinical mental distress. The International Labor Organization (ILO) report states as well that women were 7% to 4% more likely to show anxiety or depression, respectively. This could be due to the possibility that women are more subject to stress-inducing responsibility at home [15]. This becomes especially bleak in countries like India, where mental health resources are sparse and suicide rates by women are already double the global suicide death rate. The United Nations (UN) has reported increased rates of violence against women and children, especially girls during COVID-19 [16]. In India, the

National Commission for Women (NCW) recorded 123 complaints of Domestic Violence from 27 Feb-22 March, 2020, whereas after imposition of the first lockdown in late March, the number of cases rose to 250 complaints by 22nd April [17].

- Adolescents and children are also at risk. Children are facing the same fears as adults but without the maturity to deal with such stress. In the midst of the fear of infection, dying, loss of loved ones, there is loss of structure, stimulation, and support provided by schools and peers. In homes where inter-personal violence takes place, children are more exposed to the same. Data from Italy and Spain show that parents reported a 31% increase in feelings of loneliness, 38% increase in nervousness, 39% increase in restlessness, 39% increase in irritability and 77% increase in concentration difficulties, in their children during COVID-19 times [31]. In the case of adolescents, problems such as closure of schools, diminishing economic opportunities, loss of routine and social connections have resulted in higher stress. A study of young people from the UK who had pre-existing mental health conditions showed that 32% reported aggravation their mental health situation [18]. The rise in deteriorating mental health conditions also leads to substance abuse and increased alcohol consumption [19, 20].
- People in humanitarian and conflict settings have a higher burden of mental health issues. In a 2019 report, estimates for people who had been forcibly displaced by violence and conflict stood at more than 70.8 million people [21]. The huge number of displaced people has a bigger intangible aspect to it; evidence suggests that one in five persons in such crises already have a mental health condition [22]. This condition is worsened in situations where internally displaced people are living in close and crowded camps and settlements where preventive guidelines are next to impossible to follow, leading to higher chances of spreading the virus and consequent rise in stress levels. In addition to this, such individuals had limited access to "quality, affordable mental health care." The pandemic has further diminished the availability of such services by disrupting chains around the world.

8.2.1 ALLOCATION OF RESOURCES ON MENTAL HEALTH

Even before the pandemic, the global state of mental health affairs was grim. The UN Policy Brief on Mental Health noted that the global economy lost more than $1 trillion every year due to depression and anxiety. Depression affects more than 264 million people in the world, and suicide is the second leading cause of death for the age group 15 to 29 years. In low- and middle-income countries, between 76% and 85% of people with mental health problems receive no treatment at all. Moreover, globally there is less than one mental health professional for every 10,000 people. This is because of low spending on mental health resources globally [31]. On an average, countries spend only 2% of their health budgets on mental health. The coronavirus aid, relief, and economic security act (CARES Act) worth almost 2 trillion dollars was passed by the US congress. With one of the highest number of cases and deaths in the world, a mere sum of 425 million dollars has been allotted for substance abuse and mental health services administration. In comparison, the airline industry has been allotted 75 billion dollars, and health providers have been allotted 185 billion dollars respectively [23].

8.3 COVID-19 AND MENTAL HEALTH IN INDIA

In India, a stringent nationwide lockdown was declared by the Prime Minister on 24th March, 2020 [24], which was further extended till 31st May, by the National Disaster Management Authority. Even the unlock phases that followed were subject to various restrictions on movement and travel, as well as restrictive measures pertaining to various sectors of the economy. The lockdown and the economic crisis that ensued pushed millions into unemployment. With the onset of the crisis, several surveys were conducted in India which revealed mental health repercussions. However, the subject of mental health is yet to gain priority in India [33]. Reports reveal that even with hundreds of psychiatrists graduating each year, India will have 0.75 psychiatrists per 100,000 persons, which would still fall short by around 27,000 doctors from the figure in high income countries [34]. This account coupled with specific features of the country draws an even darker picture. In a recent independent study conducted in India, the number of recorded suicides committed by people till June 2020, due to various reasons related to the pandemic, stood at 133 [25]. The Department of Psychiatry, National Institute of Mental Health and Neurosciences, set up a task force under the Ministry of Health and Family Welfare, Government of India to delve into the mental health impact of COVID-19 in India. Its report published in April 2020, lays down detailed guidelines for effective mental health management [16]. Initiatives have also been taken by states to provide support through tele-counseling. A notable example is Kerala where *Sanjeevni* or tele-medi-cine e-portals and "*Ottakala Oppamundu*" have been established throughout the state to provide psychosocial support. Under the scheme, 1143 mental health personnel, including psychiatrists, psychiatric social workers, clinical psychologists, and counselors have provided support to 11,68,950 people [26].

8.4 IMPACT OF COVID-19 ON MENTAL HEALTH OF THE MIDDLE AND UPPER MIDDLE CLASS OF INDIAN METROPOLIS

Initially, the infection was considered to be an imported one, as it was brought to the country by people belonging to more affluent sections of society who had returned to India from abroad. However, from the time India reported its initial cases, there has been a shift in perception about the spread of the virus. Now the virus has spread from rich neighborhoods to the poor and more densely populated ones, which are worse off. This shift in class character of disease is not uncommon. Even before there was any medicine for tuber-culosis, its character as a fashionable upper-class disease soon changed to that of an infection widespread amongst people living in squalid conditions, in 19th century England. Polio in India followed the same trajectory as it continued to infect people who lived in neighborhoods without adequate potable water and sanitation, even after the discovery of a vaccine, till its aggressive administration in these areas. The repercussions of the COVID-19 pandemic on the poor, in both rural and urban areas have been severe, and much has been written about them. However, there is also a perception that the urban middle class and above benefitted more from the lockdown and associated social distancing measures [35].

Though the effect of the COVID-19 crisis is felt by everyone, there is still not enough research to test its psychological impact on different sections of society. The author has conducted a brief survey to assess the mental health impact of COVID-19 on a section of people living in metropolitan cities (Delhi, Mumbai, Bangalore, and Kolkata) to find out how persons from the so-called privileged sections of society who have access to basic necessities/facilities/infrastructure and more-have reacted to the pandemic. The findings reveal that the psychological impact of COVID-19 on the middle class and above, is also considerable. People in metropolitan cities are experiencing myriad psychological problems in adjusting to the current lifestyle, or the "new normal." This appears to be in line with the reasoning that the psychological impact of COVID-19 will be faced in varying degrees by the general population, the rich as well as the poor, across professions and occupations, age, gender, and religion [36].

8.5 MENTAL HEALTH SURVEY CONDUCTED BY THE AUTHOR

8.5.1 AIM AND METHOD

The survey was conducted to evaluate the psychological impact of the COVID-19 pandemic and lockdowns on people belonging to the middle class and above, across different ages, occupations, and genders, in metropolitan cities. The study was conducted in English, through an online survey using Google Forms, with the link forwarded through Email or WhatsApp Messenger. Each person could fill up the response only once and submit it using Google Forms. The responses were visible only to the person conducting the survey, not to others. Moreover, only the responses were visible, not the names of persons sending the responses. The survey questionnaire consisted of 24 closed-ended questions and a total of 139 responses were received.

8.5.2 DATA ANALYSIS

In order to evaluate the psychological impact of COVID-19 on people residing in metropolitan regions of India, the author chose a few cities, namely, Mumbai, Delhi, Kolkata, and Bangalore. The convenience method of sampling was used in the survey. Convenience sampling is a non-probability-based method of sampling whereby the researcher draws samples from people who are easy to contact or reach. The survey questions were mostly closed-ended, therefore the respondents had to choose the option most appropriate for them. The author conducted the survey to understand the overall psychological impact of COVID-19 on the respondents hence did not select any particular variable(s) or factor(s) which could be considered more important than the others. The author however did take into account age and gender as two separate criteria to give readers a better understanding of how these attributes may have an impact on an individual's mental health. The survey responses were first compiled in MS-Excel and then tabulated and tallied. A pictorial description of some of the data that was gathered is given below. The data generated is graphically represented in most places, through Bar-diagrams and Pie-charts, to give readers a clearer understanding of the general findings of the survey. The analysis is mostly done through numbers. Percentage values are only mentioned where Pie-charts are given.

The data derived from the survey can be divided into three broad themes:

1. The Demographic Profile of Respondents Who Took the Survey: At the very onset of the survey, respondents were asked their age, gender, and occupation. The responses received were used to construct the demographic profile of the respondents who participated in the survey. Separate methods of graphic representations were used to summarize the data.

2. People's Initial Response to the COVID-19 Crisis: Three broad questions were asked in the second part of the survey to gauge the respondents' initial responses to the COVID-19 crisis. These questions attempted to understand reactions to the sudden lifestyle changes brought about by the pandemic and the worries faced by the respondents regarding their physical and financial health. Respondents were also asked about the impact of COVID-19 related news on their mental health.

3. The Physical, Psychological, Emotional Indicators of Stress and Mental Well-Being of the Respondents: Eleven questions were asked in the third and final section of the survey. These questions attempted to measure different indicators of stress to evaluate the overall psychological impact of COVID-19 on people. Both physical and emotional indicators were used here to understand the presence or absence of stress in respondents.

8.5.2.1   PART ONE: DEMOGRAPHIC PROFILE

When considering the demographic profile of the respondents, certain attributes were taken into consideration, such as:

- Gender of the respondents;
- Age of the respondents;
- Occupations respondents may be engaged in.
- A total of 139 people responded out of which 71 (51%) of the respondents were female, 66 (48%) were male while only 2 (1%) were transgender.

1. Age-Based Distribution of the Respondents: For convenience, the sample was distributed into four major age categories-10 to 18 years of age, 19 to 30 years of age, 31 to 50 years of age and above 50 years of age. Among the 139 respondents who took part in the survey, 32 (23%) belonged to the 10 to 18 years of age group, 34 (24.5%) belonged to the 19 to 30 years age category, 41 (29.4%) belonged to the 31 to 50 years of age group and 32 (23%) belonged to the above 50 years age group. So, the majority of the respondents were 19 to 50 years in age, with a slight inclination on the higher end of the age category.

2. Occupation of the Respondents: Out of 71 female respondents, 27 were students, 8 were homemakers, 11 were self-employed and 8 pursued other career options. Out of the 2 transgender respondents, 1 was self-employed and 1 was engaged in part-time/full time work. Out of 66 male respondents, 13 were students, 27 were self-employed, and 14 were engaged in full-time/part-time work, and 13 were engaged in other kinds of work. So, it may be observed that there are 27 (71%) self-employed males as against only 11 (29%) females. There are no male homemakers, only 8 female homemakers. In terms of being engaged in part-time/full-time jobs, females have a slightly higher number 16 (53.3%) as opposed to males 14 (46.7%). Finally, 13 (62%) males, as opposed to 8 (38%) females, are engaged in other occupations.

8.5.2.2   PART TWO: GENDER AND AGE-BASED INITIAL RESPONSES TO THE COVID-19 CRISIS

Several questions were asked in this part, to observe how respondents reacted to the COVID-19 crisis. Some responses are depicted graphically below. The questions included the following:

• Respondents were asked about their initial reaction to the COVID-19 crisis. They had to choose between whether they felt it is a pandemic and will pass, whether it is the end of the world, whether it is a conspiracy theory, or whether they have nothing to fear because it does not affect the fit or the young. A two-fold analysis of these questions has been done (see Figures 8.1 and 8.2). Figure 8.1 represents responses of female interviewees across all age categories, and

Figure 8.2 represents responses of male interviewees across all age categories. The age-gender nexus has been considered to comprehend if there might be any noticeable changes in responses across these categories. Respondents were also asked about the biggest lifestyle change they had to go through, due to the crisis.

- Respondents were asked how worried they were about their own health and safety, along with those of their family members, and how often they worried about their job or financial health. The respondents were given a similar set of responses for these questions. They were asked if they worried sometimes, on most days, every day, or not at all. Both male and female respondents across all four age categories were asked these questions. Their responses were noted and compiled to provide a clearer picture.
- The survey also addressed their concerns about the world in general and the nation in particular due to the pandemic, and also their reactions to COVID-19 related news in the media.

The graphical representations of some of these concerns have been made in the following section, in numeral values (Figures 8.1–8.4).

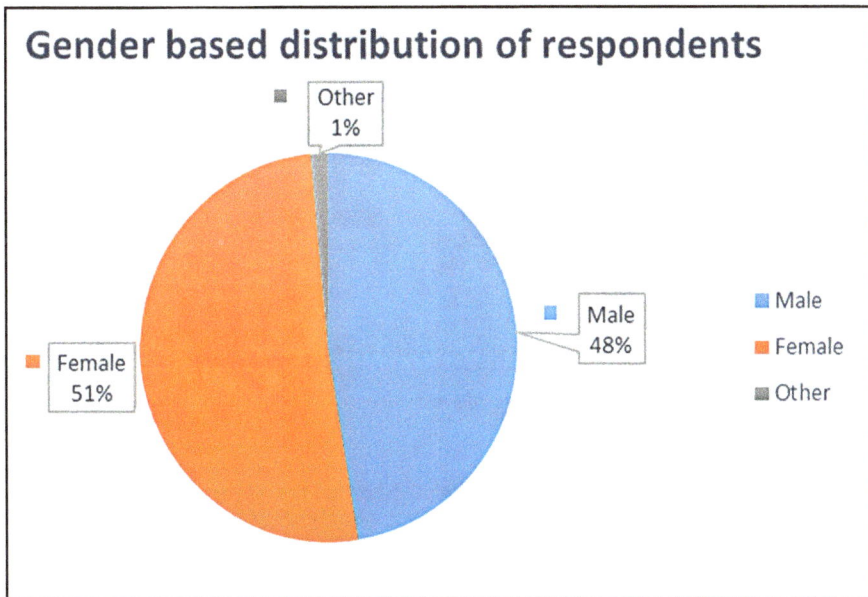

FIGURE 8.1 Gender-based distribution of the respondents.

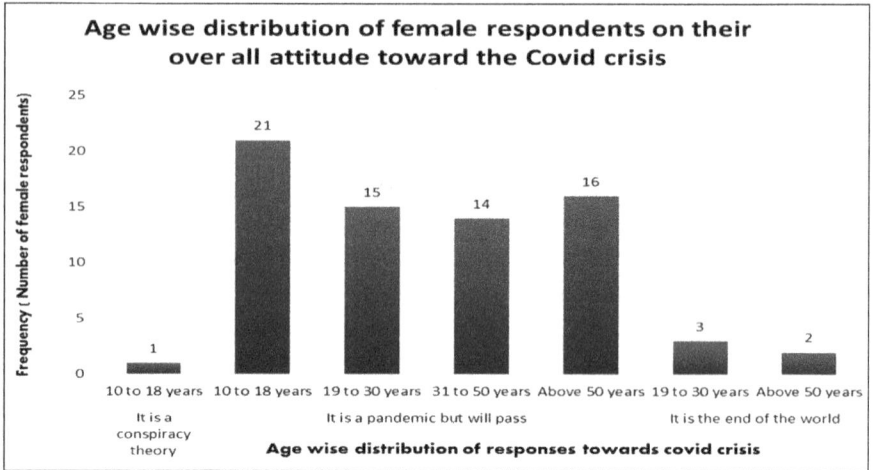

FIGURE 8.2 Age-wise distribution of female respondents and their attitude towards the crisis.

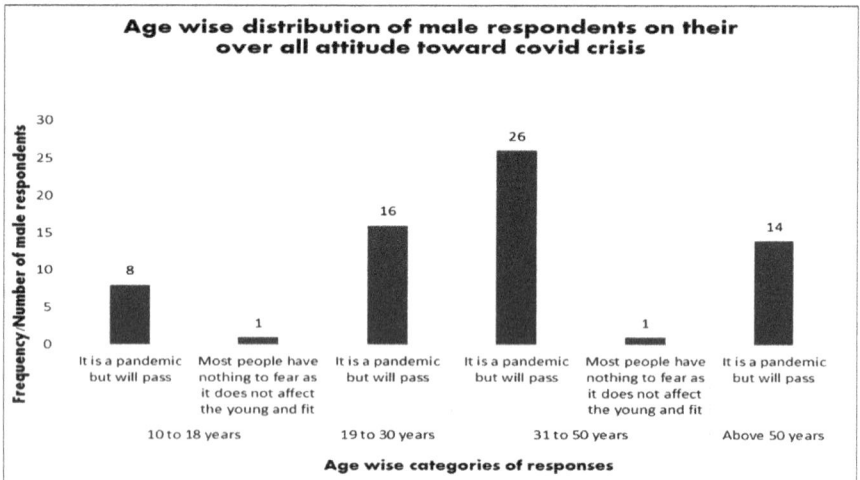

FIGURE 8.3 Age-wise distribution of male respondents and their attitude towards the crisis.

- **Analysis:** Out of 71 female respondents, 66 feels that the COVID-19 crisis is a pandemic, and that it would pass eventually. The maximum numbers of these female respondents belong to the 10 to 18 years of age group. One female respondent believes that the pandemic is a conspiracy theory and 5 female respondents believe that it is the end of the world.

- **–Analysis:** Majority of male respondents (64 out of a total of 66) feel that the crisis is temporary and it will eventually pass. Most of these respondents belong to the 31 to 50 years age category. No male respondent feels that the pandemic is either a conspiracy theory or the end of the world. However, 2 male respondents in the age brackets 10 to 18, and 31 to 50 believe that the disease does not affect the young and fit.

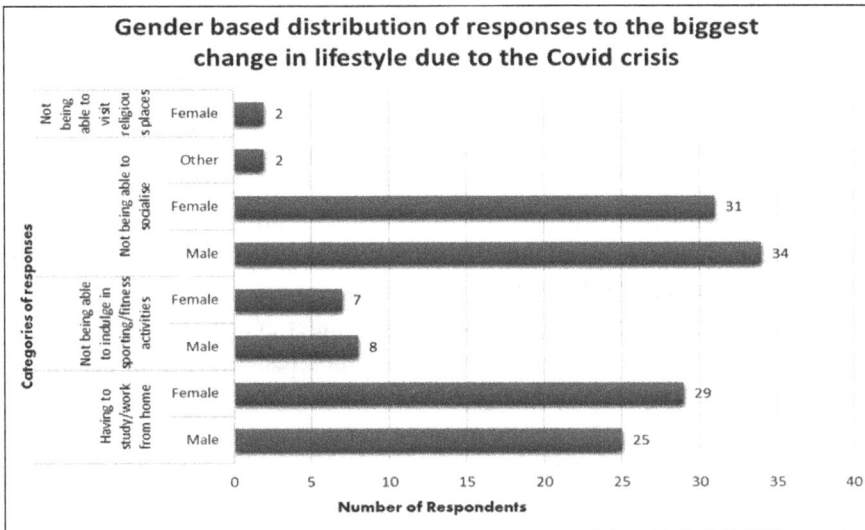

FIGURE 8.4   Gender-based distribution of responses to the biggest change in lifestyle.

- **Analysis:** 67 people in total (31 females, 34 males and 2 transgender) have reported that the biggest lifestyle change they had to make due to the COVID-19 crisis was not being able to socialize. Around 54 respondents (29 female and 25 male) have reported that the biggest lifestyle change they had to make was studying or working from home. Around 15 respondents (8 male and 7 female) reported that they could not indulge in sporting activities. Only female respondents (2) reported that they could not visit religious places.

If we choose to comprehend how the response to COVID-19 has been across the gender categories, we observe a difference. More male respondents felt that the most important lifestyle change they had to go through was limited socialization, whereas for women, everyone staying at home meant more pressure on the household front. Hence more women experienced additional pressures of having to juggle office and household work simultane-ously, and this was their biggest lifestyle change. The pre-existing differential distribution of labor at home and prevalent gender roles exerted more pres-sure on women during the crisis. When respondents were asked about how often they worried about their own health and safety, most respondents (79) across age and gender categories, appeared to worry "sometimes." Within this category, male respondents were more in number (43) than women (36). Only 7 respondents reported that they did not worry at all about the impact of COVID-19 on their health.

Two observable facts that draw attention with respect to this query is that more women (5) as opposed to men (2) did not worry about the effect of COVID-19 on their health at all. There could be several probable reasons for this; one could be that these women were genuinely unconcerned about their health or, under the circumstances, they got very little time to worry about their own health. Around 7 respondents within the 19 to 30 years of age category and 7 respondents within the 31 to 50 years of age category worried about their health every day. The 19 to 30 age bracket emerges as a bit of a surprise as it is anticipated that the younger generation would worry less. Similarly, another unexpected result is that 7 respondents falling above the 50 years of age category appeared to be least concerned about their own health.

When respondents were asked how often they worried about the health and safety of their family, the responses revealed the following:

- Across gender categories, female respondents worry more than males. Around 20 female respondents as opposed to 18 male respondents worry about this every day. Around 22 female respondents as opposed to 18 male respondents worry about it on most days. Male respondents appear to worry less about the effect of COVID-19 on their family's health than their female counterparts.
- Across age categories, the respondents falling within the 10 to 18 years of age category seem the least worried about their family's health and safety. The 19 to 30 years and 31 to 50 years seem the most worried. Around 24 respondents belonging to these age categories worry about the effect of COVID-19 on their family's health and safety almost every day, while 22 respondents worry about it on most days.

Regarding how often respondents worried about their job and financial health, the arguments are supported with Figures 8.5–8.8.

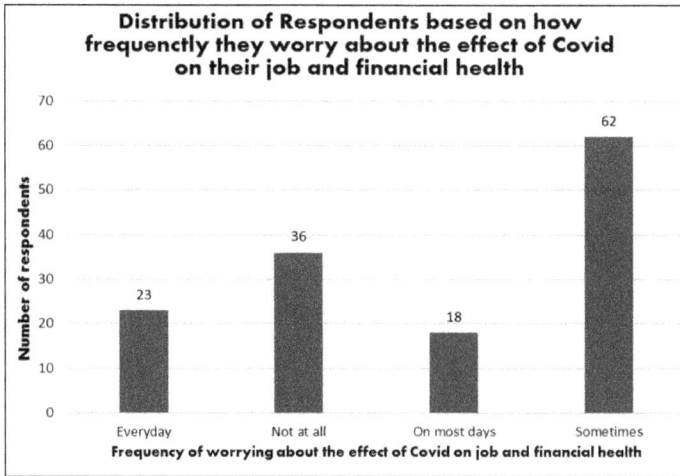

FIGURE 8.5   Distribution of respondents is based on the frequency with which they worry about their jobs and financial health.

- **Analysis:** 62 respondents reported worrying about the effect of COVID-19 on their job and financial health. Around 36 reported not worrying about it at all. Around 23 reported worrying about it every day, and 18 reported worrying about it on most days.
- **Analysis:** As revealed, more female respondents (21) as opposed to male respondents (15) do not worry about the effect COVID-19 might have on their job and financial health. More male respondents (12) as opposed to female respondents (9) worry about this every day. The same number of males and females worry about it on most days and sometimes.

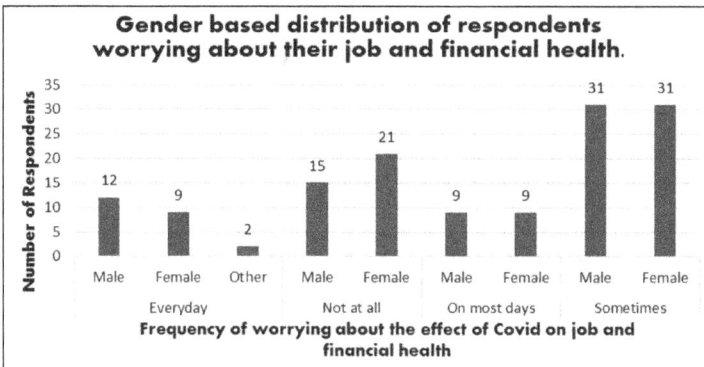

FIGURE 8.6   Gender-based distribution of respondents based on the frequency with which they worry about their jobs and financial health.

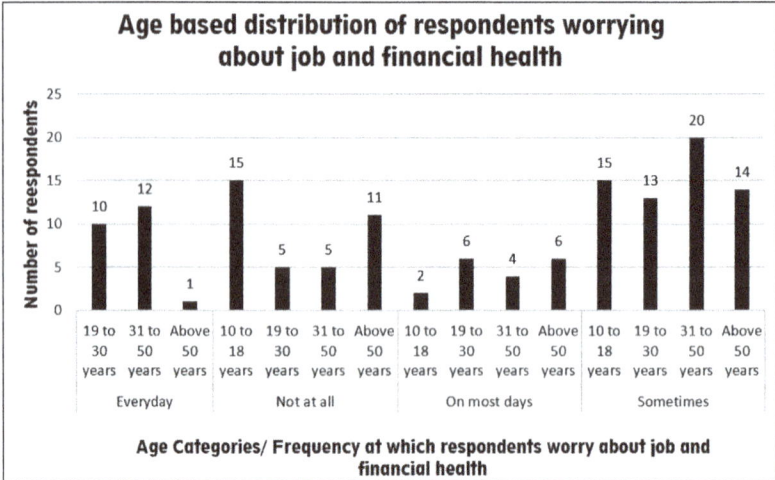

FIGURE 8.7 Age-based distribution of respondents based on the frequency with which they worry about their jobs and financial health.

- **Analysis:** The age group category that seems to worry more about their job and financial health is 31 to 50 years. As this group is typically in the life stage which involves earning occupations, this finding does not come as a surprise. Around 12 respondents belonging to this category worry about it every day, while 20 respondents worry about it sometimes. The below 18 years age category and above 50 years category seem to worry the least about it which is possibly an expected result.

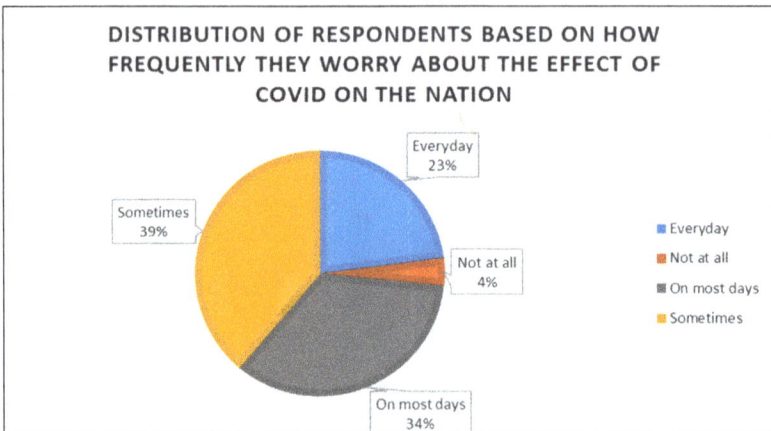

FIGURE 8.8 Distribution of respondents based on the frequency at which they worry about the effect of COVID-19 on the nation.

- **Analysis:** 39% of the total respondents sometimes worry about the effect of COVID-19 on the nation, followed by sizeable 23% respondents who worry about it every day and a substantial 34% who worry about it on most days. Only 4% do not worry about it at all. When considering this distribution across gender and age categories, the following observations emerge:
  - In numerical terms, 29 male respondents as opposed to 25 female respondents worry about the effect of COVID-19 on the nation only sometimes. Around 16 female and 14 male respondents worry about it every day. Around 27 female and 21 male respondents worry about it on most days, while 3 male and 2 female respondents do not worry about it at all.
  - It has been observed that the respondents falling within the 19 to 30 years and 31 to 50 years age category worry about the effect of COVID-19 on the nation every day. The majority of respondents above 50 years of age worry about it on most days. More respondents belonging to the 31 to 50 years age category tend to worry about it "sometimes." So, it may be concluded that across age categories, there is worry about the impact of COVID-19 on the nation, with varying intensity.
  - Respondents were asked how often they worried about the impact COVID-19 would have on the world. The replies showed that 57 respondents worried about the effect of COVID-19 on the world sometimes, followed by a sizable 44 respondents who worried about it on most days. A substantial 32 respondents worried about it almost every day while only 6 did not worry about it at all.

Towards the end of this discussion, the respondents' attitude towards COVID-19 related news in the media was also considered (Figure 8.9).

- **Analysis:** Figure 8.9 provides a graphical representation of the responses obtained when asked how frequently respondents watched COVID-19 related news (the source of this news primarily being the electronic media). Around 74 respondents reported watching only the important updates on COVID-19. Around 55 respondents reported watching COVID-19 news every day. Around 7 reported that COVID-19 is the only news they follow, while 3 reported they do not follow any COVID-19 news at all.

Distribution showing how frequently respondents follow Covid related news

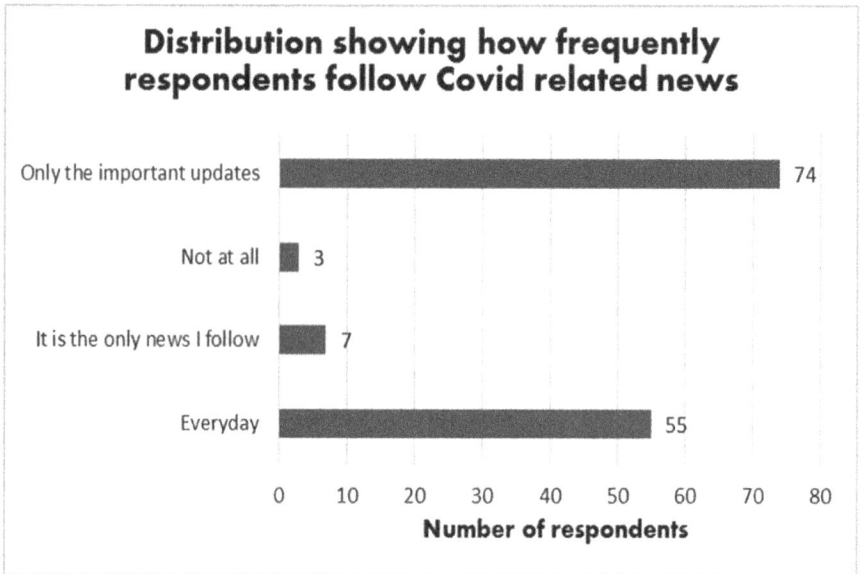

FIGURE 8.9 Distribution showing how frequently respondents followed COVID-19 news.

Interestingly, the survey also examined the emotional reaction of participants to COVID-19 related news. Out of the 136 respondents who answered this question, 50 respondents feel angry that the government and health officials are not doing enough and another 50 feel negative and depressed. Only 24 respondents do not bother about COVID-19 news, while 12 respondents responded with a sense of gratitude towards a higher deity towards not having been affected by COVID-19.

8.5.2.3 PART THREE: THE PHYSICAL, PSYCHOLOGICAL, EMOTIONAL INDICATORS OF STRESS AND MENTAL WELL-BEING OF THE RESPONDENTS

The third and final part of the survey pertains to physical, psychological, and emotional indicators of stress that individuals might experience during the crisis. For this reason, several questions addressing issues of mental well-being have been asked in the survey.

Some of the broad questions are:

1. How often do respondents feel nervous, anxious or on the edge?

2. How often do respondents feel annoyed or irritable during this crisis?
3. How often do respondents feel scared that something awful might happen?
4. How often does one feel demotivated or lose interest/ pleasure in doing tasks?
5. Whether respondents have trouble falling asleep, or have irregular sleeping patterns?
6. Do respondents feel tired or have less energy during the COVID-19 crisis?
7. Whether one tends to over eat or has developed a change in appetite since the crisis began?
8. Whether one has trouble concentrating while performing daily tasks?
9. Respondents are asked to describe the most common emotion they feel during the crisis and also estimate their own vulnerability to the COVID-19 crisis.
10. How is one looking after his/her mental health during the COVID-19 crisis, if at all?
11. What has been the biggest problem faced by the respondents during the COVID-19 crisis?

The analysis attempts to comprehend the emergent data in three ways, firstly, an overall understanding of the full data set, and subsequently through a more detailed analysis factoring in the gender and the age of the respondent. The author has presented only the relevant data that throws light on the indicators of stress taken into consideration for the study. The author has included age and gender-based analysis only when the data has indicated important findings (Figure 8.10).

- **Analysis:** Respondents were asked how often they felt nervous, anxious or on the edge during the COVID-19 pandemic. They were given four options to choose from, namely every day, not at all, on most days and sometimes. Out of 139 respondents, 78 reported feeling anxious only sometimes. Around 27 reported feeling anxious or nervous on most days. Around 22 reported feeling not anxious at all, while 12 reported feeling so every day. Across all frequency categories, females appear to feel more anxious, nervous or on the edge during the COVID-19 crisis (see Figure 8.10). Among those who do not feel anxious at all, males (14) are more in numbers than females (8).

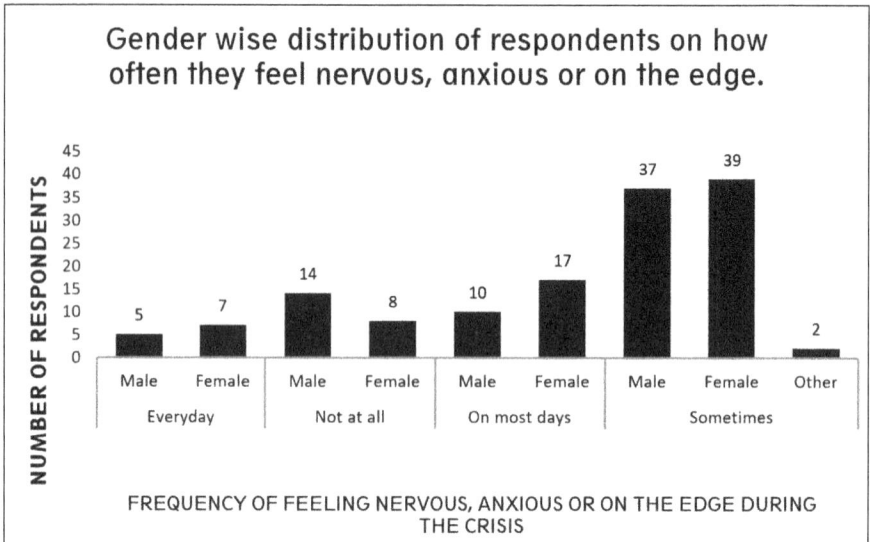

FIGURE 8.10 Gender wise distribution of responses on how often respondents feel nervous, anxious or on the edge.

Coming to the second question mentioned in the theme, majority of the respondents (90) feel annoyed or irritable during the COVID-19 crisis sometimes. Around 8 respondents feel annoyed or irritable during the COVID-19 crisis every day. Around 23 respondents do not feel annoyed or irritable at all. Around 9 female respondents as opposed to 14 male respondents do not feel annoyed at all. The 31 to 50 years age category records the highest number of respondents who feel annoyed or irritable. When asked how frequently respondents worry that something bad might happen to them, 78 respondents sometimes worry that something bad might happen. Around 30 respondents do not worry at all, 22 respondents worry on most days, while 9 respondents worry about it every day. Again, the 31 to 50 years age group worries the most about something bad happening to them. Among those who do not worry at all, the youngest (10 to 18 years and the oldest above 50 years) seem to worry the least. Around 41 female respondents, as opposed to 37 male respondents tend to worry sometimes that something bad might happen to them. However, 5 male respondents as opposed to 4 female respondents tend to worry about it every day (Figures 8.11–8.15).

Distribution showing how frequently respondents feel demotivated or have lost interest in doing things during the pandemic

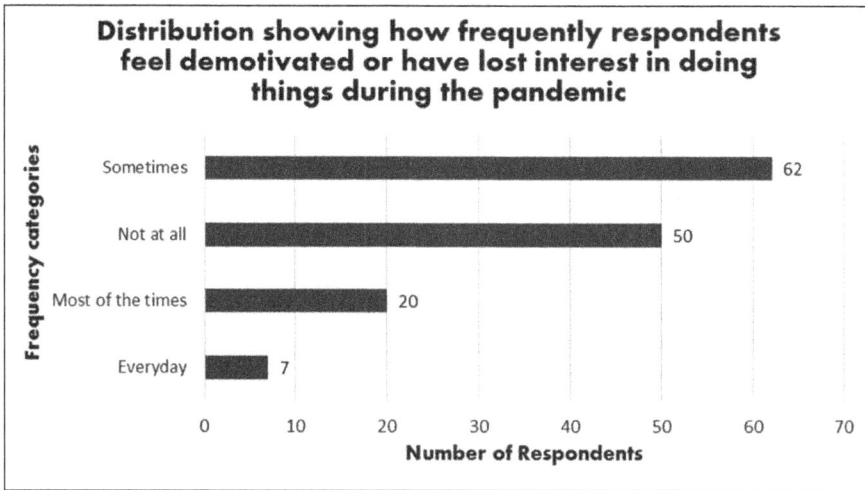

FIGURE 8.11 Distribution of respondents based on how frequently they feel demotivated or have lost interest in doing things.

- **Analysis:** 62 respondents reported that they feel demotivated to do anything, sometimes. Around 50 have reported that they do not feel so at all. Around 20 have reported they feel so on most days while only 7 have reported feeling so every day. Maximum respondents who feel demotivated belong to the 19 to 30 years age category and are females.

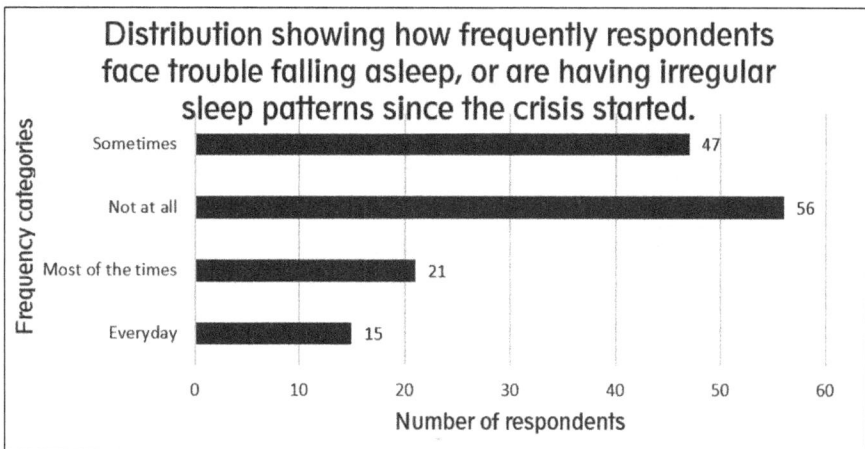

Distribution showing how frequently respondents face trouble falling asleep, or are having irregular sleep patterns since the crisis started.

FIGURE 8.12 Respondents on how frequently respondents face trouble falling asleep or have irregular sleeping patterns with the onset of the COVID-19 crisis.

- **Analysis:** When respondents were asked if they faced lack of sleep or irregular sleeping patterns, most respondents (56) reported not experiencing any trouble falling asleep or having irregular sleeping patterns. However, a greater number of males (22) as opposed to females (12) have reported trouble falling asleep or having irregular sleeping patterns.

Further, 61 respondents (34 females and 27 males) also reported feeling tired sometimes during the COVID-19 crisis. Around 51 reported not feeling tired at all. Around 27 respondents reported feeling tired on most days or every day.

- **Analysis:** 58 respondents reported that they did not over-eat or notice a change in their appetite. Again, a sizeable 52 reported doing so sometimes, 20 reported doing so most of the time. Around 9 people reported over-eating, or experiencing a change in appetite, every day. Those who reported over-eating sometimes belonged mostly to the 31 to 50 years of age group. Those who over-ate on most days belonged to the 19 to 30 years of age group.

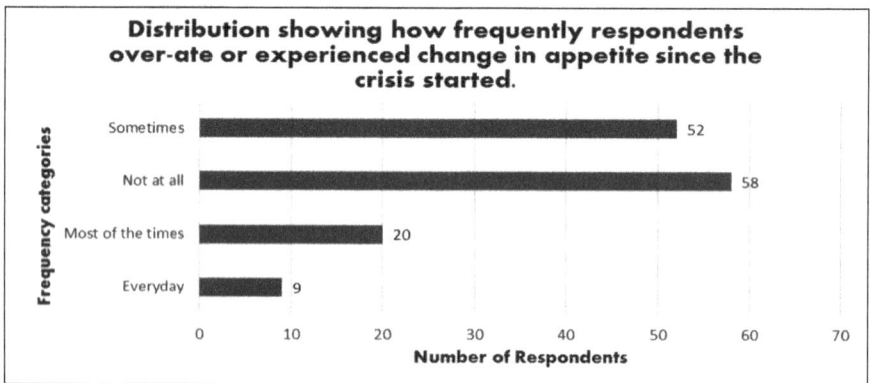

FIGURE 8.13   Distribution showing eating pattern and appetite during the COVID-19 crisis.

Respondents were also asked whether they have trouble concentrating while performing daily tasks. Around 75 reported facing no problems in concentrating while taking up simple household activities. Around 37 respondents reported experiencing so sometimes. Around 11 felt so on almost all days, while 16 felt so every day. Around 8 females as opposed to 3 males reported experiencing so on all most days.

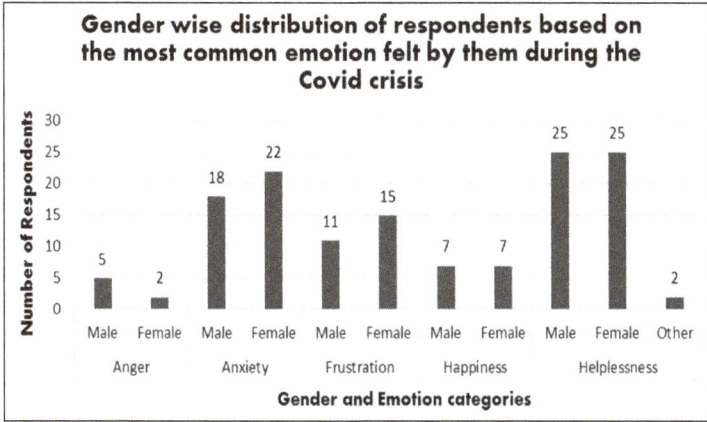

FIGURE 8.14   Gender-wise distribution of respondents based on the most common emotion felt by them during the COVID-19 crisis.

- **Analysis:** Respondents were asked about the most common emotion they felt during the pandemic. Five options were given. These were anger, anxiety, frustration, happiness, and helplessness. Responses could be presented in the form of a bar graph (see Figure 8.14). The predominant feeling about the crisis is helplessness. Around 52 respondents reported feeling helpless during the COVID-19 crisis. Around 40 respondents felt anxiety, 26 felt frustrated, 14 said they felt happiness (perhaps as a respite from their usual, busy lives) while 7 felt angry. While an equal number of male and females felt helpless during the COVID-19 crisis, more females as opposed to males felt anxious and frustrated. More males as opposed to females felt angry.

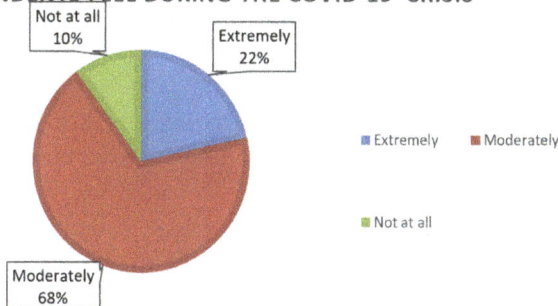

FIGURE 8.15   Distribution showing how vulnerable respondents feel during the COVID-19 crisis.

- **Analysis:** Respondents were asked how intensely they felt vulnerable during the pandemic, and they had to choose from three options. These were moderately, extremely, or not at all. The responses received are presented through a pie-chart in percentages (see Figure 8.15).

Majority of respondents, 95 (68%) felt moderately vulnerable during the COVID-19 crisis. Out of 95 respondents, 29 (31%) belonged to the 31 to 50 years age category (highest frequency/percentage). Among 95 respondents who felt moderately vulnerable there are 50 (53%) female and 45 (47%) male respondents. Around 30 (22%) respondents felt extremely vulnerable during the COVID-19 crisis. Within the 19 to 30 years of age category, 9 (30%) respondents mentioned feeling extremely vulnerable, while in the above 50 years of age category, 9 (30%) respondents reported feeling most vulnerable. Across categories, female respondents felt more vulnerable than male respondents. Around 15 (50%) female and 13 (43%) male respondents felt most vulnerable. Around 14 (10%) respondents did not feel vulnerable at all. Out of this, 8 (57%) were males and 6 (43%) were females.

Further analysis reveals, there is a clear gender difference in how people have been trying to take care of their mental health during the COVID-19 crisis (Figure 8.16) (respondents were given seven options to choose from):

1. 53 respondents reported keeping in touch with their family and friends as a way of taking care of their mental health. Out of this, there are 29 male, 1 transgender and 23 female respondents.
2. 22 respondents reported exploring new hobbies as means of taking care of their mental health, out of which there are 17 female, 4 male and 1 transgender respondent.
3. 16 respondents reported eating well and drinking sensibly as a way of taking care of their mental health, out of which 11 were female and 5 were male respondents.
4. 16 respondents reported keeping fit as a way of taking care of their mental health. Out of this, 11 were male while 5 were female respondents.
5. 14 respondents considered doing yoga and meditation as a means of taking care of mental health. Out of this, there were 10 females as opposed to 4 male respondents.

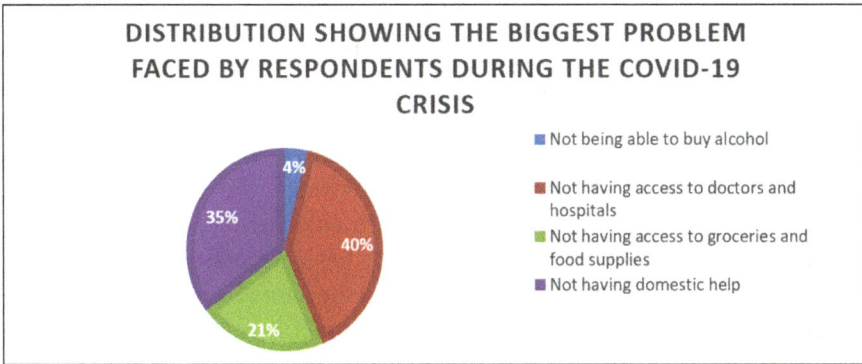

FIGURE 8.16   Distribution showing the biggest problem faced by respondents during the COVID-19 crisis.

6. 9 male and 4 female respondents took to social media to take care of their mental health.
7. 3 male and 1 female respondent did not seem to be bothered about mental health at all.

- **Analysis:** When asked what was the biggest problem faced by respondents during the COVID-19 crisis, 128 out of 139 respondents reported the following:

  1. 40% of 128 respondents reported not having access to doctors and hospitals as a major problem, out of which 46% were female while 54% were male respondents.
  2. 35% of the total respondents reported not having a domestic help as a major problem. Out of this, 60% were female while 40% were male respondents.
  3. 21% reported not having access to groceries and food supplies was a major problem.
  4. Out of the 4% who reported not being able to buy alcohol as a major problem, all were male respondents.

8.6   CONCLUSION

Considering the fact that several studies have already been conducted and many more in the process, each study attempts to grasp different aspects of the world during the COVID-19 crisis and the impact it might have thereafter. In the present study, too, the author makes an attempt to envisage the extent of impact COVID-19 might have had on the mental health of individuals. The conclusions drawn hence-forth are non-exclusive for they can only be representative of the sample used in the study. The author does not make any claims of extending the conclusions drawn from this study to a wider population. The sample is representative of people who have certain common attributes like access to the basic necessities, access to the internet and can read and write in English (as the survey was administered in English). It is important to clarify that the chapter relies on a small sample convenience-based survey, and consequently the results discovered are primarily indicative and serve as a guide for future research in this field.

Nevertheless, certain important conclusions may be drawn from the survey. Some of these findings comply with the existing body of literature, while others bring out some very intriguing facts about the impact of COVID-19 on the mental health of individuals residing in metropolitan cities of our country. The study is divided into three broad themes, namely the demographic profile of those who took part in the survey, secondly, how respondents across different age groups and gender responded to the COVID-19 crisis and finally, the nature of impact COVID-19 had on the mental health of individual respondents who took the survey. A total of 139 respondents took part in the survey, out of which 51% of the respondents were female, 48% were male, while only 1% were transgender. The majority of the respondents were 19 to 50 years in age with a slight inclination on the higher end of the age category. Majority of the male respondents were either self-employed or engaged in part-time, full-time work. Women were mostly homemakers; few self-employed and still others were engaged in part-time/ full-time work.

Respondents who took part in the survey felt that COVID-19 was a pandemic but would eventually pass by. The young generation, especially those belonging to the 10 to 18 years of age group were more optimistic. When attempting to comprehend how respondents react to the COVID-19 crisis, a significant difference could be observed across the gender categories, male respondents feel that the most important lifestyle change they had to go through was the limited social interaction they could have, however for women, everyone staying at home meant more pressure on the house-hold front. The pre-existing differential distribution of labor at home and prevalent gender roles exerted pressure on women during the crisis. This is in compliance with the existing body of literature which talk about how women bear the brunt of excessive pressure at home having to balance work and domestic chore.

In addition to the excessive pressure they face, women in general are more stressed due to the crisis as they worry about the health of their family. This is true for the present survey as well. Women, when asked if they worried about their own health answered mostly in the negative. Men worried more about their own health than women. The women however, worry more about the health of the family than their men counterparts. In the case of job and financial health, the 19 to 30 years and 31 to 50 years seemed the most worried while females tend to be less worried than males about job and financial health. Women, more than men, tend to worry about the effect of COVID-19 on the nation. From the survey is can be observed that the 31 to 50 years age category seem to be more receptive to the myriad changes that the COVID-19 crisis has brought with it.

While existing studies talk about the vulnerability of certain sections of the population more than others, especially the old, the above 50 years age category of the present survey did not present excessive signs of vulnerability. This could be due to the fact that the sample size was small and would require more in-depth study, which falls beyond the purview of the present one. Some very intriguing findings surfaced with the survey. Most respondents felt the psychological, emotional, or physical indicators of stress up to a moderate level. However, a majority of respondents reported feeling helpless during the COVID-19 crisis. While an equal number of male and female respondents felt helpless during the COVID-19 crisis, females felt more anxious and worried and males felt angrier than their female counterparts. Majority of respondents felt moderately vulnerable to the COVID-19 crisis. The 31 to 50 years age category felt extremely vulnerable during the COVID-19 crisis, and across gender categories, female respondents felt more vulnerable than male respondents. A few important things that could be mentioned here is that, for the present sample, there may be no apparent physical, psychological indicators that could prove the presence of extreme stress, however, the study found varied degrees of stress in most people. Further, feelings of vulnerability and helplessness are indicators of stress. One has to remember that the feeling of stress is subjective and may be dependent on various factors.

While the respondents may experience some level of stress, the survey tried to understand how respondents who were in stress took care of their mental health. Around 38% respondents reported keeping in touch with their friends and family as a way of taking care of their mental health, while

16% reported exploring new hobbies and interests as a way of taking care of mental health. Here too, we find a gender-based segregation, men found keeping in touch with their families and friends and remaining connected to social media as an effective way of taking care of mental health, while more women preferred pursuing hobbies, engaging in yoga and other forms of exercises as a means of taking care of their health. At the concluding section of the survey, respondents were asked about the biggest problem they faced during the crisis. While most reported not having access to doctors and hospitals as a major problem faced by the, 35% reported not having a domestic help as a major problem. Around 21% reported not having access to groceries and food supplies was a major problem, and only 4% reported not being able to buy alcohol as a major problem, all of who were males. Here too we find a gender difference, those who reported not having domestic help were mostly women.

Finally, an important thing that must be mentioned is that the survey was undertaken in metropolitan cities. What is most interesting to observe is that respondents who live in metropolitan cities usually have access to almost all amenities that a city would have to offer, however, the COVID-19 crisis made many basic amenities inaccessible to the respondents. In these cities too, inaccessibility to resources, uncertainty about the future along with the feeling of anxiousness and vulnerability made things difficult for most respondents. If this is the situation among the more privileged sections of society, one can only imagine the situation of people living in rural areas who lack basic resources. In conclusion, it may be said that COVID-19 is affecting the mental health of most people, in varied degrees. The pandemic is unlike any event experienced in living memory. The data available indicates that governments and policymakers need to prioritize the issue of mental health and help populations cope with the far-reaching psychological consequences of the pandemic before they accelerate.

ACKNOWLEDGMENT

The author would like to thank Ms. Sayanti Ganguly, PhD Scholar at WBNUJS Kolkata and Ms. Sneha Sanyal, 4th Year, B.A. LL.B (Hons.) student of NLIU, Bhopal for their excellent research assistance.

KEYWORDS

- **acquired immune deficiency syndrome**
- **coronavirus aid, relief, and economic security act**
- **human immunodeficiency virus**
- **international labor organization**
- **severe acute respiratory syndrome**
- **united nations**

REFERENCES

1. WHO Bulletin, (2020). https://www.who.int/bulletin/volumes/89/7/11-086173.pdf (accessed on 13 July, 2021).
2. Liu, C. H., Stevens, C., Conrad, R. C., & Hamn, H. C., (2020). Evidence for elevated psychiatric distress, poor sleep, and quality of life concerns during the COVID-19 pandemic among U.S. young adults with suspected and reported psychiatric diagnoses. *Psychiatrist Research, 292*.
3. Pfefferbaum, B., & North, C., (2020). Mental health and COVID-19 pandemic. *Perspective, 383*, 510–512. https://www.nejm.org/doi/full/10.1056/NEJMp2008017 (accessed on 26 June 2021).
4. De Roo, A., Ado, B., Rose, B., Guimard, Y., Fonck, K., & Colebunders, R., (1998). Survey among survivors of the 1995 Ebola epidemic in Kikwit, Democratic Republic of Congo: Their feelings and experiences. *Trop. Med. Int. Health, 3*(11), 883–885 [PUBMED].
5. Xiang, T., et al., (2020). Timely mental healthcare for the 2019 novel coronavirus outbreak is urgently needed. *The Lancet Psychiatry, 7*(3), 228–229 available at https://www.thelancet.com/journals/lanpsy/article/PIIS2215-0366(20)30046-8/fulltext (last accessed on 21/07/2020).
6. Lee, A. M., Wong, J. G., McAlonan, G. M., et al., (2007). Stress and psychological distress among SARS survivors 1 year after the outbreak. *Can Journal of Psychiatry, 52*(4), 233–240. doi: 10.1177/070674370705200405.
7. WHO Health Topics, Coronavirus, (2020). *Advice for the Public*. https://www.euro.who.int/en/health-topics/health-emergencies/coronavirus-covid-19/novel-coronavirus-2019-ncov (accessed on 13 July 2021).
8. Nicho, J., (2013). The SIR epidemiology model in predicting herd immunity. *Undergraduate Journal of Mathematical Modeling: One + Two, 2*(2). doi: 10.5038/2326-3652.2.2.8.
9. Qui, J., et al., (2020). A nationwide survey of psychological distress among Chinese people in the COVID-19 epidemic: Implications and policy recommendations. *General Psychiatry, 33*(2).
10. Mukhtar, S., (2020). Mental health and psychosocial aspects of coronavirus outbreak in Pakistan: Psychological intervention for public mental health crisis. *Asian Journal of Psychiatry, 51*, 102069. https://doi.org/10.1016/j.ajp.2020.102069.

11. Rana, U., (2020). Elderly suicides in India: An emerging concern during COVID-19 pandemic. *International Psychogeriatrics*, 1, 2. doi: 10.1017/S1041610220001052.

12. Rana, U., & Singh, R., (2020). Emotion analysis of Indians using google trends during COVID-19 pandemic. *Diabetes & metabolic syndrome, 14*(6), 1849–1850. https://doi.org/10.1016/j.dsx.2020.09.015.

13. *Centers for Disease Control and Prevention (CDC)* (2020). https://www.cdc.gov/coronavirus/2019-ncov/need-extra-precautions/older-adults.html (accessed on 26 June 2021).

14. Sareen, J., et al., (2013). *Depress Anxiety, 30*(4) 321–327. https://doi.org/10.1002/da.22077.

15. ILO Survey Report, (2020). Y*outh & COVID-19: Impacts on Jobs, Education, Rights and Mental Well-Being*. https://www.ilo.org/wcmsp5/groups/public/---ed_emp/documents/publication/wcms_753026.pdf (accessed on 27 June 2021).

16. Department of Psychiatry National Institute of Mental Health & Neurosciences, Bengaluru, India (NIMHANS) Mental Health in the times of COVID-19 Pandemic Guidance for General Medical and Specialized Mental Health Care Settings, (2020). https://www.mohfw.gov.in/pdf/COVID19Final2020ForOnline9July2020.pdf (accessed on 13 July 2021).

17. NITI Aayog, (2020). https://niti.gov.in/making-homes-safer-women-during-COVID-19 (accessed on 27 June 2021).

18. *COVID-19 Summer 2020 Survey*, (2020). https://youngminds.org.uk/about-us/reports/coronavirus-impact-on-young-people-with-mental-health-needs/ (accessed on 26 June 2021).

19. Statistics Canada, (2020). https://www150.statcan.gc.ca/n1/pub/11-627-m/11-627-m2020029-eng.htm (accessed on 27 June 2021).

20. Rana, U., & Govender, J., (2020). Indian Women's mental calamity: A shadow pandemic. *Asian Journal of Psychiatry, 54*, 102308. https://doi.org/10.1016/j.ajp.2020.102308.

21. Report of the CSIS Humanitarian Agenda, (2019). *Denial, Delay, Diversion Tackling Access Challenges in an Evolving Humanitarian Landscape*. https://www.humanitarianlibrary.org/sites/default/files/2019/10/Kurtzer_DenialDelayDiversion_WEB_FINAL.pdf (accessed on 27 June 2021).

22. United Nations Office for the Coordination of Humanitarian Affairs (OCHA), (2018). *Global Humanitarian Overview*. Geneva.

23. Committee for a Responsible Federal Budget (CRFB), (2020). *A Visualization of the CARES Act*. http://www.crfb.org/blogs/visualization-cares-act (accessed on 26 June 2021).

24. Ministry of Home Affairs (MHA), (2020). Order No. 40-3/2020, Government of India, https://www.mha.gov.in/sites/default/files/MHAorder%20copy_0.pdf (accessed on 27 June 2021).

25. Thejesh, G. N., (2020). *Projects*. https://thejeshgn.com/projects/COVID-19-india/non-virus-deaths/ (accessed on 27 June 2021).

26. Government of Kerala, Health & Family Welfare Department, (2020). *COVID-19 Outbreak Control and Prevention State Cell*. https://dhs.kerala.gov.in/wp-content/uploads/2020/06/Bulletin-HFWD-English-June-23.pdf (accessed on 27 June 2021).

27. Abhijit, D., (2020). *COVID-19's Changing Class Character will Create New Borders and* Inequalities. https://thewire.in/urban/coronavirus-spread-urban-india (accessed on 26 June 2021).

28. Izaguirre-Torres, D., & Siche, R., (2020). COVID-19 disease will cause a global catastrophe in terms of mental health: A hypothesis. *Medical Hypotheses, 143*, 109846. https://doi.org/10.1016/j.mehy.2020.109846.

29. Liu, Y. C., et al., (2020). COVID-19: The first documented coronavirus pandemic in history. *Biomedical Journal*. https://doi.org/10.1016/j.bj.2020.04.007.

30. WHO Health Topics. *Coronavirus.* https://www.who.int/health-topics/coronavirus#tab=tab_1 (accessed on 27 June 2021).

31. Moldofsky, H, & Patcai, J, (2011). *Chronic widespread musculoskeletal pain, fatigue, depression and disordered sleep in chronic post-SARS syndrome; a case-controlled study, BMC Neurol*, doi: 10.1186/1471-2377-11-37.

32. Joshi, A., & Paul, S., (2020). *Phylogenetic Analysis of the Novel Coronavirus Reveals Important Variants in Indian Strains*, Cold Spring Harbour Laboratory, https://www.biorxiv.org/content/10.1101/2020.04.14.041301v1 (accessed on 13 July, 2021).

33. Ministry of Health and Family Welfare, Government of India, National Institute of Mental Health and Neuro Sciences, Bengaluru, *National Mental Health Survey of India 2015-2016*, http://indianmhs.nimhans.ac.in/Docs/Report2.pdf (accessed on 13 July, 2021).

34. Garg, K., Kumar, N. C., & Chandra, P., (2019), Number of Psychiatrists in India: Baby Steps but a long Way to Go, *Indian Journal of Psychiatry, 61*(1), 104–105.

35. Abhijit, D., (2020). *COVID-19's Changing Class Character will Create New Borders and* Inequalities. https://thewire.in/urban/coronavirus-spread-urban-india (accessed on 26 June 2021).

36. Izaguirre-Torres, D. & Siche, R. (2020). *COVID-19 disease will cause a global catastrophe in terms of mental health: A hypothesis. Medical hypotheses. 143.* 109846. https://doi.org/10.1016/j.mehy.2020.109846.

PART III

Impacts of COVID-19 on Age, Gender, and Profession

CHAPTER 9

'Making Connections': Feminist Activism in a Quarantined Chinese City

HONGWEI BAO

Department of Cultural, Media, and Visual Studies, The University of Nottingham, United Kingdom, E-mail: hongwei.bao@nottingham.ac.uk

ABSTRACT

This chapter conceptualizes the possibilities, conditions, and strategies of feminist intervention in the current global pandemic. It does so by analyzing the activist practices of a Chinese feminist named Guo Jing at an early stage of the pandemic (from January to April 2020). Using Guo's published diary as a primary source, this article illustrates how Guo's experience has highlighted the impact of the pandemic on women's lives, and how it has exemplified a form of context specific and culturally sensitive activist strategy in a predominantly masculine quarantine environment. Guo's activist practices demonstrate that feminist interventions are not only possible but also essential in a global pandemic. An effective engagement with the quarantine environment therefore requires a keen awareness of local conditions and cultural specificities; it also entails careful negotiation with spaces, places, and cultures –private/domestic and public, online and offline.

9.1 INTRODUCTION

For 77 days between 23 January and 8 April, the Chinese city of Wuhan, with a population of 11 million people, was under strict lockdown to contain the spread of COVID-19. This extreme measure was 'unprecedented' in world public health history, celebrated by some and criticized by others [1]. The total number of COVID-19 infection cases recorded in the city stood at

50,333, with 3,869 deaths, as of 17 April 2020 [2]. Guo Jing, a 29-year-old feminist activist, and social worker, was in Wuhan at the time, trapped in her small flat. In the first few days of the lockdown, she felt depressed, vulnerable, and helpless, not knowing what to do. The initial feel of helplessness soon gave way to a feeling that she should act up and do something useful for society. But what could she do as a feminist activist in a quarantined situation? She could not meet others face to face; she could not even walk out of her own residential compound for most of the lockdown period. Many of her activist experiences from the past, which relied largely on bringing people together in public spaces, were rendered impractical and even useless in a pandemic environment. What could she do?

Guo was not the only one who had to face this problem. COVID-19 has spread across the world and developed into a global pandemic, with varied ramifications in different parts of the world. Many governments have enforced strict quarantine measures such as the lockdown of neighborhoods, cities, and even entire countries to contain the spread of the coronavirus. 'Self-isolation' and 'social distancing' have become common phrases in public health policies: people are advised to stay at home and keep away from strangers. Under these circumstances, feminists from all over the world have been asking the same questions: What is the impact of the pandemic on women's lives? What is the role of feminism in such a pandemic? How can feminism effectively engage with the current situation, not only by offering a better understanding of the gendered nature of the pandemic and quarantine measures, but also by providing timely help and support for women in need? *Feminist Studies* [3], a leading feminist journal, has recently issued an urgent call for commentaries on the COVID-19 pandemic. It starts the call with an inspiring line: 'Feminist ideas can help guide us as we move through this crisis.' But how?

This chapter takes up the challenge to conceptualize the possibilities, conditions, and strategies of feminist intervention in the global pandemic. It does so by analyzing the feminist activist practices led by Guo Jing at an early stage of the pandemic (from January to April 2020). If COVID-19 accidentally pushed Chinese feminists to the forefront of the global pandemic activism, Chinese feminists' insights, experiences, and strategies at an early stage of COVID-19 need to be taken seriously by scholars and activists from all over the world, where the pandemic can potentially last longer and hit harder. I suggest that, among other things, Guo and her activist friends have highlighted the impact of the pandemic on women's lives; they have also designed context specific and culturally sensitive strategies to make women's voices heard in a predominantly masculine quarantine environment. Guo's activist practices therefore demonstrate that feminist interventions are not only possible but also essential in a global pandemic. An effective engagement with the quarantine environment requires a keen awareness of the local conditions and cultural specificities; it also entails careful negotiations with spaces, places, and cultures-private/domestic and public, online, and offline.

Methodologically, I have used digital ethnography, otherwise known as Internet ethnography, cyber ethnography, or virtual ethnography [4–6], to gather research data. Guo's activism during the pandemic mostly takes place online and on social media, and such an approach is therefore appropriate. I have primarily followed Guo's social media accounts and interviewed her informally through social media. I have also attended a couple of her online talks including her book talk organized by the Matters News website. An important part of my research data comes from Guo's diary, *Wuhan Lockdown Diary (Wuhan Fengcheng Riji)* [7] published in early April 2020 by Taipei-based Linking Publishing.[55] During the lockdown period, Guo kept a diary, which functioned like a blog, and published it online and on her social media every day. The diary kept a comprehensive account of Guo's life and her observation of the pandemic situation; it also documents her feminist activist practices and engages with her readers. The diary is an important record of the pandemic. Also, because of its explicit feminist political stance, the diary is also an exemplary piece of feminist literature, contributing to the writing of a transnational feminist history. In this chapter, I quote Guo's diary extensively to give readers a feel of her voice; this method also gives an opportunity for Guo to represent herself in her own words. I am aware of the narrative nature of the diary, which complicates our understanding of the 'objectivity' of such an account. But I suggest that Guo's diary is an important record of the pandemic narrated from her own experience and perspective. Indeed, although the diary cannot offer a comprehensive picture of the pandemic situation or feminist movements in Wuhan at the time, it was as realistic as it could be from Guo's perspective, and was therefore a reliable representation of her own activist practices.

---

[55] Guo's book title *Wuhan Fengcheng Riji*, (2020) is officially translated as *Diary of the Wuhan Lockdown* by Linking Pushing but I have retranslated the book title as *Wuhan Lockdown Diary*. It is the first 'Wuhan lockdown diary' officially published by a literary press. There are other published 'Wuhan lockdown diaries' and they mostly come from well-known writers and intellectuals, including Ai Xiaoming (2020); and Fang Fang (2020). Guobin, Yang (2020) calls these diarists 'digital radicals' because of the social critique and political potentials of these publicly circulated diaries.

9.2   FEMINIST CRITIQUE OF THE QUARANTINE

In the quarantine discourse, public health advice such as 'stay at home' and 'avoid public gatherings' often has a distinct spatial dimension, resting largely on a public space/ private space dichotomy. These spatial imaginations are usually highly gendered: public space is imagined as masculine, and private space feminine. As Fraser [8] argues, the Habermasian notion of public sphere is an intrinsically gendered concept, which often relegates women to the domestic and private space, in contrast to the valorized public space of political debate often occupied by men.

Writing in the context of China, Yang [9] charts the emergence of women's public spaces in post-Mao China, but she also observes the patriarchal, political, and commercial domination of women's spaces. After decades of socialist experiments where women were pushed out of the domestic space and into the public space of work, the neoliberal reform in post-Mao China has commodified women's bodies and sexualities for the male gaze in a market economy [10]. The state also attempts to push women back to the domestic sphere through the valorization of family, marriage, and home, together with a vilification of 'left-over women' (*shengnü*, a stigmatized term for unmarried young women) and feminists (*nüquan zhuyi zhe*) [11, 12]. Trapped between traditional family values and individual ambitions for financial independence and career success, a young generation of Chinese women are negotiating the traditional dichotomy of *nei* (inner) and *wai* (outer) spaces in different ways from the older generation [13]. In today's China, *funü*, the female subjectivity crafted by socialist revolution and state feminism is stigmatized; it is replaced by *nüxing* (female the sexed subject) and *nüren* (female, the other of man), both of which emphasize universal humanity and essentialized sexual difference [14].[56] Celebration of the International Women Day (*funü jie*) on 8 March risks being taken over by a frantic shopping season on 7 March, branded as Girls' Day (*nüsheng jie*), Queens' Day (*nüwang jie*), or Goddess Day (*nüshen jie*) [15]. Since its start in the 1980s, the dust has never settled on the debate about how to translate the English term 'feminism'-*nüxing zhuyi* (literally 'Womanism') or *nüquan zhuyi* (literally 'Women's Rights-ism') [16]. Meanwhile, a highly egoistic, selfish, and calculating version of 'made-in-China feminism' (*zhonghua*

---

[56] In Chinese-language context, all three words-*funü*, *nüxing* and *nüren*-translate the English term 'woman,' but they have different associations and denote distinct female subjectivities. For more discussion about female subjectivities in China, see Barlow (2004). Similarly, both words-*nüxing zhuyi* and *nüquan zhuyi*-translate the English term 'feminism,' but they occupy distinct discursive and political positions. For more discussion about feminism in China, see Min (2017).

tianyuan nüquan zhuyi) has emerged: by celebrating middle-class distinction and neoliberal consumption, 'made-in-China feminism' in effect stigmatizes and undoes feminism [17]. Women can enter the public space, but when they do so, their bodies and sexualities are put under the patriarchal male gaze and risk being incorporated by a state-led neoliberal discourse which further marginalizes women.

If gender and space are closely intertwined in the post-socialist public discourse, the quarantine environment has only perpetuated such a discourse: women are told to stay at home and take care of their families and children; home is imagined as the ultimate safe space for the weak. In contrast, men are compared to fearless fighters bravely going out to combat an invisible but treacherous enemy that is the virus (and this virus happens to have come from an 'oriental' and 'primitive' other). In this process, gender inequalities and hierarchies have been reinforced, and normative social orders have been restored and legitimized.

In this context, publishing a diary is a way for young women such as Guo to exit the private space of home and enter the public space to have their voices heard in a quarantine environment. Ironically, this has been achieved by making public something which is usually seen as deeply personal and private. After all, it is a feminist motto to make the private-public and to make the personal political.

The quarantine reinforces the boundary between the public space and the private space, rendering gendered division of labor more visible than before. In Guo's observation of the residential compound where she lives, usually more men than women are taking a walk around the neighborhood enjoying the sunshine. She reflects that many women have to do housework at home, and the quarantine situation has placed more burden on women in terms of cooking, cleaning, and childcare. When women do appear in the public space, they are mostly careers of children and the elderly, sometimes shoppers, and seldom spend their leisure time entirely on their own. Guo observed on 8 March, the International Women's Day:

In the morning, Tong Tong and her grandma were downstairs chatting with another family. The grandmother and the mother are like many other women who have to take care of their children even on their own holidays. How many people notice the hard and unpaid work of all these women at home, year in and year out? [7] [57]

---

[57] All the dates quoted are taken from Guo's diary (Guo 2020). The dates refer to the time when these entries were first published online. All the translations are mine unless otherwise specified. Excerpts of Guo's diary translated into English can be accessed through the BBC (2020) and *The Guardian* (2020).

Guo reflected on the reason for the invisibility of women in the public space. She attributed this to the privatization and commercialization of public services under neoliberalism.

Nowadays, there are very few public-run kindergartens. Most private kindergartens are expensive. Some of them finish school as early as three or four o'clock in the afternoon. A single woman usually must make the difficult choice between a full-time job and full-time childcare. When the state walks away from its own childcare responsibility, the family starts to take over the duty. As soon as a social or family crisis strikes, women, and children are usually victims to tragedies [7].

- **In another entry, Guo challenged gender norms such as masculinity and femininity in society:** What is normal? We often use what most people do as the criteria for being normal, but what most people do is not always right. They however become social norms and rules, and we must conform to them in our everyday life. For example, they say that a woman should behave like a 'woman;' a man must behave like a 'man;' and that a person needs to get married and have children at a certain age. Our society has little tolerance for those who do not fit into these norms, and often criticize them to maintain the so-called 'normality' [7].

- **Guo pointed out the implications of *jia* (home or family) for women:** Women cannot simply 'stay at home.' Our society never gives women an easy life. If single women stay at home, they are often forced into marriage by their families and society. They are often criticized for not doing enough housework. Many people start to escape from gender norms: men do not want to lead the traditional role of being a breadwinner for the family; women do not want to be 'good wives and virtuous mothers' (*xianqi liangmu*) [7].

- **The quarantine situation has exacerbated some deeply entrenched gender stereotypes and hierarchies:** To an extent, the lockdown gives men an idea of what women's life is like without a public life. The life of many married women revolves around their own families. Even if they work full-time, they must cook dinner, do laundry, and take care of their children at home. All the domestic work they undertake is unpaid and undervalued. Their public life gradually shrinks, as they have less and less time to talk to their colleagues and friends. They care more about their families than about themselves [7].

- **When women do go to work, they often face sexual discrimination or a 'glass ceiling' in their workplace:** Women are marginalized in the public space. They are often sexually harassed by men and discriminated against at work. However, when it comes to sexual harassment and workplace discrimination, women always take the blame. Therefore, many women often blame themselves in times of difficulty, attributing failures to their own incapability [7].

Guo herself had an experience of workplace discrimination. In 2014, she was involved in China's first lawsuit regarding gender discrimination in employment and subsequently won the case against the employer [18]. Inspired by the success, Guo set up a legal aid helpline for women facing gender discrimination in the workplace. On her social media accounts, she frequently advertises the helpline. During the Wuhan lockdown, she kept the helpline running and answered questions from callers every evening.

When Guo learned that her diary would be published by Linking Publishing soon, she initially had a sense of disbelief and insecurity, feeling that this could not have been true and that she did not deserve the achievement. She then came to realize the prevalence of 'imposter syndrome' among women.

The 'imposter syndrome' is an impact of social discrimination against women. Under patriarchy, women are marginalized by society, and their contributions are often neglected. That is why we see fewer successful women than men. We often hear of disparaging remarks such as 'being a teacher is an ideal job for women' or 'this female leader is too aggressive' [7].

Using her diary, Guo commented on the quarantine environment and society in general; she also shared these comments with her readers and followers online. Her observations and experiences shed light on the gendered nature of the quarantine discourse. In such a discourse, existing social equalities are exposed and even exacerbated; social norms are reproduced under a capitalist political economy [19]. Guo reflected that the media have an important role to play in constructing and challenging these norms.

9.3   FEMINIST CRITIQUE OF THE MEDIA

Although Guo used the Internet and social media to publish her diary and to engage her readers in feminist discussion, she was keenly aware of the role of media in commodifying women's bodies and sexualities for a largely heterosexual male audience. She commented on the deeply entrenched patriarchal ideas and stereotypes at work in news media, the Internet, as well as animation, comics, and games.

News media are like mirrors of society. There are still a lot of gender stereotypes in news media. For example, many news reports focus exclusively on male doctors and nurses in the frontline [7].

The exposure of the Nth Room case in South Korea has recently attracted much public attention to online sexual exploitation and sexual violence. Such circumstances also exist in China, but they are relatively hidden from view. The Internet is an extension of the patriarchal society. Women are continuing to be consumed and even subject to exploitation and violence in the cyberspace [7].

The world of *erciyuan* [*nijigen* in Japanese, literally two-dimensional world, including animation, comics, and games, ACG for short] is full of gender discrimination, often representing women as sexual objects [7].

As stated in the previous section, stringent quarantine measures such as the ones adopted in Wuhan often rely on a masculinist language such as the use of the 'war' metaphor to justify social cost and human sacrifice. In doing so, they downplay or ignore the duty of care. This negligence can sometimes lead to the violation of women's rights and reinforce patriarchal control over women's bodies. Guo wrote in response to a news report that some female nurses had all their hair cut off to 'facilitate their work' in a hospital in Gansu Province so that they did not have to visit a hairdresser during the quarantine period [20].

We talked about the female nurses from Gansu Province who were forced to have their hair cut; we also noticed that there was only one male nurse with short hair in the photo. Many female nurses were very unhappy when they had their hair cut; some even cried. Hair is not simply about looks; it also symbolizes dignity. Is it necessary to cut off all their hair? Have all these women given their consent? Women's bodies never truly belong to themselves. There are always people who feel more entitled to putting women's bodies at their disposal [7].

Guo compared the draconian lockdown measures to the dystopian society in Margaret Atwood's *The Handmaid's Tale* [21], where women lose their freedom in an authoritarian state and are ruthlessly exploited by a male-dominated society [7]. Guo's diary in response to the news was circulated widely by her readers, attracting widespread criticism of the practices in Gansu Province. Although Guo was not the only one to criticize the practice, her diary, published online and circulated widely, can be seen as a counter-hegemonic strategy, using social media to launch feminist critiques and to create a friendly media environment for women. Aware of the crucial role of the media in shaping and changing gender norms, Guo and other feminists have taken action to combat the 'hegemony' [22]: some started the 'seeing female workers' campaign, drawing public attention to the hard work of female workers in the frontline [7]; others reported the illegal websites that photograph or video record women secretly and without their consent [7]. Feminist activist Liang Yu started the 'Supporting Our Frontline Sisters' activist campaign (*jiemei zhanyi anxin xing dong*), raising funds to donate personal protective equipment (PPE) and tampons for female doctors and nurses working on the frontline [23]. Guo also launched an online feminist activist campaign called 'anti-domestic violence little vaccine,' raising awareness of the issue of domestic violence during the lockdown [24].

9.4   AN INTERSECTIONAL FEMINIST POLITICS

In media and government discourses worldwide, the fight against the coronavirus is often compared to fighting a war. Countries and cities have got into the 'state of exception' [25] or 'state of emergency' one after another, where normal rules are suspended, and stringent measures are imposed upon human lives. Behind all these is an unimaginable human cost, especially for marginalized social groups who are struggling with survival even under ordinary circumstances. On the first day, as a single woman who lived alone in a still strange city, Guo was keenly aware of the potential human cost of the lockdown. She queried:

"In this battle, many people can only rely on themselves, instead of on a well-developed social welfare system. I am relatively young and can take care of myself. But what about those disadvantaged social groups such as the elderly people and people living with disabilities? Can they survive the war? [7]."

After Guo had made up her mind to make connections with others, she decided to reach out to other people, not only online and through social media, but offline as well. This was not always easy during the quarantine period, and the people she met were also different from usual. Whilst most middle-class urban dwellers sheltered themselves in their private homes, countless working-class people-cleaners, drivers, deliverers, security guards and shop assistants, many of whom were migrants to the city from other parts of the country and could not go back to their hometowns-still had to risk their lives to go to work. In the first week of the lockdown, when she could still go out, Guo ventured out of her apartment every day, walking around the city or in the neighborhood talking to people whenever she could. She acted more like a journalist, asking people how they were coping with the epidemic:

I interviewed 8 sanitary workers: six women and two men. They work 7 to 8 hours every day. Their monthly income averages 2,300 to 2,400 RMB [Chinese currency]. After-tax, they can only get less than 2,000.

I asked them if they could get a pay rise during the epidemic. Some said that they could get a double wage only for three days during the Chinese New Year period. Some had no idea about this information.

They can get disinfectants and protective gloves for work. There was overall a lack of disposable face masks. If they are lucky, they can get 20 face masks at a time. One worker has only received two face masks since the start of the lockdown.

They are all very kind. Some even do not have a disposable surgical mask; they cover their mouth with a scarf. I gave them the three disposable masks that I took with me […].

They earn meager wages and are not protected from the virus. But they kept on working. Do we really deserve their hard work? [7].

The interview with the sanitary workers made Guo reflect on her own privilege as a university-educated woman living in the city. It also connected gender with other social issues such as class, migration, and the rural/urban divide. Indeed, feminism must take into consideration other social structures and issues and see these structures and identities as intersected [26], which create 'scattered hegemonies' [27] on women's lives. Guo remarked on the epidemic's differentiated impact on various social groups.

No one deserves to die. But society has divided people into different social groups and given them different values. I do not know if anyone has conducted a study of the quarantine measures and the fatalities from the perspective of class. The virus itself does not discriminate, but there are deeply embedded discriminations in our society. These already existing discriminations usually inform the decision-making of quarantine measures and their subsequent implementation, as well as the medical care those affected will receive [7].

Guo astutely pinpointed the impact of social inequalities and injustices on the making and implementation of public health policies. But she did not take a passive attitude, making complaints and venting out grudges all the time; instead, she took action to help those in need—from giving workers face masks to delivering medicine and goods to people in need. For example,

Guo successfully connected a surgical mask donor from another part of the country to a local hospital in Wuhan [7]. Guo frequently finished her diary with a signature signoff, encouraging people to get in touch with her: 'I want to become a point of connection, and I hope to establish connections with more people and act together. My WeChat number is [XYZ].' Indeed, 'making connection' (*jianli lianjie*) is important for establishing mutual support, building a community of care, and conducting social activism. As Guo makes connections with other people through writing and sharing her diary, Chinese feminism also makes connections with other intersected social issues.

Where most people could see disaster and tragedy in Wuhan during the lockdown, Guo saw and experienced the epidemic in a different way. She has noticed intensified connections between people, and that these connections have changed society and people's lives in a positive way. She has also seen that the ongoing pandemic is a gendered event and it has serious implications for women's lives, and that women should act up to change the patriarchal world. Her commitment to feminism has been strengthened along the way. Guo wrote in an early phase of the lockdown: 'The luckiest thing in my life is to have become a feminist and to be able to work with a group of like-minded friends, accompanying, and supporting each other' [7]. She wrote near the end of the lockdown: 'I will still be a feminist activist because women are still facing repression' [7].

9.5 CONCLUSION

Guo and her friends' feminist activist campaign demonstrates the necessity and significance of feminist intervention in a global pandemic. It offers a good example of the possibilities, conditions, and strategies of feminist activism in a time of crisis and a 'state of emergency.' COVID-19 has exacerbated gendered hierarchies and oppressions in a society already infiltrated by unequal power relations. Meanwhile, it also brings unprecedented opportunities and challenges to transnational feminism. The pandemic has raised the public's awareness of social issues and problems and issued an urgent call for them to be addressed. Social activism addressing these problems is therefore more likely to garner support from people and invite a wide participation in society. Although the quarantine measures have made public gatherings and physical contact between people difficult, the Internet and social media have facilitated social mobilization and political activism in significant ways. Physical isolation, therefore, does not bring an end to social activism. The collective spirit and emotional intensity generated in a time of crisis can be mobilized for activist purposes, and their impacts are likely to be greater now than in ordinary times.

Guo's activism has also highlighted the importance of space, place, and culture for feminist interventions in a quarantine environment. Through the strict demarcation of spaces and through the stratified division of labor-both of which are deeply gendered processes-the state exerts powerful control over human bodies and mobilities. This can facilitate the containment of the coronavirus, but it can also help the state to better control its population. Feminist interventions aim to disrupt this separation by strategically appropriating and transgressing these spatial boundaries, by making the private and domestic public. Meanwhile, by exploiting the potentials of the Internet and social media for the formation of a public sphere, feminists can offer support to each other, build solidarity, and even enact activist interventions into society. If the quarantine discourse is characterized by a masculine logic and a war rhetoric, it is time to recognize the insufficiency of such a rhetoric and highlight the feminist discourse of care-care for the self, the community, and the society. The feminist politics and ethics of care is likely to be more helpful and effective for a society to go through a pandemic safely and collectively. After all, we need alternative narratives about the pandemic and alternative strategies to tackle the pandemic, recognizing what feminism can offer is just the first step.

KEYWORDS

- **China**
- **COVID-19**
- **cyber ethnography**
- **digital ethnography**
- **feminism**
- **Wuhan**

REFERENCES

1. Crossley, G., (2020) *Wuhan Lockdown 'Unprecedented', Shows Commitment to Contain Virus: WHO Representative in China.* Reuters. https://www.reuters.com/article/us-china-health-who/wuhan-lockdown-unprecedented-shows-commitment-to-contain-virus-who-representative-in-china-idUSKBN1ZM1G9 (accessed on 27 June 2021).

2. Griffiths, J., & Jiang, S., (2020) *Wuhan Officials Have Revised the City's Coronavirus Death Toll up by 50%*. CNN. https://edition.cnn.com/2020/04/17/asia/china-wuhan-coronavirus-death-toll-intl-hnk/index.html (accessed on 27 June 2021).

3. Feminist Studies, (2020) The COVID-19 pandemic. *Feminist Studies*. http://www.feministstudies.org/home.html (accessed on 27 June 2021).

4. Hine, C., (2000) *Virtual Ethnography*. Sage.

5. Sade-beck, L., (2004) Internet ethnography: Online and offline. *International Journal of Qualitative Methods*, 45–51.

6. Pink, S., et al., (2015) *Digital Ethnography: Principles and Practice*. Sage.

7. Guo, J., (2020) *Wuhan Fengcheng Riji [Wuhan lockdown diary]*. Linking Publishing.

8. Fraser, N., (1989) *Unruly Practices: Power, Discourse, and Gender in Contemporary Social Theory*. University of Minnesota Press.

9. Yang, M. M. H., (1999) *Spaces of Their Own: Women's Public Sphere in Transnational China*. University of Minnesota Press.

10. Evans, H., (1997) *Women and Sexuality in China: Dominant Discourses of Female Sexuality and Gender Since 1949*. Polity Press.

11. Fincher, L. H., (2016) *Leftover Women: The Resurgence of Gender Inequality in China*. Zed Books.

12. Fincher, L. H., (2018) *Betraying Big Brother: The Feminist Awakening in China*. London: Verso.

13. Evans, H., (2008) *The subject of Gender: Daughters and Mothers in Urban China*. Rowman & Littlefield.

14. Barlow, T., (2005) *The question of women in Chinese feminism*. Duke University Press.

15. Xi, P., (2019) *How Women Got Taken Out of International Women's Day*. Sixth Tone. https://www.sixthtone.com/news/1003653/how-the-women-got-taken-out-of-international-womens-day (accessed on 27 June 2021).

16. Min, D., (2017) *Translation and travelling Theory: Feminist theory and praxis in China*. Routledge.

17. Wu, A. X., & Dong, Y., (2019) What is made-in-China feminism(s)? Gender discontent and class friction in post-socialist China. *Critical Asian Studies, 51*(4), 471–492.

18. Legal Information Institute, (2014). In: Guo, J. V., (ed.), *East Cooking Vocational Skills Training School Women and Justice*. https://www.law.cornell.edu/women-and-justice/resource/guo_jing_v_east_cooking_vocational_skills_training_school (accessed on 27 June 2021).

19. Bhattacharya, T., (2017) *Social Reproduction Theory: Remapping Class, Recentring oppression*. Pluto Press.

20. Li, J., (2020) *China is Being Accused of Mistreating Coronavirus Nurses for Propaganda*. Quartz. https://qz.com/1804040/chinas-coverage-of-coronavirus-nurses-provokes-backlash/ (accessed on 27 June 2021).

21. Atwood, M., (1985) *The Handmaid's Tale*. McClelland and Stewart.

22. Gramsci, A., (1992) *Prison Notebooks*. Columbia University Press.

23. Liang, Y., (2020) *Jiemei zhanyi anxin xingdong [Supporting Our Frontline Sisters Activist Campaign]*. Weibo. https://s.weibo.com/weibo?q=%23%E5%A7%90%E5%A6%B9%E6%88%98%E7%96%AB%E5%AE%89%E5%BF%83%E8%A1%8C%E5%8A%A8%23&from=default (accessed on 27 June 2021).

24. Bao, H., (2020) 'Anti-domestic violence little vaccine': A Wuhan-based feminist activist campaign during COVID-19. *Interface: A Journal for and About Social Movements, 12*(1), 53–63.

25. Agamben, G., (2008) *State of Exception.* University of Chicago Press.

26. Crenshaw, K., (1989) Demarginalizing the intersection of race and sex: A black feminist critique of antidiscrimination doctrine, feminist theory and antiracist politics. *University of Chicago Legal Forum, 1*, 139–167.

27. Grewal, I., & Kaplan, C., (1994) *Scattered Hegemonies: Postmodernity and Transnational Feminist Practices.* University of Minnesota Press.

28. Ai, X., (2020) Wuhan diary. *New Left Review*, 122 https://newleftreview.org/issues/II122/articles/xiaoming-ai-wuhan-diary (accessed on 27 June 2021).

29. BBC, (2020) *Coronavirus Wuhan Diary: Living Alone in a City Gone Quiet.* BBC. https://www.bbc.co.uk/news/world-asia-china-51276656 (accessed on 27 June 2021).

30. Fang, F., (2020) *Wuhan Diary: Dispatches from a Quarantined City.* Translated by Michael Berry. Harpervia.

31. Feng, J., (2020) *COVID-19 Fuels Domestic Violence in China.* SupChina. https://supchina.com/2020/03/24/covid-19-fuels-domestic-violence-in-china/ (accessed on 27 June 2021).

32. Fumian, M., (2020) *To Serve the People of the Party: Fang Fang's Wuhan Diary and Chinese Writers at the Time of Coronavirus.* MCLC. https://u.osu.edu/mclc/online-series/marco-fumian/ (accessed on 27 June 2021).

33. The Guardian, (2020) *'We Were Trapped for too Long: Coming Back to Life After Lockdown in Wuhan.'* The Guardian. https://www.theguardian.com/world/2020/apr/06/we-were-trapped-for-too-long-coming-back-to-life-after-lockdown-in-wuhan (accessed on 27 June 2021).

34. Wu, G., Feng, Y., & Lansdowne, H., (2018). *Gender Dynamics, Feminist Activism and Social Transformation in China.* Routledge.

35. Yang, G., (2020) Digital radicals of Wuhan. *Centre on Digital Culture and Society.* https://u.osu.edu/mclc/2020/02/07/digital-radicals-of-wuhan/ (accessed on 27 June 2021).

CHAPTER 10

COVID-19 Pandemic and the Plight of Women Migrant Workers: Gendered Issues Involved and the Strategies Required

NEHA MISHRA[1] and ANINDYA J. MISHRA[2]

[1]*PhD Research Scholar, Department of Humanities and Social Sciences, Indian Institute of Technology, Roorkee, Uttarakhand, India, E-mail: neha.mishra1293@gmail.com*

[2]*Full Professor of Sociology, Department of Humanities and Social Sciences, Indian Institute of Technology, Roorkee, Uttarakhand, India*

ABSTRACT

The current coronavirus pandemic has exacerbated the existing inequalities in society. While all the marginalized sections are undergoing suffering amid the COVID-19 situation, a gender lens is required as women, in particular, suffer the most in the hierarchy, cutting across caste, class, and religion. For female migrant workers, the economic, social, and health implications are far more severe. In light of this, the present study focuses on the myriad issues involved, exploring how female migrant workers' lives have changed in the face of COVID-19 in the case of developing country India. Primarily focusing on the impact of the COVID-19 pandemic on the lives of female migrant workers and discussing how the gender inequality that persists in labor force participation further gets more intensified amid the pandemic. This has led to higher deprivation, exploitation, and discrimination due to the various social constraints on mobility and patriarchal barriers. The chapter also outlines the lessons learned from the current pandemic and the different strategies required to accompany the long-term recovery efforts.

10.1   INTRODUCTION

"The COVID-19 pandemic is a public health emergency-but it is far more. It is an economic crisis. A social crisis. And a human Crisis that is fast becoming a human rights crisis."
         —Antonio Guterres (Secretary-General, United Nations, 2020)

The current coronavirus pandemic has resulted in a significant dislocation of India's migrant population since the central government announced a nationwide lockdown. United Nations (UN) stated that migrant workers worldwide are at higher risk and are marginalized to a greater extent amid the pandemic [1]. In India's case, the shopkeepers, restaurant workers, taxi drivers, and the poor migrant laborers working in big cities, capitals, towns, and other segments of the society belonging to impoverished areas were the innocent receivers of the recent outbreak of the coronavirus pandemic. Migrant workers stay in a crowded slum with poor living conditions where maintaining physical distancing is practically impossible. Also, they have limited access to health care, resources, and essential services. The print reported that in India, more than 200 people who mainly comprised of migrant workers, died during the COVID-19 crisis due to hunger, suicide, lack of access to medical care, and vigilant killings [2]. In India, around 40 million migrant workers involved in the informal sector got impacted owing to the pandemic [3]. Since the lockdown was announced in India, there is a flood in media regarding the news coverage related to the migrants' plight, covering their horror and terrifying experiences. Nevertheless, another segment that is equally impacted but has received very little coverage by media is looking at the current migration crisis from the lens of gender. Undoubtedly, all vulnerable people have undergone suffering, but a gender lens is required as women face discrimination and oppression, cutting across class, caste, or religion. It is vital to understand that for the women who work in the informal economy, gender inequality exists in a multifold manner. They get fewer wages; the burden of care is on them, and fewer resources are available to them.

The current study tries to unravel the plight of women migrant workers through a gendered perspective. It explores how society responded to the earlier pandemic through the literature review and analyzes the impact of the pandemic on the lives of migrant women workers, and discusses the various issues involved. It also focuses on strategies needed amid the pandemic concerning the female migrant workers. It is essential to explore the crisis through a gendered perspective, as pointed out by UN Women [4], that women who are the daily wage earners, owners of small businesses, and those involved in the informal sector are greatly affected amid the pandemic. "Crisis always exacerbates gender inequality," says Maria Holtsberg, an advisor of disaster risk at UN Women Asia and Pacific [24]. Still, the narratives and stories of these poor female workers were hardly covered by the media. They become disadvantaged as traditional roles become more rapidly diffused from high income to low-income societies. As women constitute a large proportion of migrant workers, they became significantly affected during long-sustained lockdowns. It is so because the social taboos and social distancing made it very difficult for them to hold on to their work and dignity. When it comes to migrant women, they are the most vulnerable section in the informal sector. They are dealing with the increased risk of gender-based violence due to mobility restrictions and lack of social safety nets available for them. Additionally, these vulnerable women have to face the ideological and social conditioning of patriarchal values that operate at multiple levels. Thus, one could see how a pandemic is intersecting with the already existing inequality in society, leading to discrimination and violence against vulnerable women in the developing country India. People's moral responsibilities towards their communities in which they live are getting questioned by the situations created due to epidemics. The difficulties in balancing public and private interests and the repercussions of having inadequate development in public infrastructure, especially in the health and welfare sector, are also emphasized by such situations.

10.2 LITERATURE REVIEW

Wallis [5] narrated people's responses against plagues in early modern Europe and identified the nucleus of this tension in America and Europe. Since the 19th century, there had been the proper imposition of quarantines or physical distancing by putting restrictions on trade and travel to limit disease spread [5]. Spinney [6] had further suggested the role of comparative methodology in combating and containing the epidemics and states that Quarantine, handwashing, isolation, and the wearing of masks were the methods of ensuring that the sick and the healthy keeps apart, thereby minimizing the possibility of the disease transmission. John Hopkins, who is a sociologist, put forward that the pandemic has changed the way different society's function that can be seen from the 14th century bubonic to the outbreak of Spanish flu in 1918, and this holds true in COVID-19 pandemic times too [7]. He also elaborated that the current pandemic has widened the economic and social divisions within society, and the consequences of this can last for years. Similarly, Fisher and Bubola [8] argue that inequality and poverty can exacerbate mortality and transmission rates during pandemic times. As both reinforce each other, it results in the rise of virus cases and the deepening of society's socio-economic divides. Moreover, the history of pandemics tells us that in the most of the cases, the development of networks has been created because of trade and commerce, migration of people, conquest, and explorations that further resulted into the growth of diseases and spread of epidemics into different parts of the world [9]. He also states that most importantly, the poor people became the "innocent passive recipient" indirectly and became the "compelled carrier" of these contagious diseases. The unchecked and aggressive growth of capitalism and colonialism, in one sense, fuel the growth of epidemics in human society. The class of rich and economically powerful people could become mobile, which exposed the clutches of outbreaks to the otherworld. Thus, directly and indirectly, infecting the poor and the vulnerable people. Migration and further movement in various forms and stages of history imported culture, money, and diseases together to the native land. Anthropologist Vigh [10] stated how the ethnographies of the crisis in the Latin American and African societies depicted the 'constant prospect' of the societies, which suggests that in the contemporary times, there is a 'constant prospect' of the crisis that is intrinsically woven into the social fabric of the existing society. This could offer a productive lens in understanding how the migrant workers in Mumbai, Delhi, and other Indian cities respond to the crisis, one after the other.

Further, on the nature of the state and government in times of the crisis is highlighted by the Walter Benjamin's in his essay 'The Concept of History' (1968) where he states that how in times of emergency and unforeseen circumstances, the state act as a 'state of exception' where even the bare lives of the citizens become subject to the state power [22]. Similarly, Agamben's [11] stated the current response in western countries to the coronavirus outbreak is just another example of this. In such a crisis-like situation, citizens are left with no options other than accepting the bare minimum of existence. Restrictions are put on liberty due to the suspension of the majority of laws in emergencies. Agamben [11] also stated that the current pandemic is further exacerbated by the media and conjured by the authorities. The Citizens respond by adapting to the changing reality, which becomes new normal for them. Similarly, Foucault [12] points out how plague in the past was controlled by a proper order and system of surveillance. However, Foucault also noted that this order provoked disorder through "suspended laws, lifted prohibitions, the frenzy of passing the time, bodies mingling together without respect, individuals passing the time and going their statutory restriction." According to Foucault, the plague's disorder gave legitimacy to use regulations related to the everyday lives of the general public. The pandemic's chaos and complexity give rise to 'biopolitics,' which involved consistent monitoring, and surveillance gave rise to imminent government control over the people's lives, which indirectly led to the further marginalization of pre-existing deprived and vulnerable sections of the society. Further, pandemics' history has shown that the measured morbidity was far more significant in numbers for women than others. Literature has also pointed out that the marginalized and the poor people routinely face the abridgment of their human rights due to a lack of safety measures and discriminatory policies [26].

Today, UN Women [4] warned that migrant laborers worldwide are disproportionately at risk and most vulnerable from the impact of the pandemic due to their crowded living conditions (where physical distancing is practically not possible), extended-lasting lockdowns, and harsh containment measures, their narrower reach to healthcare and essential services, poor, and exploitative working conditions and labor systems. They become disadvantaged as traditional roles become more rapidly diffused from high-income to low-income societies.

10.3   COVID-19 PANDEMIC AND THE VOICES OF FEMALE MIGRANT WORKERS

According to the International Labor Organization [13], around 81% of women work in India's informal sector. As the informal economy is hit hard due to the COVID-19 pandemic, economic costs are borne disproportionally, affecting the vulnerable migrant women to a greater extent. In any situation of physical threatening, women suffer the most, leading to an increase in the level of gender inequality in society. Moreover, as hospitality and caregiving are considered traditionally to be part of women's jobs, they are called upon to give care to the sick either at home or outside with little or very little preventive support. In one of the interviews conducted by Global Voices [14], with Aarti, who stays in one of Delhi's housing societies, Aarti says that Shaila, a migrant worker from Kolkata, asked for resuming work in her housing society. However, as domestic workers were not allowed in housing society amid the pandemic, Shaila was left with no option. She lost her only source of livelihood. Similarly, Laila, a migrant worker from Uttar Pradesh, worked as a domestic worker in Delhi. However, due to lockdown, she was not allowed to work in gated communities. Laila feared that whatever she has earned till now would be swept away due to the crisis and would not be able to look after her three children. Shaila and Laila's stories are echoed in the stories of around 45 million migrant workers who live in different parts of the country. Apart from that, there are also heart-wrenching images and videos covered by media of pregnant women covering miles to reach their native villages as they have no option left. For instance- how pregnant migrant women workers have borne extra pain, as highlighted in one of the news by Hindustan Times [15], where it reported how a woman who was 8 months pregnant and her husband walked more than 100 Kilome-ters towards their home without any food. In the National Capital of Delhi, the situation was even worse. In Delhi, these migrants' women are involved mostly in the informal sector and often work as street vendors, housemaids, construction workers, security guards, etc. The COVID-19 pandemic led to a stampede-like situation in Delhi. When the Delhi government arranged a bus for them, more than 15,000 workers were at Anand Vihar bus station. Added to that, thousands of people were seen walking in foot towards Ghaziabad, Bihar, and Uttar Pradesh. They tried to employ every possible means to reach their hometown. However, many of these migrants got stuck in the district and state border areas. Those who could not afford to return to their villages struggle to manage food for their family. COVID-19 has created an existential threat for these women migrant workers. They suffer from economic distress, and looking from a health perspective, women migrant workers suffer from greater risk. Further, they had to deal with the uncertainty and loss of livelihood and income with limited infrastructure facilities and resources available for them [16]. Living in a substandard environment and dealing with social inequities like health, safety, and gender-based violence during the pandemic times made them more vulnerable. Due to a lack of resources, most of them dealt with health and menstrual hygiene issues. They also suffer from social stress due to restrictions on traveling, leading to anxiety among them. The subsequent and unplanned lockdowns made it more difficult for them to seek help from others.

10.4 COVID-19 PANDEMIC AND THE FEMALE MIGRANT WORKERS: AN INTROSPECTION OF THE ISSUES INVOLVED

Though the coronavirus does not discriminate people based on class, gender, race, or nationality, the critical factor that plays a crucial role in avoiding infection is physical distancing. However, for many physical distancing is a privilege and is not possible for one and all. Migrant workers in general and female workers, in particular, are not in the position of maintaining such physical distances. For poor women migrant workers, it makes no sense at all. They live in crowded slums, where they have to share the same water tap, washroom, and lanes. Thus, they are not among those who can afford to maintain social distance. They constitute the most vulnerable population to these diseases mainly because of their poor immunity, limited food availability, lack of awareness and health facilities, poor living conditions, work losses, and dependency over daily living wages. In these circumstances, when these female migrant workers have lost their livelihood sources, their survival in the cities has become unmanageable. They are left with no option other than going back to their hinterland. Chinmay Tumbe, the author of 'India Moving: A History of Migration,' highlights these migrants' mass exodus towards their villages. He argues that the city promised them economic security, but their villages provided them social security, where they are assured that they will get food and accommodation [17]. Moreover, in the struggle of choosing an option between lives and livelihood, these vulnerable female workers chose lives over livelihood. It is survival and existence that matter the most for them in the pandemic times. The situation in quarantine centers is not much better.

Mohanty [18] reported that there are cases of death of female migrant workers in the quarantine center, especially in Odisha and Telangana. There is also coverage of women in media who travel miles with their children and lots of luggage. The logic is simple-with no employment and money left, they cannot pay rent and manage food for their family. These issues and insecurities forced these poor women to go back to their villages. The pandemic impacts on the life of urban poor are not gender-neutral. They become more vulnerable because of multiple discrimination and disadvantages that they face in their life. First, being a woman, second due to being poor, and third, being an informal worker. Apart from that, most of them belong to the socially backward castes and disadvantageous communities. Another section of migrant women workers includes women from India's northeastern part who come to cities searching for work. These women have to deal with various struggles. They have to stay in a hostile and unfamiliar environment, mainly when they belong to a religious or racial minority. They are vulnerable to sexual violence, especially young migrant workers from the northeastern people. These women sometimes are harassed due to their looks and are often teased due to their facial looks. This situation represents the worst form of gender and racial prejudice. These poor, migrant women workers have gone into suffering and uncertainty gyre. They are also visible in the present crisis finding the way to return. They are left with no income, cannot pay rent, and cannot get transport to return to their home. There is a strongly hierarchical and caste connotation that is attached to these female migrant worker's lives. For example-In a study conducted in Bangalore, it was found that around 75% of the workers that were interviewed belong to the scheduled caste group, and just 2% belong to upper castes. Apart from that, due to the financial crisis, many of these poor women could not afford to buy sanitary pads. For instance, Laxmi, a migrant worker, reported to the Indian Express [23] that amidst the crisis, she had been forced to use unsanitized cloth pieces as she could not afford to buy pads. She added that there is no privacy where they could change it. To make it worse, sometimes she has no access to running water. Therefore, the unavailability of water and toilets and inaccessibility in purchasing sanitary pads have worsened their overall health.

Furthermore, the current crisis has reinforced the patriarchal setup of Indian society. Women in the informal sector with no employment left have lost the status of being independent. This has reduced women's status again as a 'depender' on her male partner, thereby leading to male domination. Sadly, these are those women who keep the wheels of the Indian economy going, but still, they have minimal social protection in these challenging times. Furthermore, as the lockdown was extended time and again, most of them left with no savings to sustain themselves in difficult times. Those who tried to go back home faced the police's wrath, stigma by the village people, and the disinfectant was thrown on them. Amidst the coronavirus pandemic, migrant workers are often perceived as carriers of the virus, a threat, and a spreader of contamination in their villages and hinterland. The poor migrant female workers faced challenges like-social stigma, ostracizations, and social boycott. Sociologically, we can say that the 'gaze' of the local village population is now on the migrant's body. Migrant female workers are stereotyped as virus suspect. It becomes crucial to analyze this aspect in India's context as the stigma of ostracization is associated with its social history. Even the 'social distancing' is accentuating a new kind of fault line in society. The existing social structure is already hierarchical, cutting along the class, gender, caste, etc. The current crisis may unleash newer forms of untouchability and new ways of maintaining purity and pollution. Thus, the repercussions of the pandemic on migrant workers involved in an unorganized sector were devastating. Not only their fundamental right to live with dignity was abridged amidst the coronavirus-induced lockdown, which highlights how the government did not take into consideration while imposing the lockdown again and again. At the same time, it also highlighted the ill and selfish responses of these migrant workers' employers. The employers just got their work done without giving any future security for unforeseen circumstances to them. Thus, inadequate social safeguards and 'othering' of them result in more exploitation of them.

10.5 LESSONS LEARNED AND THE STRATEGIES NEEDED

The current pandemic situation has given visibility to the poor migrant workers who have been ignored during regular times [27]. It is prime time now that we focus more on social security measures, especially on the capacity building to deal with the heath and existential crisis that migrant workers are facing today. The ILO has estimated that India has more than 400 million informal workers at high risk. It is a possibility that they may sink further amid the COVID-19 crisis. To deal with these issues, both central and state governments have to come with a comprehensive solution to the problems faced by these migrant workers. From a social perspective, it becomes significant to analyze various government policies, efforts, and practices to solve their plight. It would help us to identify people and groups where government intervention is required. All national and state-level responses must represent rights, economic outcomes, protection, inclusion, and equality at the center concerning women [4]. Responses and actions have to be local in nature to identify the necessary interventions on a need and bases easily. It is equally imperative that the policy-makers adopt a gender perspective in understanding the effects of the COVID-19 outbreak and the lockdown on female workers' livelihood and the social structures of society. "The differential needs of women and men in long-and-medium-term recovery efforts also need to be considered. It is equally essential to ensure that women's voices are heard and recognized, says Mohammad Naciri, the regional director of UN Women Asia and the Pacific" [24]. The one truth is that this crisis has revealed the significant role these informal workers play and are actually 'essential workers' and not what they were earlier treated as 'unskilled workers' [19]. The first step to that end would be evolving a gender-appropriate response that leaves no one behind. An ecosystem should be created prioritizing the transfer of food, shelter, cash, and health. The rural economy has to be revived to ensure the wellbeing of the vulnerable. It is crucial to update migrant workers' data and categorize the data into gender skills and states to ease the transfer of benefits to them. Voice of the vulnerable women should be heard while making policies and solutions against the COVID-19 pandemic dealing with the myriad issues of inequality, poverty, stigma, and unemployment that these vulnerable groups face. Again, it is essential to note that it is not the government's sole concern to care for these vulnerable women. Media and society have a more significant role to play in it. For instance, the director Das [20] recently released a short film named "listen to her," supported by UNESCO, UN Women, and UNICEF. The key lines of the film are "whisper speak shout. Your voice will be heard." The film has added to the voice that is much needed in public space, especially related to domestic violence. This shows how media has a more significant role in spreading awareness among the masses and conveying the message and lessons we need to learn for the future. This pandemic has taught us that our lives are deeply intertwined, and so we must respond to the realities beyond ours. As emphasized by the UN Women [4], domestic and social solidarity is needed at all levels. All of us should help those who are ultra-vulnerable in society and are greatly affected due to the current pandemic prevailing situation. If this issue remains unaddressed and the needs of the vulnerable sections are not taken into account, it may result in a more profound social crisis that may increase inequality, unemployment, discrimination, and exclusion. As pandemic has presented asymmetrical risks to migrant workers, a just and comprehensive response is needed at the government and society level. At the societal level, an alteration in the mindset and perception regarding migrant workers is imminent. At the government level, the rights of these marginalized sections need to be protected. A commitment to their betterment and amelioration of the vulnerable section is required because, in times of corona when there are left with no income and employment, the central question remains how are they going to sustain themselves, whether they are staying in cities in cities or at home.

10.6   CONCLUSION

The pandemic has revealed the enormity of the crisis in women migrant women's workers' lives where they are suffering from multilayered vulnerabilities. The situation has demonstrated an urgent need to provide economic and social security to the needy women migrant workers. Although the government provided a $ 22.6 billion relief package, it started shramik trains alongside other government initiatives like Public Distribution System and Direct Benefits Transfer. Still, hardly a few of the women workers got benefitted by these interventions of the government. The critical challenge is that there is a lack of comprehensive and robust data on internal migration patterns. Thus, the benefits failed to reach to the needy ones. Therefore, the government has to ensure that authentic information is available related to the interstate migrant workers so that a properly planned roadmap can be drawn. However, the current cataclysmic crisis has also provided an opportunity. It has made visible the most overlooked sections of the society and jarringly exposes the lacunas and fractures in governmental approaches. The government has to ensure that these vulnerable sections do not face an existential crisis in the future. The government should have a strong political will to build a just society by providing social protection to society's most vulnerable. Further, at the broader level, the perception related to migrant workers need to be changed. Migrant Workers should not be viewed as objects of patronage or charity; instead, they are to be seen as the builder of the economy.

KEYWORDS

- **abusive head trauma**
- **COVID-19 pandemic**
- **economic distress**
- **female migrant workers**
- **gendered issues**
- **strategies required**

REFERENCES

1. Dutta, S., (2020). *India: Migrant Workers' Plight Prompts UN Call for 'Domestic Solidarity' in Coronavirus Battle*. UN News. https://news.un.org/en/story/2020/04/1060922 (accessed on 27 June 2021).
2. Mishra, D., (2020). *No One Wants to Go Near Them' in Bihar face Social Boycott*. The print. https://theprint.in/india/no-one-wants-to-go-near-them-returning-migrant-workers-in-bihar-face-social-boycott/392081/ (accessed on 27 June 2021).
3. Patel, C., (2020). *COVID-19: The Hidden Majority in India's Migration Crisis*. Chatham House. https://www.chathamhouse.org/expert/comment/covid-19-hidden-majority-indias-migration-crisis (accessed on 27 June 2021).

4. UN Women, (2020). *The First 100 Days of COVID-19 in Asia and the Pacific: A Gender Lens*. Bangkok. UN Women Asia. https://asiapacific.unwomen.org/en/digital-library/publications/2020/04/the-first-100-days-of-the-covid-19-outbreak-in-asia-and-the-pacific (accessed on 27 June 2021).

5. Wallis, P., (2006). Plagues, morality, and the place of medicine in early modern England. *English Historical Review, 121*(490), 1.

6. Spinney, L., (2020). *Closed Borders and Black Weddings: What the 1918 Flu Teaches us About Coronavirus*. The Guardian. https://www.theguardian.com/world/2020/mar/11/closed-borders-and-black-weddings-what-the-1918-flu-teaches-us-about-coronavirus (accessed on 27 June 2021).

7. *How Pandemics Shapes Society?* (2020). Johns Hopkins University. https://hub.jhu.edu/2020/04/09/alexandre-white-how-pandemics-shape-society/ (accessed on 27 June 2021).

8. Fisher, M., & Bubola, M., (2020). *As Coronavirus Deepens Inequality, Inequality Worsens its Spread*. The Newyork Times. https://www.nytimes.com/2020/03/15/world/europe/coronavirus-inequality.html (accessed on 27 June 2021).

9. Samaadar, R., (2020). *Borders of an Epidemic: COVID-19 and the Migrant Workers*. Kolkata. Mahanirban Calcutta Research Group.

10. Vigh, H., (2008). Crisis and chronicity: Anthropological perspectives on continuous conflict and decline. *Ethnos, 73*(1), 5–24.

11. Agamben, G., (2020). *The Invention of an Epidemic.* Quodlibet. https://www.quodlibet.it/giorgio-agamben-l-invenzione-di-un-epidemia (accessed on 27 June 2021).

12. Foucault, M., (1995). *Discipline and Punish: The Birth of the Prison* (2nd edn., Vintage Books). New York: Vintage Books.

13. ILO, (2018). *Women and Men in the Informal Economy: A Statistical Picture* (3rd edn.). Geneva. ILO Office. https://www.ilo.org/wcmsp5/groups/public/---dgreports/---dcomm/documents/publication/wcms_626831.pdf (accessed on 27 June 2021).

14. Verma, A., (2020). *COVID-19 Creates More Uncertainty for Migrant Workers in India*. Global Voices. https://globalvoices.org/2020/04/23/covid-19-creates-more-uncertainty-for-migrant-workers-in-india/ (accessed on 27 June 2021).

15. Raju, S., (2020). *Coronavirus Update: Pregnant Woman, her Husband Forced to Walk over 100km Without Food, Rescued by Locals*. Hindustan Times. https://www.hindustantimes.com/india-news/locals-help-pregnant-woman-her-husband/story-s9QEWktmfZ4sKXDx3KUkYI.html (accessed on 27 June 2021).

16. *More than 21,000 Camps set up for Over 6,60,000 Migrants: State Governments,* (2020). The Economic Times. https://economictimes.indiatimes.com/news/politics-and-nation/more-than-21000-camps-set-up-for-over-660000-migrants-state-governments/articleshow/74920798.cms (accessed on 27 June 2021).

17. Biswas, S., (2020). *Coronavirus: India's Pandemic Lockdown Turns into a Human Tragedy*. BBC News. https://www.bbc.com/news/world-asia-india-52086274 (accessed on 27 June 2021).

18. Mohanty, D., (2020). *Women Migrant Worker Found Dead Near the COVID-19 Quarantine Centre in Odisha*. Hindustan Times. https://www.hindustantimes.com/india-news/woman-migrant-worker-found-dead-near-covid-19-quarantine-centre-in-odisha/story-Dr8KqAv5Wg0IOA9yx4nI3K.html (accessed on 27 June 2021).

19. Sinha, S., (2020). *How India Can Ensure that Women in the Informal Sector Get the Protection they Deserve*. Scroll.in. https://scroll.in/article/961181/

covid-19-how-india-can-ensure-that-women-in-the-informal-sector-get-the-protection-they-deserve (accessed on 27 June 2021).

20. Das, N., (2020). *Listen to Her [Video].* YouTube. https://www.youtube.com/watch?v=scwYray2Dsk (accessed on 27 June 2021).

21. Agamben, G., (2005). *State of Exception.* Chicago. University of Chicago Press.

22. Benjamin, W., (1968). Theses on the philosophy of history. In: Hannah, A., (ed.), *Illuminations.* Edited by New York. Schocken Books.

23. Josh, D., (2020). *Period, an Added Worry for Migrant Women on the Move.* The Indian Express. https://www.newindianexpress.com/states/telangana/2020/may/27/period-an-added-worry-for-migrant-women-on-the-move-2148440.html (accessed on 27 June 2021).

24. Owen, L., (2020). *Women's Affairs East Asia, BBC World Service Coronavirus: Five Ways Virus Upheaval is Hitting Women in Asia.* BBC News. https://www.bbc.com/news/world-asia-51705199 (accessed on 27 June 2021).

25. United Nations (2020). *We are All in this Together: Human Rights and Response Recovery.* https://www.un.org/en/un-coronavirus-communications-team/we-are-all-together-human-rights-and-covid-19-response-and (accessed on 27 June 2021).

26. Yamin, E. A., (2020). *Power, Suffering, and the Struggle for Dignity: Human Rights Frameworks for Health and Why They Matter.* Pennsylvania. University of Pennsylvania Press.

27. Chatterjee, P.(2020). *The Pandemic Exposes India's Apathy Toward Migrant Workers.* The Atlantic. https://www.theatlantic.com/ideas/archive/2020/04/the-pandemic-exposes-indias-two-worlds/609838/ (accessed on 27 June 2021).

CHAPTER 11

The Impacts of the Novel Coronavirus 2019 on Vulnerable Groups of Society: The Case for Mauritius

ASHWINEE DEVI SOOBHUG,[1] NAUSHAD MAMODE KHAN,[2] and DEEPA GOKULSING[3]

[1]Department of External Trade/Statistics Mauritius, Ministry of Finance, Economic Planning and Development, Mauritius, E-mail: soobhugn@gmail.com

[2]Department of Economics and Statistics, University of Mauritius, Mauritius

[3]Department of Social Studies, University of Mauritius, Mauritius

ABSTRACT

The emergence of the Novel Coronavirus 2019 brought unforeseen changes in the predominant norms of the Mauritian society, ranging from the sudden shift in socialization to self-isolation, replacement of the traditional classroom learning to technology intensive learning processes, changes in the expenditure and saving patterns of individuals, and more focus on strengthening family ties than succumb to work pressures. The forefront is on the members of the vulnerable groups of the society namely women, children, sex-workers, prisoners amongst others who are usually marginalized and stigmatized. During the economic crisis linked to the COVID-19 pandemic, their societal distress went beyond endurance thus the involvement of concerned authorities is required. A situational assessment of the impact of COVID-19 pandemic, as elaborately discussed in this chapter, allows a better and thorough understanding of the negative impact of COVID-19 pandemic on the lifestyles of the vulnerable groups in Mauritius and the roles of the concerned authorities to prevent further aggravation of the current situation. Based on the stated facts and through timely comprehensive policies, it should be ensured that no individual, irrespective of the social class, be unfairly treated, especially during unprecedented crisis.

11.1   INTRODUCTION

The prospective position of a country on the world map depends, undeniably, on the health of its economy. Nations cannot have successful reforms if the economic drivers of its economy are not strong enough to face the wrath of unprecedented crisis and economic shocks. In line with David Cameroun's quotes, this belief is nothing but the ultimate truth [1]. The global economy, health, socialization norms, global connectivity have altogether been put into a turmoil after an egregious mismanagement of laboratory biosafety and biosecurity ethics. The novel coronavirus-2019, baptized as COVID-19, suddenly appeared, in Wuhan, China, on the 31st December 2019, and since then the entire human race residing on the planet Earth, irrespective of being part of a developed or developing country, has been witnessing an unprecedented yet disruptive crisis. Due to its highly contagious yet complex nature, this newly discovered zoonotic virus propagated in every nation at the speed of light and the WHO declared the novel coronavirus as a pandemic in March 2020. In the beginning of August, more than 17 million confirmed cases and around 675,000 deaths were recorded, bringing most countries and international agencies working for the betterment of humanity, like the WHO, to their knees [2]. Sanitary measures like mass isolation and quarantine that were implemented in the mid-14th century, during the medieval epidemics of Black Death (bubonic plague), have been re-introduced and are successfully curbing down the pandemic. For instance, in the case of Mauritius, the national confinement, strict sanitary restrictions in public places and excessive marketing strategies with slogans like 'stay-at-home' and 'stay safe' have significantly helped in reducing the number of COVID-19 cases. Re-enforcement of the law and order through frequent road blockages has minimized frequent movement of people, leading to fewer community events, ultimately less propagation of the virus. The availability of adequate hydroxychloroquine tablets to treat COVID-19 and the number of quarantine centers eliminated the risk of spreading the virus into the local community. All these factors have worked successfully due to the timely implementation of the policies [3]. However, more research on the coronavirus should be conducted so that the authorities are well guided when drafting the action plans. In this globalizing world, all societies have lately witnessed a sudden change in its norms-an unpredictable shift from socialization to confinement, social distancing, and isolation and undeniably like other countries, the Mauritian society could not be spared from the impacts of COVID-19.

This chapter highlights the impacts of COVID-19 on the society, more specifically on members of the vulnerable groups in Mauritius.

The chapter is structured as follows: Section 11.2 provides an overview of the situational analysis of COVID-19 in Mauritius whilst Section 11.3 emphasizes on the positive and negative impacts of COVID-19. Section 11.4 sets out the discussion of all the issues raised in the previous section. We finally conclude with some lessons learnt during this pandemic.

11.1.1 SITUATIONAL ANALYSIS OF COVID-19 IN THE MAURITIAN CONTEXT

Located in the Indian Ocean, Mauritius has a population of around 1.3 million and is a multi-ethnic society. Mauritius initially termed as a 'doom' country, has developed miraculously from a monocrop, heavily dependent on the sugarcane industry, into a well-diversified economy, evolving around the financial services, tourism, manufacturing, Fintech, international merchandise trade, communication, and technology (ICT) and seafood hub sectors. In a minimal lapse of time, Mauritius moved from a low-income country to an upper-middle-income one, ultimately bringing in a more equitable distribution of income and economic resources, improved Human Development Index, and better economic and infrastructural development [3]. As of date, Mauritius wears the crown among the African countries, with a praiseworthy World Bank Ease of Doing Business index and Mo Ibrahim Index of African Governance. Compared to other African countries, Mauritius has a strong footing than many sub-Saharan countries since its social protection systems are well structured. As such, the government can sustain the most vulnerable households during this unprecedented health and economic crisis. However, there is a need to improve the quality of the health and education services. As of now, Mauritius can trust its strong social protection systems as it crosses the coronavirus desert. But will welfare be enough to protect the societal rights of its people? In fact, whatever the restructuring plan is, equal income distribution, the right to live and protection of every member of the society against all social pains, should be ensured as it is known to the world that the vulnerable households which are part of the society, are facing major dilemma. The pandemic disrupted the normal functioning of the society and worrisome scenarios like a soaring unemployment rate in most countries, an elevated crime rate due to unavailability and limited sales of illicit drugs and alcoholic drinks respectively, thus leading to an outrage in the number of sociological abuses and violence. People living below the poverty line have lately been facing financial problems and have been neglected by the authorities. It is known to the world that the human race should be treated equally, but with the current pandemic and lockdown, the society is unveiling several social pains, enlarging further the inequality gap between the rich and the poor. With the quest to have a fruitful economy, authorities should ensure that the essence of humanity is not lost, especially for the case of Mauritius, which has been blessed with a multicultural society, the rights for humans and empowerment of the younger generation should be valued and encouraged. On the one hand, with the pandemic, a surge in negative vices has been witnessed, for instance, most traders, with the aim to reap more profits, are exploiting consumers and violating their rights. Pornography is booming during the COVID-19 lockdown, and children who are locked home due to school closures, may get access to such content, impacting negatively on their psychological state. On the other hand, the pandemic has helped in strengthening the family ties which were lately slowly being detached due to hectic lifestyles but unfortunately, due to the current challenges which our society is facing, the negative impacts are much more deficient, thus outweighing the positive consequences.

From an economic perspective, the COVID-19 pandemic has been labeled as the "black swan" in the already unstable economic environment. Most countries are expected to face a recession in 2020, moving off many countries from achieving the sustainable development goals (SDGs) and pulling around tens of millions of people back into extreme poverty [5]. Another lucrative sector which has largely been upended by the current novel coronavirus-2019 (COVID-19), is international trade. Globally, unavoidable declines in trade and output, worse than those experienced in the global financial crisis (2008–2009), are expected due to the prevailing unprecedented health and economic crisis. For the first two quarters of 2020, restrictions on travel and transport and slowdown in production will lead to a decline of 32% in trade of goods across international boundaries, subject to the effectiveness of preparedness and response strategies of the countries [6]. For small economies with huge dependence on international trade and tourism sector, like Mauritius, a huge downturn in their economic growth is expected. As per the latest estimates published by Statistics Mauritius, an economic contraction of around 13.0%, as expected, for the year 2020. This is due to decline in the textile manufacturing sector due to poor demand from exporters (–45%) and in accommodation and food service activities due to lower tourist arrivals (–70%) partly offset by an increase of 1% in financial and insurance activities [7]. It is however agreed that a rebound in trade performances is possible, depending on the government's fiscal and monetary policies to counter the downturn as well as on the duration of the outbreak. But undeniably, the positive externalities related to the economic restoration will be reaped in the long run. Based on the recent merchandise trade data compiled by the Statistics Mauritius, as shown graphically below, the Mauritian economy is slowing picking up post confinement (Figure 11.1).

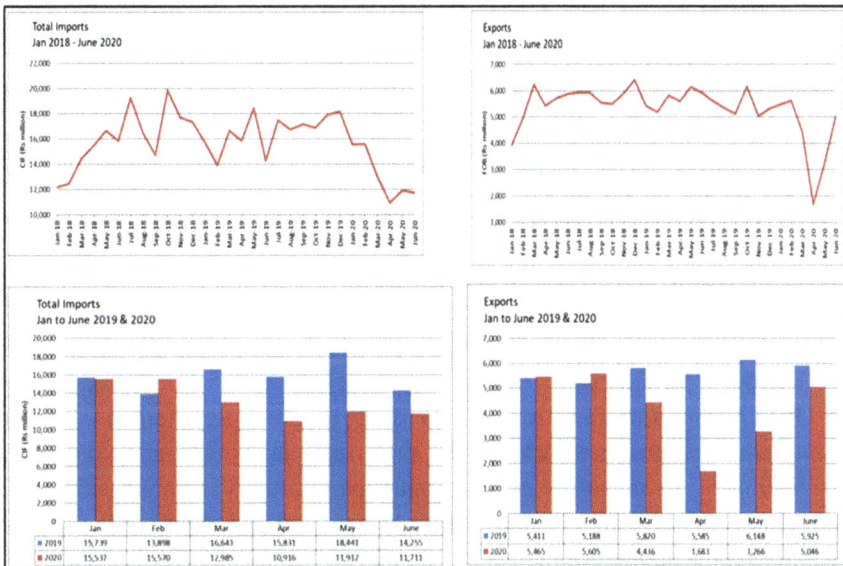

FIGURE 11.1   External merchandise trade, January 2018 to June 2020.
Source: Statistics Mauritiu [34].

From the above chart, it can clearly be seen that in March 2020 and April 2020, trade dropped drastically as compared to the corresponding period of 2019. Reason obviously was slowdown in economic activities due to confinement imposed to curb down the coronavirus which is currently ravaging the whole world. From the line graphs, both exports and total imports are picking up as from May 2020. As compared to April 2020, exports rose by 108%

whilst imports still shows a decrease of 0.7% since 60% of the countries still have travel restrictions, thus limiting supply from main markets. It is expected that total exports, which includes ships stores and bunkering, will increase in the following quarters given that there is currently an appreciation of the US dollars, thus, export earnings will be higher, ceteris paribus. As for imports, an improvement is expected as from 2021.

From an environmental perspective, Mother nature is recovering while humanity stays at home. During the lockdown, air pollution has decreased, sprouts are growing, and the animals are living freely and roaming in their natural habitat without fearing for any gut shots. In Mauritius, based on lessons learnt from this sanitary and health crisis, concerned authorities, under the guidance of experts in United Nations (UN) SDGs, are re-framing the action plans regarding achievement of the SDGs. Therefore, it is high time for authorities to act towards *"#planetoverprofit"* rather than just *"#profit."*

The following sections explain the positive as well as the negative impacts of COVID-19 on Mauritius.

11.2   POSITIVE AND NEGATIVE IMPACTS OF COVID-19 ON MAURITIUS

11.2.1   UNEMPLOYMENT DURING COVID-19

As a matter of fact, in the United States, the unemployment rate reported in the first three months of COVID-19 was higher than that reported during the Great Depression, and in South Africa, the unemployment rate soared to around a worrisome 30%. With this, the claims for unemployment benefits are rising as well as government expenditure. As a consequence, the inequality between the rich and the poor is expected to widen. For the case of the US, black workers are facing much more economic and health insecurity from COVID-19 than white workers. The latest data indicates that the black unemployment rate is 16.7%, compared with a white unemployment rate of 14.2%. COVID-19 is just worsening the racial disparities that exist in the US [8].

For Mauritius, from March to April 2020, that is the confinement period, a total of 1,107 workers complained about unfavorable and untimely termination of employment, 983 workers did not receive any payment as remuneration for work done whilst 339 workers received only part of their wages. This was mainly due to the sudden closure of private firms which were unable to recover their production costs due to lower sales or exports. Also, lower demand from foreign markets is envisaged following prevailing recession thus as most manufacturing firms prefer to temporarily close down [9].

Unemployment of such type is referred to as cyclical unemployment, and since most of these workers specialize on one particular task out of the whole manufacturing process, they may remain unemployed for a longer time due to mismatch of skills or until government intervene through expansive monetary and fiscal policies. This type of unemployment should be triggered immediately as with lower income, the laid-off workers' have a reduced purchasing power, and this results in lower demand for goods and services in the economy. This can also lead to indebtedness from borrowing money to support one's needs, use of savings to cover costs, and in case no other source of finance is found, these unemployed people may get trapped into the vicious cycle of poverty. Several societal pains are chained with unemployment and will be discussed in the following sections.

11.2.2   WOMEN IN DANGERS DUE TO COVID-19

"For many women and girls, it is their beloved homes that proved to rather be a selcouth mirage. The sole place which is considered to be the safest for them, has ironically, become worse than the fire of hell. We know that sanitary lockdown and self-isolation are important during the COVID-19 pandemic to prevent propagation of the SARS-CoV-2 virus. But we cannot ignore that during this phase, unfortunate women are trapped with abusive partners, under one roof and for a long time" said the UN Secretary-General António Guterres. It is well documented that many women face interpersonal violence during times of crisis, but less than 10% seek help. In the United Kingdom (UK), the figures are frightening. In the first three weeks of COVID-19 lockdown, 14 women and 2 children were assassinated. A well-known non-profitable organization, Respect, recorded increases of 97%, 185%, and 581% in calls, e-mails, and website visits, respectively [10]. In Mexico and Brazil, the number of grievance calls peaked and most of them related to domestic abuse [11]. In China, the number of domestic violence calls in February 2020 tripled, as compared to the corresponding month of 2019 [12].

Inevitably, an unemployed person is expected to be psychologically and physically affected. A disturbed person is most likely to disrupt the normal functioning of his family, and consequently, abusive behaviors in the domestic setting is expected. For Mauritius, as compared to the corresponding period, the number of domestic violence escalated by 47% in May 2020. During the period 20 March to 30 May 2020, that is during the peak national lockdown, 520 cases of which 481 were female and 39 were male victims, have been registered by the officials. Out of 520 cases reported, 208 were physical assaults, 173 verbal abuse and 139 other types of problems. A worrisome, 111 female victims, have filed grievances against their abusive partners and quitted the conjugal roof during the lockdown. Now, as a result of such actions, younger children of those particular households may experience physiological reactions related to stress, harming to a great extent their brain development [9].

11.2.3   IMPACTS ON CHILDREN OF COVID-19 OUTBREAK

During the confinement period, since many nurseries and schools were closed, many children were trapped with their offenders, be it at home or in out-of-home care, because of a mental or physical disability or a situation of dependence. Child abuse, in terms of sexual abuse, physical abuse, and psychological abuse, has been a matter of concern given that pedophilia and other dangers are becoming more frequent in our modern society. Entrapped in the daily quest for a better status, a better standard of living, a better revenue, parents trust relatives for taking care of the younger children. But are they safe in the hands of their own ones? In France, the police intervened in 92 child abuse cases and more than 20% of child abuse cases were reported via the helpline "Allo Enfance en Danger" [13]. During the lockdown period, in Mauritius, higher occurrences of child abuses were in households with threatening environment. Some cases of abuse were unheard by the parents, and some were unreported due to fear of being neglected in this vicious society. The child sexual abuse case, that recently surfaced post lockdown, has shook the whole Mauritian community. An 11-year-old innocent girl trusted her uncle but little did she know that the latter was in quench to satisfy his sexual desires. Mauritius, indeed has been blessed by a paradise-like landscape and a diversified society, but when such despicable cases of abuses occur, especially on children, these acts stigmatize Mauritius.

International agencies like UNICEF [14] already predicted cases of child maltreatment due to lockdown measures [14]. Parents are the ones with whom a child feel safe, but they are also viewed as the main perpetrators.

It is argued by Lindo et al. [35] that when unprecedented crisis like the COVID-19 strikes and many heads of the families, especially fathers, lose their jobs, then physical abuse of children like nonaccidental injury (NAI) including abusive head trauma (AHT) arises [15, 16]. In fact, Brown and De Cao [36] proved that child neglect is very well present when the male employment increases [16]. An unemployed father is often frustrated thus may vent out his anger or depression on the child. For some children, staying at home may be a good means for enhanced educative learning and more quality time with family, but for some, it can be an emotional torture. Children, under the guardship of abusive caregivers, may be facing frequent abuses, and due to the temporary suspension in social work and related legal and protective services for children, these abuses may go unnoticed. Due to current online pedagogy obligation, children may not have access to teachers to report any incident that occurred at home [22].

11.2.3.1 *CONFINEMENT MAY LEAD TO SEXUAL EXPLOITATION, CYBER-BULLYING, AND SEXUAL EXTORTION OF CHILDREN*

During the confinement period, as a result of school closures, many children, some of earlier ages, are increasingly surfing the internet, especially social media, with the aim to interact with their friends, for online schooling, and for distraction. Social offenders may take advantage of such situations and try to sexually extort the children. According to the child online safety index [17], sexual exploitation or cyber bullying may also occur and with cyber-bullying comes suicidal thoughts.

In Mauritius and in many other nations, the *TikTok* application, a video-sharing social networking service, has gained the attention of many children. As a result, many cyber-bullying videos whereby many of these children are being mocked are circulating on the social media. During this pandemic, along with the implementation of restorative economic strategies, there should be re-enforcement of the child protection and cyber risks laws as well as encourage digital citizenship to make the children, independent, and responsible thinkers.

11.2.3.2   *CHILD MENTAL HEALTH AND NEW LEARNING TECHNIQUES DURING LOCKDOWN*

The traditional classroom teaching was replaced by virtual schooling during the pandemic. Many children were able to catch up their studies. However, some were still deprived of technological accessibility. WhatsApp, Zoom, Google classroom and Skype were some of the virtual platforms used to conduct online classes, yet not all children had equal access to internet connectivity and electronic gadgets. The fear of lacking behind may have devasting effects on the child's mental health. Children with disturbing family background and unpleasant past, are prone to commit suicide.

Conversely, during the pandemic, it is questionable whether the children living with foster families, have had adequate access to education. In Mauritius, the SOS Village, a non-governmental organization which works to provide family care, education, and support to children who are no longer able to live with their parents, does help in re-integrating the children into the society but during this crisis, did it have enough infrastructure especially in terms of connectivity, for more than 150 children? Also, in case the children are following virtual classes, are they well supervised in order not to fall prey to any cases of cyber-bullying? All these should be addressed to avoid any future repercussions on the child's mental health and education level.

11.2.4   **THE DILEMMA OF SEX WORKERS DURING COVID-19 PANDEMIC**

A red umbrella! A sigh of distress and a call to authorities for better conditions of work and security in the sexual service industry. Since time immemorial, paid sexual labor is viewed as a taboo in the society, but despite that and the associated limited job security, many choose this easy way of making money. During this pandemic, authorities have marginalized the sex workers and most of them are witnessing a sudden decline in their income level since with strict sanitary restrictions in place, the demand for paid sex is at its lowest level. Most of them are surviving with minimum access to basic necessities, with no assurance of a better life in the future. It is most probable that with uncertainty evolving around the pandemic, the sex industry will take time to return to normal. Some sex workers even feared of losing all clientele and returning to the hustle and bustle when they started.

Another issue is that of financial assistance. Sex workers are often self-employed and many unregistered sex workers may find themselves in severe financial problems. Teela [37] a criminology professor at the University of Leicester, argued that the government aims to provide social security benefits to the majority of its people [18], but unfortunately, sex workers are excluded. Sex workers are not eligible for any COVID-19 reliefs, put into place by the local authorities, to sustain the working class and at-risk populations. For instance, in Canada, most sex workers are not eligible to postulate for the Canada Emergency Response Benefit (CERB) because their annual income level remains undisclosed [19]. In some countries, prostitution is criminalized and due to this fear, even those who can provide proof of being eligible for COVID-19 reliefs are afraid to apply for financial assistance from the authorities as by doing so, there are associated risks, for example, surveillance, arrest, and fines which can further aggravate the circumstances. As such, these sex workers find themselves in financial distress, which ultimately may entail much more devastating societal pain.

During this pandemic, world's biggest brothel, Daulatdia in Bangladesh, is still trading with 1,300 female sex workers. The latter choose to work despite the risk of hefty fines and exposure to the virus because of their need for finance. Many of the sex workers are mothers and need to nurture their children. As a matter of fact, Daulatdia is also home to around 400 children [18, 20].

Due to circumstantial events, children whose mothers are engaged in prostitution may reportedly be forced to get into sex trafficking at a young age or in other criminal offenses to earn easy money. This put into danger the physical and as well as mental health of children. Even the education of the children is hindered, and it is most likely that the children of the lower-class population are unable to get out of the quagmire of poverty; thus, they may remain under privileged for a longer time or even for a whole lifetime. Frustrated parents, may even physically abuse of the children of their households, and the latter, out of fear, may not even seek advice or help from third parties.

In Mauritius, sex workers are facing the same dilemma as those in Canada and other nations, but non-governmental organizations (NGOs) like 'Parasol Rouge,' are working to offer shelter and healthcare services to the sex workers. Many of them are living with communicable diseases like HIV or non-communicable diseases like diabetes mellitus; thus anti-viral or anti-anxiety medicaments should be provided to them on time. In Nairobi, Professor Sanders is already working on an "Uber-style" app that will enable sex workers to electronically purchase pharmaceutical products and have it delivered [18]. Hopefully, Mauritius can benefit from such technological advancements.

Sex workers, even though they are devoted to titillation and are stigmatized in the society, should be supported during this pandemic. Just like other members of the society are afraid to go near a sex worker with fear of getting infected by the coronavirus or any other communicable disease, a similar fear of the unknown is felt by the sex workers. Also, it is known to the world that even when most brothels start operating normally, it will take a long time for the sex industry to return to its normal functioning. As such, from a humanitarian perspective, exclusion of sex workers from the COVID-19 reliefs funds may be unethical since the former deserve financial support from the authorities but do not receive them. Concerned authorities should revise their rights charter and recognize the rights of most marginalized members of society.

11.2.5 CONSUMER PROTECTION DURING COVID-19

The sudden health and economic crisis have provoked a disruption in the supply chains as well as caused violation of consumer rights. The UN Food and Agriculture Organization forecasted uncertainty and disruption in the global food markets until 2021. Worse, within 6 months, from 1st January to 6th August 2020, the number of complaints lodged by consumers was 81,108 which represented a loss of $99.85 million. Most frauds occurred via online shopping and travel transactions which ultimately caused loss of $13.98 million and $34.23 million, respectively [23]. It is to be highlighted that during the peak periods, that is, between April to May 2020, when most countries were under lockdown, the number of complaint reports was at its highest-say around 38,000 reports were lodged. Even in Mauritius, a developing country, consumers had to pay a high price for the basic necessities and sanitary products. It was after the intervention of the local authorities that the rights of consumers were restored. In fact, the prices of the earlier mentioned products have been controlled by allowing a maximum mark up. Traders engaged in illegal trade practices, that is non-abiding of price control measures imposed by the authorities, have been fined. During the pandemic in Mauritius, more than 2500 retail shops were inspected, and 2352 contraventions [24] were issued for breaching the consumer protection regulations.

Every region of the world came up with actions plans in order to ensure consumer advocacy and consumer protection. From the Asian pacific regions, Australia, New Zealand, and China are principally supporting consumers by encouraging banks and financial institutions to offer some debt repayment reliefs. In Europe, due to the mass manufacturing of masks, there is a risk of supplying masks of lower quality. Health authorities in Romania are alerting consumers on the circulation and use of poor-quality sanitary masks. To avoid digital scams, Denmark and the UK came up with scam tracking applications and are taking actions to limit the prices of commodities on the online platforms. American regions have lately been using the radio, TV, and social media in order to disseminate reliable information and clarity regarding refunds for travel bookings and are ensuring that all consumers have accessed to sufficient medicines. African and Middle Eastern countries, on the other hand, are building on good environmental practices and sustainability projects on social media and are coming up with action plans to tackle food shortages and price gouging [25]. All these government actions are mainly to protect the consumer's rights and help curb down the negative impact of COVID-19 on the consumer market. In a nutshell, the consumer remains the king.

11.2.6   THE CONSUMPTION OF PORNOGRAPHY IS HIGH DURING THIS PANDEMIC

With the pandemic, came isolation rules and with the latter came boredom. With eyes glued on their screens and alone most of the time, people are looking for ways to alleviate boredom by either indulging into something artistic or into something not so good. During the lockdown, even though most business were facing a downturn, one industry which is still flourishing is the pornography industry. Undeniably, pornography is having a good pandemic. Pornhub, have lately published statistics regarding consumption patterns during quarantines and lockdowns across the world. The figures are intriguing. On average, the global number of visits to these sites have witnessed a rise of almost 20% as compared to standard operating in February. Italy and Spain topped the chart with an increase of more than 50% whilst, traffic in Australia was above 30% [26]. The pornography industry is so lucrative that Pornhub, when most businesses were struggling to survive this global recession, is promoting "premium service" during lockdown. During lockdown in European countries, people preferred watching sexual content online, rather than educative or entertaining soap operas on Netflix [38].

Now, apart from personal satisfaction, pornography is linked to other negative consequences. India, for instance, registered a record-breaking 95% increase in pornography consumption during the 3-week lockdown [28]. Now, it is known to the world that India is one of the countries, where a woman reports a rape every 15 minutes, and with such high consumption of pornography, the fear of a rape crisis is very well prevalent. In fact, pornography acts like a drug in the brain and Love et al. [29, 39] proved that excessive viewing of internet pornography activates the brain region and encourage similar cravings and drug cue reactions as for alcohol, cocaine, and nicotine. India lately recorded worse cases of rapes and with such sexual content, available free of charge on the internet, the women and most importantly the young girls are not safe. Most porn content clearly depicts violence and abuse on women, and as a bored man is already irritated and frustrated, he can easily vent out his anger on family members. Worse, the children are also isolated at home, and since they are already following online courses and teaching, if left unsupervised, they may get trapped in those negative vices at an early age. Exposure to adult content at a young age may result in depression, most of the time or provoke the immature and young children to indulge in sexual activities, out of curiosity. Conversely, parents may use pornography as a sex education for their children. But in this modern society, it is known that pornography brings in more devastating consequences than positive ones. Sexting, virtual intimacy, sharing of explicit images online or over text and erotic online games have surfaced during this lockdown. The teenagers have been well exposed to teen sexting since most of them were looking for ways to connect outside social distancing and gathering restrictions. Now, these teens may not anticipate the dangers associated with circulating of explicit images online [26, 32]. Thus, legal consequences may be faced as such sexual acts by teenagers are perceived as child pornography.

Conclusively, with the emergence of technology, new areas of research, namely, erobotics, a field intersecting sexuality and technology, are being surfacing even in times of worldwide health crisis [32]. It is however debatable whether such sudden changes in norms and practices regarding intimacy will be accepted in society. Pornography, consequently, has been present for many years but is still viewed as a taboo, though ironically is much consumed, especially when lonely and bored.

11.2.7   RIGHT TO HEALTH AND PROTECTION FOR PRISONERS

Prison health are part of public health thus, the state should ensure that at all times, the rights of prisoners to minimum food requirement, adequate medical support, life security and the fundamental personal freedom, are adhered. In fact, the prisoners are amongst the most vulnerable individuals. Most of them live in close proximity, and given the highly contagious nature of the novel coronavirus, the prisoners are more at risk. As per the research findings by Johns Hopkins and University of California, Los Angeles (UCLA) [30], the COVID-19 is 5.5 times more likely to infect prisoners and chances for the latter to die from it, is three times more than an average normal individual. UNAIDS, the Office of the UN High Commissioner for Human Rights, the World Health Organization (WHO) and UN Office on Drugs and Crime have been urging policymakers in each country to release prisoners with favorable long-term conduct in prison and who were condemned for trivial offenses. During the pandemic, in the light of reducing overcrowding in many places of detention, the Islamic Republic of Iran has released 40% of its total prison population, and Chile was set to release around 50,000 people [31].

During this pandemic, the world has seen unusual situations, but luckily, the rights of every people, be it those in liberty or deprived of liberty, have, and are being preserved.

11.3   DISCUSSION

Based on the prevailing situation, it is clear that all countries, whether with cases of COVID-19 and with no case, will face a "social recession" but the pandemic also made us aware of "who we are and what we value in the next few months." It is now time to do something to make the world better.

During the pandemic, as discussed earlier, several negative facets of COVID-19 on the society have been revealed. It is through frequent collaboration between concerned authorities and NGOs and the principal actors of the private sector that these social pains can be mitigated on time. For instance, with regard to domestic and child abuses, the ombudsperson for children and the authorities working for the betterment and equality of women, should ensure that the rights of these vulnerable beings are protected. Especially, in shelters and foster homes for children, frequent surprise visits by authorities and access to connectivity for educative purposes only should be done. NGOs should ensure that during COVID-19, the children in foster homes have access to online teaching platforms so that they do not lag behind in comparison to other better off children. Private firms, post-pandemic, may consider the provision of educational facilities and useful stationaries to deprived children and financial support to women, victims of domestic abuse, as part of their Corporate Social Responsibility (CSR) scheme. Pornography, on the other hand, should be consumed moderately. Here, providers of telecommunication services may limit access to some outrageous sites and authorities in the education sector should rather bring in sex education in the syllabus to make the child more at ease with sexual content and make them aware of the devastating consequences in case of indulgence in sexual activity at an early age. Finally, international agencies fighting for equality in the human race, for instance L 'Amnesty International, should ensure that the rights of every individual, be it sex workers, white-collar officers, or a pensioner, are respected. The animal species have not been spared. Thus, PAWS in Mauritius or other NGOs with the help of skeleton of veterinary, may provide full support to cure these innocents who fell prey to the novel coronavirus.

Historically, it has been proved that societies are deeply transformed by great pandemics. The novel coronavirus-2019 surely has brought a great surge of interest in socialism, and a decline in capitalism. Hopefully, the changes witnessed during the pandemic will be the new "normal" post the pandemic.

11.4   CONCLUSION

During this pandemic, the human race has fallen on the wrath of God. The world consists of several intellectuals, but for a subsequent period of time, humans were unable to come up with reliable solutions and medications to counter attack the virus. More intriguing is that the coronavirus originated from animal species, most probably from bats, and we, as humans, tend to control, overpower and kill domestic and wild animals, thinking that the latter are weak. What a misconception? Today, the entire humanity is in a weakened state due to the novel coronavirus, a tiny particle with 65 to 125 nm diameter. Humans should learn lessons from this pandemic and try to amend their way of living as well as their priorities.

Luckily, humans were confined with their families for more than 3 months, hence the relations between parents and children have been strengthened. Work, which was prioritized pre-pandemic, has moved to the second position.

People, be it the rich or the poor, have learnt to survive on basic necessities, avoiding excessive and unnecessary purchase of commodities. With social distancing norms and other sanitary measures implemented to curb the virus, every individual was taught the law of discipline and the power of law and order, and it was found that these positive behavioral traits do make things work out efficiently in a short lapse of time. An example is Mauritius, whereby Mauritians, bounded by the COVID-19 Bill, which emphasizes on the importance of sanitary measures and the contraventions and fines associated with breach of the "sanitary" laws, have respected the confinement strictly. Panic buying and consumer exploitation were controlled through the imposition of additional price control strategies. All workers engaged in the provision of essential services to the public, have respected their obligation to serve the nation during this pandemic, and this is indeed praiseworthy. All these positive behaviors have eventually led to the complete eradication of COVID-19 in Mauritius as of mid of August 2020.

With more than 25 million confirmed COVID-19 cases and more than 900,000 deaths by mid-September 2020, as citizens of the global village called Planet Earth, we all should pray for a better future with good environmental and economic successes for the young generation. As Michael Jackson sang, "It's high time that the entire human race stops existing and concentrate on living. Together, we can heal this heavenly world, make it a better place and save it for our children" [33].

The study of vulnerable in the Mauritian society remains unexplored, and given its importance, academic researchers should add value to the limited literature. As such, concerned authorities through efficient policies and the support of non-governmental agencies, can work for the betterment of the vulnerable. It is also important to instill rays of hope for better condition of work, job security, sufficient food and for financial assistance as and when required and equal respect in the society, in the young generation living in the unfavorable environment so that they, with the support of education, can escape the vicious cycle of poverty.

ACKNOWLEDGMENTS

We would like to highlight that this research is part of the CY Initiative of Excellence ("Investissements d'Avenir" ANR-16-IDEX-0008), Project "EcoDep," PSI-AAP2020-0000000013. We also extend our appreciation towards the Higher Education Commission (HEC) of Mauritius for the bursary granted to Ms. Ashwinee Devi Soobhug, MPhil/PhD student.

KEYWORDS

- **communication and technology**
- **corporate social responsibility**
- **COVID-19**
- **higher education commission**
- **Mauritius**
- **nonaccidental injury**
- **non-governmental organizations**

REFERENCES

1. *David Cameron Quotes,* (n.d.). BrainyQuote.com. Retrieved from: BrainyQuote.com. Retrieved from: https://www.brainyquote.com/quotes/david_cameron_745058 (accessed on 27 June 2021).
2. Tim, W., (2020). *First Thing: Coronavirus has Brought the US 'to its Knees'*. The Guardian. Retrieved from: https://www.theguardian.com/us-news/2020/jun/24/first-thing-coronavirus-brought-us-knees (accessed on 27 June 2021).
3. Naushad, M. K., Ashwinee, D. S., & Heenaye-Mamode K. M., (2020). Studying the trend of the novel coronavirus series in Mauritius and its implications. *PLOS One.*
4. CIA World Fact Book and Other Sources, (2019). *Mauritius Economy*. Retrieved from: http://theodora.com (accessed on 27 June 2021).
5. The World Bank, (2020). *The Global Economic Outlook During the COVID-19 Pandemic: A Changed World.* Retrieved from: https://www.worldbank.org/en/news/feature/2020/06/08/the-global-economic-outlook-during-the-covid-19-pandemic-a-changed-world (accessed on 27 June 2021).
6. Press Release, (2020). *Trade Set to Plunge as COVID-19 Pandemic Upends Global Economy*. Retrieved from: https://www.wto.org/english/news_e/pres20_e/pr855_e.htm (accessed on 27 June 2021).
7. Statistics Mauritius, (2020). *National Account Estimates*. Retrieved from: https://statsmauritius.govmu.org/Pages/Statistics/ESI/National_accounts/NA/NAE_Jun20.aspx (accessed on 27 June 2021).
8. Elise, G., & Valerie, W., (2020). *Black Workers Face Two of the Most Lethal Pre-existing Conditions for Coronavirus- Racism and Economic Inequality*. Economic Policy Institute. Retrieved from: https://www.epi.org/publication/black-workers-covid/ (accessed on 27 June 2021).

9. *Statistics Mauritius - Amid the Pandemic,* (2020). Website: https://statsmauritius.govmu. org/Documents/Homepage/Covid19/SM_amid_the_Covid_19_pandemic.pdf (accessed on 27 June 2021).

10. United Nations, (2020). *COVID-19 Response. UN Supporting 'Trapped' Domestic Violence Victims During COVID-19 Pandemic.* Retrieved from: https://www.un.org/en/coronavirus/un-supporting-%E2%80%98trapped%E2%80%99-domestic-violence-victims-during-covid-19-pandemic (accessed on 27 June 2021).

11. World Health Organization, (2020). *The Rise and Rise of Interpersonal Violence - an Unintended Impact of the COVID-19 Response on Families.* Retrieved from: https://www.euro.who.int/en/health-topics/disease-prevention/violence-and-injuries/news/news/2020/6/the-rise-and-rise-of-interpersonal-violence-an-unintended-impact-of-the-covid-19-response-on-families (accessed on 27 June 2021).

12. Bettinger-Lopez, C., & Alexandra, B., (2020). *A Double Pandemic: Domestic Violence in the Age of COVID-19.* Council on Foreign Relations. Retrieved from: https://www.cfr.org/in-brief/double-pandemic-domestic-violence-age-covid-19 (accessed on 27 June 2021).

13. AFP, Paris, (2020). *Coronavirus: France's Child-Abuse Hotline Sees Spike in Calls During Lockdown.* Retrieved from: https://english.alarabiya.net/en/coronavirus/2020/04/09/Coronavirus-France-s-child-abuse-hotline-sees-spike-in-calls-during-lockdown (accessed on 27 June 2021).

14. UNICEF. Coronavirus (COVID-19) Global Response, (2020). Retrieved from: https://www.unicef.org/appeals/covid-2019.html.

15. Polina, M., Lise, L. L., Græsholt-Knudsen, T., Gitte, H., Michel, B. H., Karin, K. P., Møller-Madsen, B., & Jan, D. R., (2020). Physical child abuse demands increased awareness during health and socioeconomic crises like COVID-19. *Acta Orthopaedica.*

16. Elisabetta De, C., & Malte, S., (2020). *The Potential Impact of the COVID-19 on Child Abuse and Neglect: The Role of Childcare and Unemployment.* Retrieved from: https://voxeu.org/article/potential-impact-covid-19-child-abuse-and-neglect (accessed on 27 June 2021).

17. Kate, W., (2020). *An Expert Explains: The Digital Risks Facing our Children During COVID-19.* Retrieved from: https://www.weforum.org/agenda/2020/05/children-digital-risks-cybersecurity-screentime-covid19/ (accessed on 27 June 2021).

18. Vivienne, N., (2020). *Coronavirus: Sex workers Fear for Their Future.* Retrieved from: https://www.bbc.com/news/business-52821861 (accessed on 27 June 2021).

19. Jacqueline L., (2020). *Sex Workers are Criminalized and Left Without Government Support During the Coronavirus pandemic.* The Conversation. Retrieved from: https://theconversation.com/sex-workers-are-criminalized-and-left-without-government-support-during-the-coronavirus-pandemic-141746 (accessed on 27 June 2021).

20. Susannah, B., (2020). *A Sex Worker Reveals How the COVID-19 Pandemic Has Changed Sex Work.* Retrieved from: https://www.forbes.com/sites/susannahbreslin/2020/05/14/a-sex-worker-reveals-how-covid-19-has-changed-sex-work/#c5807723a81b (accessed on 27 June 2021).

21. Natasha, M., (2020). *The Impact of COVID-19 on Sex Workers.* LSE. Retrieved from: https://blogs.lse.ac.uk/covid19/2020/06/08/the-impact-of-covid-19-on-sex-workers/ (accessed on 27 June 2021).

22. Jameela, J., (2018). *Child Abuse: The Despicable Side of our Paradise*. Retrieved from: https://defimedia.info/child-abuse-despicable-side-our-paradise (accessed on 27 June 2021).

23. *Federal Trade Commission*, (2020). Retrieved from: https://public.tableau.com/profile/federal.trade.commission#!/vizhome/COVID-19andStimulusReports/Map (accessed on 27 June 2021).

24. Le Journal, (2020). *Commerce Minister Announces Price Control on Additional Basic Goods Amid COVID-19 Pandemic*. Retrieved from: https://allafrica.com/stories/202004270541.html (accessed on 27 June 2021).

25. *Consumer Protection and Consumer Advocacy During the Pandemic*, (2020). Retrieved from: https://www.consumersinternational.org/what-we-do/covid-19/ (accessed on 27 June 2021).

26. Carmen, O., Lluís, B., & Lluc, N., (2020). *COVID-19 and Pornography Traffic in Spain: How to Prevent the Social Effects of its Consumption in Families*. Retrieved from: https://advance.sagepub.com/articles/preprint/COVID-19_and_Pornography_Traffic_in_Spain_How_to_Prevent_the_Social_Effects_of_its_Consumption_in_Families_/12326372/1 (accessed on 27 June 2021).

27. Jon, R., (2020). *Pornhub Traffic Spikes as Free 'Premium Service' is Offered to Lonely People Stuck in Coronavirus Lockdowns*. Retrieved from: https://www.the-sun.com/news/566180/pornhub-free-premium-service-italy-spain-france-coronavirus/ (accessed on 27 June 2021).

28. Saikiran, K., (2020). *Pornography Gets a Pandemic Boost, India Reports 95% Rise in Viewing*. Retrieved from: https://www.indiatoday.in/news-analysis/story/pornography-gets-a-pandemic-boost-india-reports-95-per-cent-rise-in-viewing-1665940-2020-04-11 (accessed on 27 June 2021).

29. Thomas, G. K., (2020). *Why Pornography is So Powerfully Addictive*. Retrieved from: https://thedoctorweighsin.com/why-is-pornography-so-powerfully-addictive/ (accessed on 27 June 2021).

30. Alexandra, S., (2020). Prisoners 550% more likely to get COVID-19. 300% more likely to die. *New Study Shows*. Retrieved from: https://www.forbes.com/sites/alexandrasternlicht/2020/07/08/prisoners-550-more-likely-to-get-covid-19-300-more-likely-to-die-new-study-shows (accessed on 27 June 2021).

31. *UNODC - The United Nations Office on Drugs and Crime*, (2020). Retrieved from: https://www.unaids.org/en/keywords/unodc-united-nations-office-drugs-and-crime (accessed on 27 June 2021).

32. Simon, D., Dave, A., & Maria, S., (2020). *Cybersex, Erotic Tech and Virtual Intimacy are on the Rise During COVID-19*. Retrieved from: https://theconversation.com/cybersex-erotic-tech-and-virtual-intimacy-are-on-the-rise-during-covid-19-141769 (accessed on 27 June 2021).

33. Michael, J., (1991). *Heal the World*. Dangerous. Retrieved from: https://www.youtube.com/watch?v=BWf-eARnf6U (accessed on 27 June 2021).

34. *Statistics Mauritius, COVID-19 Data Series, External Trade*, (2020). Retrieved from: https://statsmauritius.govmu.org/Documents/Homepage/Covid19/Covid_doc_External_Trade.pdf (accessed on 27 June 2021).

35. Lindo, J., Schaller, J., & Hansen, B. (2018). Caution! men not at work: Gender-specific labor market conditions and child maltreatment. *Journal of Public Economics, 163*, 77–98.

36. Brown, D., & De Cao, E. (2020). *Child Maltreatment, Unemployment, and Safety Nets,* Available at SSRN: https://ssrn.com/abstract=3543987 or http://dx.doi.org/10.2139/ssrn.3543987 (accessed on 27 June 2021).

37. Sanders, T. (2020). *Protecting sex workers: Developing policy where sexuality, law and society meet,* University of Leicester, Retrieved from: https://le.ac.uk/research/stories/social-justice/sex-workers (accessed on 27 June 2021).

38. Concern, C. (2020). *Coronavirus lockdown and the devastating grip of porn,* Retrieved from: https://christianconcern.com/comment/coronavirus-lockdown-and-the-devastating-grip-of-porn/ (accessed on 27 June 2021).

39. Love, T., Laier, C., Brand, M., Hatch, L., & Hajela, R. (2015). *Neuroscience of Internet Pornography Addiction: A Review and Update, Behavioral sciences (Basel, Switzerland),* Volume. *5,* 388–433.

CHAPTER 12

Impact of COVID-19 on Interpersonal Relations and Behavioral Aspects of the People

T. SOWDAMINI

GITAM Institute of Management, GITAM (Deemed to be) University, Visakhapatnam, Andhra Pradesh, India, Mobile: + 91-9885532350, E-mail: sthatta@gitam.edu

12.1 INTRODUCTION

COVID-19, this had become the buzzword in 2020. On 11th March 2020, World Health Organization (WHO) has confirmed the outbreak of 'Novel Coronavirus Disease (in short known as coronavirus)' as a pandemic and called upon all the countries around the world to take appropriate measures to save humanity [52]. Currently, the COVID-19 is the most prevalent worldwide event, which has evenly impacted the societies across the world, where the governments and organizations have compelled to take necessary actions in protecting their people [1].

What has caused this change? Coronavirus causes respiratory complications similar to that of flu, which can spread through the air. The pandemic had made the Educational Institutes, Work Places, Eateries close their businesses; people have called off or deferred their societal commitments, which have impacted the mental state of the people [2]. The whole world is under lockdown, which has undoubtedly interrupted the lifestyle of humans and some studies show that this disturbance of lockdown, social distancing, and isolation has increased the impact on physiological factors of an individual to a large extent. Apart from these, the tumbling economies, loss of jobs, loss in business, or no trade has impacted their mental behavior and interpersonal relations too [3].

Due to lockdown, people unable to socialize, which has led to loneliness, anxiety issues, stress, mental breakdowns, which influenced behaviors and thereby crushing interpersonal relations between them [2]. This pandemic not only impacted business but also resulted in a change in the attitude and behaviors of human beings [53].

The global economy has been impacted by COVID-19 majorly in three different systems; firstly, it will affect the production / the manufacturing of goods by interrupting the supply chain, secondly on the financial markets, and finally on the public and their response to the epidemic [4]. On the other hand, there is an immense pressure building up between the government and scientists due to this pandemic where the former wants rapid results, and the latter wants accurate results.

Researchers and funding agencies must mobilize their resources to comprehend the "psychological, social, and neuroscientific" impacts of COVID-19 on humanity. Thus, the knowledge gained will help in identifying the issue and providing solutions for the metal imbalances caused by such epidemics [5].

The COVID-19 will not show any economic disparity. It is like the justice of Thanos- "indiscriminate and randomized." It will latch upon to you irrespective of you being rich or poor, black, or white, unless you are careful (News 18, n.d.). This chapter is bifurcated into six sections. Section 12.1 deals with the introduction part. Section 12.2 elucidates on interpersonal relations and how COVID has impacted the same; Section 12.3 talks about the changes brought by COVID in the behavioral patterns of the people; Section 12.4 discusses how the COVID has altered the course of life; Section 12.5 being the back to basics. Finally, the chapter concludes with the findings and concluding remarks.

12.2   INTERPERSONAL RELATIONSHIPS

Interpersonal skills entail the ability to share and construct relationships with others. Interpersonal relationships often need two individuals who are dependent on each other, where the behavior of one is affected by others. Humans are social beings who are continuously in touch with their friends and relatives by influencing one another. Relationships like kith and kin, friendships, and professional relations, may vary from person to person based on their needs and perceptions [6]. The learning of an individual is often influenced by the quality of the relationships they had. The quality of relationships imbibes specific values and beliefs, which will last longer and will have a more significant impact on the individual's performance and career [7]. For example, a student having a good relationship with his /her teacher reflects on their behavior and academic records. Thus, these good attributes transfer to one another like a baton in a race. Offices and Education Institutes will create an environment for people to socialize. Most of the people socialize not just to learn or to work but also to enhance their interpersonal relations. More often, interpersonal relations are described as an alliance between two or more persons, which extends from informal communication to formal arrangements such as wedlock.

Before COVID-19, the interpersonal relationships were not that good too. Unfortunately, relationships between families were deteriorating due to excessive digitization, usage of social apps like WhatsApp, and games like PUBG. However, the relationship with friends and at the workplace was flourishing. This unprecedented pandemic situation has restructured multiple relationships. Due to social distancing and lockdowns, people started living in closed quarters, mostly with their family members that have resulted in isolating their friends [8]. According to a survey amid COVID-19, more than half of the senior citizens felt that health and relationship with their children are weakening [9]. Already 70% of the elders had health problems or developed new complications amid the pandemic. An increase in anxiety, loss of appetite, insomnia disorders were also witnessed in the elders that had a more significant impact on their interpersonal relations with the family [10]. On the other hand, the lockdown had a troublesome experience for the children and youngsters. Indefinite closure of schools, fear of elders getting infected, inadequate personal space, mounting financial load on parents, frequent quarrels between parents will have long-term consequences on their interpersonal relations with family members [11, 12].

The COVID-19 has created an immeasurable psychosocial disturbance among the population, which has drastically changed the relationships between them. Due to the isolation, most of the time, the families are staying inbound and in closed circles. In the initial days of lockdown, people were happy as they are getting time to spend with their families. After some days, homemakers were getting restless due to (a) increase in household work, (b) demands from the family for the variety of foods which were previously being ordered from outside, and (c) above all, the absence of servant maid [13]. This stress is even more on working women. For some, Work from Home (WFH) is a boon, and for some, it is a bane. WFH is very new for most of the people in India; usually, while people are at the office, daily chores and kids at home will least bother them; however, that is not the case while performing WFH. Sometimes it so happens those individuals working from home need to attend to numerous non-work burdens such as helping the kids in completing the homework, attending to the needs of the elders as they are advised to stay at home, and help the spouse with the daily chores [14]. Due to WFH, individuals are spending long hours on systems, and staying at home for extended hours is taking a toll on their minds [15]. These tensions between spouses have impacted their married life, and they were going for divorces [8].

Not only have the relationships between families been rotten, but they were clashes seen between neighbors and owners of the houses in the midst of the COVID-19. Issues with landlords, as a lot of individuals have lost their jobs due to lockdown and were unable to pay the rent. Some of the landlords have announced a waiver of rent or provisioned deferred payments to the tenants, which is a noble gesture. However, not all the landlords can afford it, especially those whose primary income is rent [16, 17]. Apart from the economic issue, the fear of uncertainty towards COVID-19 has bought bizarre changes in people's relations. Some examples of those behaviors are where the landlord has locked the COVID-19 positive tenants inside the house or drove them out of the house [18].

Further, the lockdown and the fear of disease have created tensions between neighboring countries, states, towns, and villages. Factually, issues like mob clashes, stone-pelting, and even sealing/building walls at borders were seen. Hostile situations were observed in the Indo-Pak and Indo-Nepal borders. Even the migrant works returning from the cities were not allowed inside their native places [19]. The unprecedented change due to the pandemic has caused people to panic, increased stress levels on them, which impacted their interpersonal relationships with family, friends, relatives, and neighbors. These changes have affected their communication, mental stability, and even the thought process [20]. In other words, change in behavior was observed in people and in their relationships, were often influenced by the actions of others.

In order to cope up with, one should be emotionally vigilant, respect others, and be empathic. When the family members are stressed out, give support, and try to cheer them out, have a fixed routine. Make most of the mornings, as the elders say, waking up early in the morning gives you an extra time which can be utilized for meditation, morning stroll for vitamin D, and exercise, which will be beneficial for the whole day. This routine will help the students to concentrate on their studies. In order to eliminate the misunderstanding between the family and friends, listen, and talk carefully (Hassaan Ahmed, n.d.). Since people are unable to socialize physically, they can have group video calls and group chats with friends and relatives to hang out [21, 22]. Across the globe, governments have come forward to help those who are financially burdened by rescheduling the lending, leveraging rules on tax and PF (Pension Fund) contributions, etc., [23].

12.3 BEHAVIORAL CHANGES

Theoretically, behavioral change means the alteration or transformation in the behaviors of human beings, which is classified as Optimistic, Pessimistic, Trusting, and Envious [24]. It is evident from the studies that in the event of infectious diseases, there are negative impacts on society vide sickness, rise in the death toll, unemployment, and discrimination. Historically it was viewed that the individuals changed their habits and accustomed to use masks in public places, wash hands regularly, avoid the public/crowded places when an outbreak of severe acute respiratory syndrome (SARS) and the pandemic of A/H1N1 influenza was occurred in 2003 and 2009, respectively [25]. This kind of change can be considered positive (optimistic) in nature.

The COVID-19 is a new virus that humanity has not encountered before, which has terrible effects across the world, which has created panic, chaos, and anxiety within the public. Due to lockdown, people were sitting at their houses and continuously checking all digital platforms, which has increased the panic levels among the population. Among that, one of the notified issues was Doom Scrolling, which is defined as "the act of endlessly scrolling down on news app for the bad news." Following negative news and watching the screen always will affect mental stability and physical health, respectively [54].

As per UNESCO, approximately 1.6 billion students, around 160 countries have been affected by the school closures. In a typical situation shutting educational institutes can be considered as a boon for the students. As the transmission in the closed quarters is higher, the closing of schools was obligatory for the governments to curtail the pandemic but also to save the lives. Educational institutes are not only for enlightening but also act as a place where the children socialize themselves, respect elders and at the same time have a physical exercise, which is very important for their growth [11]. Due to this lockdown, children developed unhealthy food habits, inconsistent sleep patterns, hostile diet plans, longer durations with the smartphone, and television, which in the long run, have negative impacts on their physical and mental health (Figure 12.1) [26].

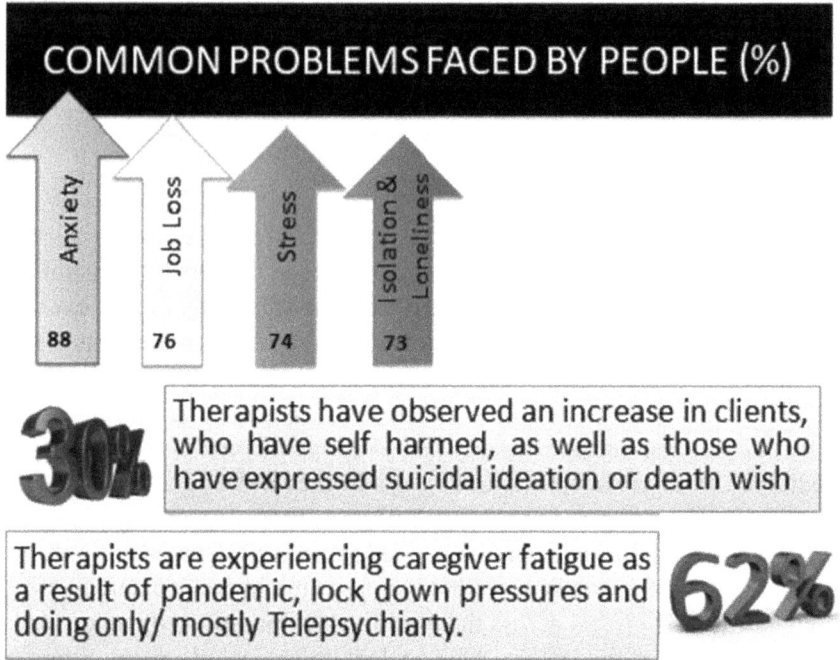

FIGURE 12.1 Common problems faced by people.
Source: https://timesofindia.indiatimes.com/india/spike-in-self-harm-suicide-ideation-amid-covid-19-pandemic/articleshow/77142884.cms.

COVID-19 has touched every walk of life, business, and industry irrespective of their size; unemployment is off the charts due to increased furloughs. Insecurity has increased, and family finances are out of balance as the breadwinners have lost their livelihood [27]. As per the report by the International Labor Organization (ILO), 54% of the youth lost their jobs due to their companies ceased to conduct business or the employees were laid off. Employees, especially in the fields of admin services, sales, and marketing, handicrafts, and other ancillary businesses, have ceased functioning [28]. Among those who lost their jobs, the migrant laborers and informal workers are those who have been asked to move to their home town within a short period, which is a very strenuous task in the lockdown period. Deprived of work, lack of transportation facilities and starving family has created so much stress on their mind, which provoked them to attack others [9, 55, 56]. From the industry, perceptive travel and tourism and Hospitality were majorly hit by COVID-19, which had a direct impact on middle and lower-income groups. Multiple eateries have closed permanently, which had an immediate effect on unskilled and semiskilled laborers and an indirect effect on their families [29]. If the effect of the epidemic on labor and job can be valued aptly, then it will be easy to guide those employees out of the situation.

As said earlier, the loss of jobs indirectly impacted the families of the breadwinners, especially the caregivers (women/housewives). At the same time, the economies have slowed down where people are not allowed to go to their workplace due to the lockdown restriction. However, women did not have this comfort (even applicable to the working women), as they need to take care of their family needs; most of the time, their efforts are considered to be unpaid jobs [30]. The hectic household work and the bleak sources of income have thrown out the mental stability of caregivers. The schedule of homemakers has been altered, due to which an increase in the level of frustration and frequent loss of temper was observed [31].

The current pandemic situation can intensify the anxiety issues and uncontrollable behaviors of those who had a previous history of mental health conditions and can view sensitive traumatic responses in this outbreak [32]. The change of behaviors has been noticed in the front liners (Doctors, Public Servants, Sanitation Staff, Nurses, Health Workers, Policemen, and others) due to long hours of working, wearing personal protective equipment (PPE), missing their families, which resulted in mental break downs, abnormal behaviors, and fatigue.

The biggest enemy of the individuals is fear-fear of getting infected or fear of dying or fear of losing dear ones, or fear of the future. Like fuel to the fire, the fake news has intensified the terror in public [33]. The fear has made specific individuals make absurd decisions such as taking life (suicide). There are cases found where the COVID-positive persons committed suicides due to fear of suffering, and on the other family members of COVID-19 have committed suicide in fear of pain their loved ones going thru [3]. The suicidal tendencies have increased in youngsters too, as per the recent report, 66 youngsters (below the age of 18) have committed suicide since the lockdown where the reasons are ridiculous, for example, parent scolding the child for not attending the online classes or for downloading a shady video (Figure 12.2) [34, 35].

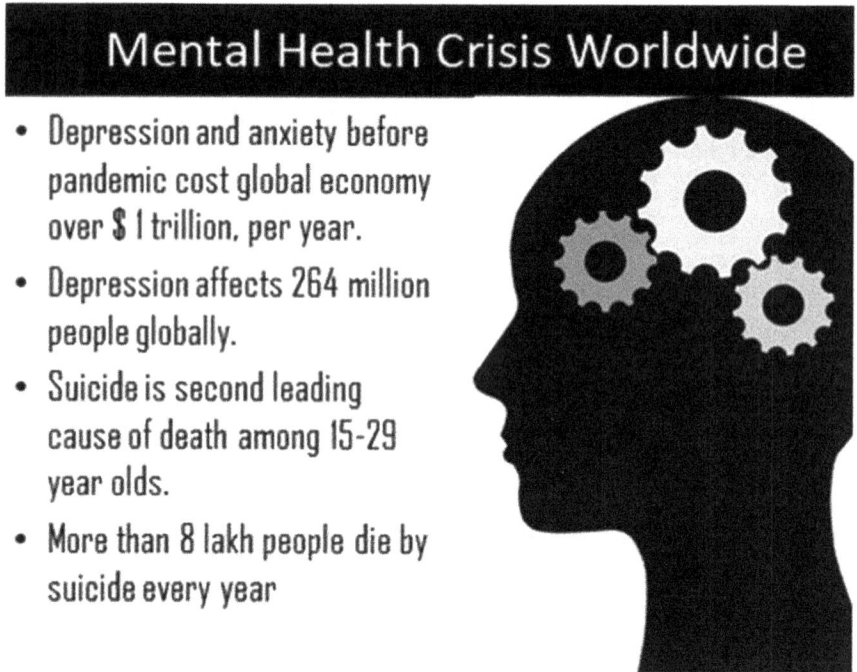

Mental Health Crisis Worldwide

- Depression and anxiety before pandemic cost global economy over $ 1 trillion, per year.
- Depression affects 264 million people globally.
- Suicide is second leading cause of death among 15-29 year olds.
- More than 8 lakh people die by suicide every year

FIGURE 12.2   Mental health crisis worldwide.
Source: WHO.

Discrimination is the prejudicial action of people basing on their creed, color, caste, or sex. Often, society's endangered with the communal disease is allied with ethnicity. People have shown a high level of intolerance and corrective actions towards these groups [36]. For example, people have barged onto Chinese and their companies blaming them for the epidemic.

Most of the epidemics have taught us something or the other. Initially, there may be negative behavioral changes observed among the population; however, after some time, the mind will make an alliance with the situation and will try to think positively. In the future, some optimistic behavioral will persevere. In the "New Normal," we can see many working and operating their businesses remotely, online shopping, watching online content vide OTT. Online food delivery will increase to reduce public exposure, and on the health front rise in access to health websites, well-being apps, and the purchase of fitness tracker products like Fitbit can be seen [37].

12.4 CHANGING LINES

It is quite evident in the history that any significant event had a drastic transformation on the humankind. Initially, the pandemic took the population by surprise, which has stalled the business, closed the schools and colleges and traveling was banned. Everything in life comes in sets like day and night, strength, and weakness, and so on; on one side, the COVID-19 threatened our existence and on the other showed opportunities [38]. Immediate changes were seen are the WFH and people concentrating on hygiene habits; however, the million-dollar question of how long this will sustain. As said earlier, people have lost jobs in the pandemic; however, some have not lost their hope and shifted their talent to other jobs. A software engineer from Orissa has lost a job, which has changed is the course of life. After returning home, he has used his idle time to reshape this future, and without any remorse, he has started "Biofloc fish farming." On the same lines, a software engineer from Telangana began selling vegetables. She states that "she does not believe false prestige and thus is doing her best to survive the economic crisis" [39, 40].

On the other hand, there was a drastic change seen in the climate around the world. Due to lockdowns, a massive reduction of global carbon emission was noticed as transportation and industries were stalled globally. There was a positive change observed in the behavior and attitude of individuals towards the environment. The upturn is temporary, which has only a partial consequence on the carbon emissions in the environment [41]. Globally the power consumption was dropped by 6%; there were fewer vehicles in the air and on-road, due to which the demand for petrol and diesel was reduced by 5% [42].

The COVID-19 had a devastating impact on trade where the businesses have permanently closed their shutters, reduced their manpower, and moved to digitalization. To passable this phase of uncertainty, certain businesses have adopted diversification as the mantra. Some retail stores have taken the most accessible option of moving to groceries, food, and health, which is safe and a sound idea. The main reason for the businesses to diversify is to maintain income and to sustain in these dire times. Some of the entities have gone a mile extra and started manufacturing medical kits such as PPE, which helped the governments in tackling the COVID situations [43, 44]. Some diversifications were like a double-edged sword giving business opportunities for both parties involved. For example, MOMO foods, after encountering the business loss, have diversified into groceries by collaborating with ITC, Nestle, and

P&G. Some of the fashion houses and breweries have divulged into making masks and sanitizers, respectively, in order to recoup some losses [45, 46].

12.5 BACK TO SQUARE ONE

Before COVID-19, the lifestyle of people was lavish, careless, and things were taken for granted. A lot of unnecessary expenses were identified like food wastage, weekend outings, less time spent with family and elders—more junk food consumed than healthy food. The youngsters were not listening to their elders on good and healthy habits. However, all these have been changed by the pandemic, which has set the time backward. In Hindi, there is a saying *"sau sunaar kee ek lohaar kee"* which translates to "A single blow of a blacksmith is equal to 100 blows of a goldsmith" in a way, we can relate this to the pandemic which has set the things like compassion and environmental protection where other movements of the 20th century have failed [47].

Generation X must have seen the basics coming into the habits of society, which are not new to them. Now people have started washing their hands before and after eating, changing clothes after coming from outside, maintaining social distance, wearing masks, however these hygienic habits which were part and parcel of certain cultures and creeds. In rural India, many families have a habit of washing their feet and hands before going into the house; the same is not evident in the urban areas for which there may reason like the dwelling we live, which do not encompass the comfort of the open space (Table 12.1) [48].

TABLE 12.1 Benefits from Hygienic Habits

Habits	Benefits
Washing hands before and after eating	Reduction in paper wastage
	Being hygienic
Avoiding eating outside	Reduction in unnecessary expenditure
	Healthy food habits
Social Distancing	Reduction in infection of corona and other commutable diseases
Using Masks	Reduces the direct exposure towards airborne infections

Source: Authors own elaboration.

Unfortunately, in urban areas, people are so accustomed to walking in with footwear inside the house, sense of dragging the dust and infections from outside lacks in the people. The simple thing of purification of themselves with water before entering any holy shrine is vital in many religions. Factually these hygiene practices have saved a lot of rural people from being infected in the time of the epidemic. Personal hygiene and tidiness in the community are indispensable and interdependent, too [49]. Even though India is viewed as an unclean country, but historically Indians are known for meticulously following hygienic methods. In Ancient India, the discipline of sanitation is enforced very rigorously, and those who do not obey are disconnected and deprived.

The COVID-19 outbreak has shown the gaps in the human behaviors and lifestyles, but happy to learn that the hygienic habits have returned to the people, which is evident from the increase of the purchase of sanitizers and other hygienic products. Further, even governments are also taking enough precautions and maintaining a sanitized environment.

12.6   CONCLUDING COMMENTS

The pandemic coronavirus or COVID-19 has ruthlessly disrupted the way of life we are living. The chapter has elucidated how COVID has impacted the interpersonal relations and brought the behavioral change in human beings. Though the COVID-19 has hindered the way we live, it has not blocked our existence. In these dire times, we need to understand how important it is to support each other mentally and physically. It is quite eminent that the people lose their temperament when something big like this occurs; however, others should understand and empathize with the situation.

Further, in this chapter, we comprehended that the biggest enemy is not the disease but the fear of getting infected or dying. Many were disturbed and diluted due to the pandemic; at the same time, some showed bravery and humanity by helping others, such as providing food and amenities. The governments globally have come with schemes and initiatives to assist the business bounce back on to the track. Most of the predicaments that were existing between family members were resolved in the lockdown, which is a positive sign. Due to job losses, there was uncertainty in people's minds; however, some have shown courage and determination in finding new jobs and careers to support their families. On the climatic front, we were able to see a reduction in oil consumption, which in turn reduced the pollution, and see clear skies, which is evident by the visibility of the Himalayas from "smog-choked towns" in India. The pandemic made its mark on interpersonal relations and behavior aspects of the public, where some were cracked, and some are healing. Except in a few places, the lockdown has been lifted and is now being called "New Normal." The positive side of the epidemic is that it has taught humanity the significance of being hygiene, to be positive in thinking and negative to Corona. The current hygiene makeover was a movement driven by the epidemic, and one day the coronavirus will be contained; however, hygienic habits should not be. In future studies, we hope more researchers will dwell on the intricacies of interpersonal relations and behavioral aspects at the micro-level.

KEYWORDS

- COVID-19
- hygiene
- interpersonal relationships
- mental health
- pandemic
- social distancing

REFERENCES

1. Accenture, (2020). *How Organizations Should Respond to the Never Normal Now Next.* https://www.accenture.com/_acnmedia/Thought-Leadership-Assets/PDF-2/Accenture-COVID-19-New-Human-Truths-That-Experiences-Need-To-Address.pdf (accessed on 27 June 2021).
2. Singh, J., & Singh, J., (2020). Electronic research journal of social sciences and humanities ISSN: 2706 – 8242. *Electronic Research Journal of Social Sciences and Humanities, 2*(I), 168–172. www.eresearchjournal.com (accessed on 27 June 2021).
3. Dsouza, D. D., Quadros, S., Hyderabadwala, Z. J., & Mamun, M. A., (2020). Aggregated COVID-19 suicide incidences in India: Fear of COVID-19 infection is the prominent causative factor. *Psychiatry Research, 290*, 17–20. https://doi.org/10.1016/j.psychres.2020.113145.
4. Bachman, D., (2020). *The Economic Impact of COVID-19 (novel coronavirus).* Deloitte Insights. https://www2.deloitte.com/us/en/insights/economy/covid-19/economic-impact-covid-19.html (accessed on 27 June 2021).
5. Holmes, E. A., Connor, R. C. O., Perry, V. H., Tracey, I., Wessely, S., Arseneault, L., Ballard, C., et al., (2020). Position Paper Multidisciplinary research priorities for the

COVID-19 pandemic: A call for action for mental health science. *The Lancet Psychiatry*, 547–560. https://doi.org/10.1016/S2215-0366(20)30168-1.

6. Sravanti, L., (2018). Interpersonal relationships: Building blocks of a society. *Indian Journal of Psychiatry, 59*(1), 2017–2018. https://doi.org/10.4103/psychiatry. IndianJPsychiatry.

7. Martin, A. J., & Dowson, M., (2009). Interpersonal relationships, motivation, engagement, and achievement: Yields for theory, current issues, and educational practice. *Review of Educational Research, 79*(1), 327–365. https://doi.org/10.3102/0034654308325583.

8. Yi-Ling, L., (2020). *As Many Countries Around the World Begin to Emerge from Lockdown, What Can We Learn from how People's Relationships and Friendships Have Fared in China, Where Coronavirus Began?* https://www.bbc.com/future/article/20200601-how-is-covid-19-is-affecting-relationships (accessed on 27 June 2021).

9. Joy, S., & Jitheesh, P. M., (2020). *Relationship Between Elderly and Younger Family Members Deteriorating During COVID-19 Lockdown: Survey.* https://www.deccanherald.com/national/north-and-central/relationship-between-elderly-and-younger-family-members-deteriorating-during-covid-19-lockdown-survey-829454.html (accessed on 27 June 2021).

10. Kanojia, A., (2020). *Impact of COVID-19 on Mental Health in India*. PsyArXiv. https://doi.org/doi.org/10.31234/osf.io/fkjsx.

11. Ghosh, R., Dubey, M. J., Chatterjee, S., & Dubey, S., (2020). Impact of COVID-19 on children: Special focus on the psychosocial aspect. *Minerva Pediatrica, 72*(3), 226–235. https://doi.org/10.23736/S0026-4946.20.05887-9.

12. Xiang, M., Zhang, Z., & Kuwahara, K., (2020). Impact of COVID-19 pandemic on children and adolescents' lifestyle behavior larger than expected. *Progress in Cardiovascular Diseases*. https://doi.org/10.1016/j.pcad.2020.04.013.

13. Khevna, P., (2020). *A Day in the Life of a Housewife Amid the COVID-19 Lockdown*. https://www.sakaltimes.com/maharashtra/day-life-housewife-amid-covid-19-lockdown...-49207 (accessed on 27 June 2021).

14. Cho, E., (2020). Examining boundaries to understand the impact of COVID-19 on vocational behaviors. *Journal of Vocational Behavior, 119*(xxxx), 2011–2013. https://doi.org/10.1016/j.jvb.2020.103437.

15. Sourabh, D., (2020). *COVID-19 Impact: Is Work from Home the New Normal?* https://www.financialexpress.com/lifestyle/covid-19-impact-is-work-from-home-the-new-normal/1981037/ (accessed on 27 June 2021).

16. Chandwani, S., (2020). *How to Avoid Landlord-Tenant Dispute Amid COVID-19 Crisis*. https://www.financialexpress.com/money/how-to-avoid-landlord-tenant-dispute-amid-covid-19-crisis/1946639/ (accessed on 27 June 2021).

17. Srivastava, N. K., (2020). *To Pay Rent, or Not? Tenant-Landlord Conflict in the Time of Coronavirus Legally Explained*. https://www.financialexpress.com/money/legal-view-on-tenant-landlord-conflict-rent-relationship-during-coronavirus-covid-19-pandemic-in-india-explained/1938353/ (accessed on 27 June 2021).

18. Express News Service, (2020). *While People Clapped for Those in Front line Fighting Virus, Telangana Landlords Leave Doctors Homeless*. https://www.newindianexpress.com/states/telangana/2020/mar/24/while-people-clapped-for-those-in-front-line-fighting-virus-telangana-landlords-leave-doctors-homele-2120839.html (accessed on 27 June 2021).

19. Bhaskar, S., (2020). *Fresh Tension at Border After Indian Villagers Thrashed by Nepal's Armed Police Force*. Hindustan Time. https://www.hindustantimes.com/india-news/fresh-tension-at-border-after-indian-villagers-thrashed-by-nepal-s-armed-police-force/story-LF6SCFg5agrDxts7Crii1M.html (accessed on 27 June 2021).
20. Frydrychowicz, S., (2005). The influence of interpersonal communication on human development. *Psychology of Language and Communication, 9*(2).
21. Kleptsova, E. Y., & Balabanov, A. A., (2016). Development of humane interpersonal relationships. *International Journal of Environmental and Science Education, 11*(8), 2147–2157. https://doi.org/10.12973/ijese.2016.585a.
22. Waldron, T., & James, W., (2020). *No Title*. https://hbr.org/2020/04/ensure-that-your-customer-relationships-outlast-coronavirus (accessed on 27 June 2021).
23. Adhil, S., (2020). *Six COVID-19 Relief Measures by Modi Govt Which Can Benefit Your Personal Finances*. Financial Express. https://www.financialexpress.com/money/6-covid-19-relief-measures-by-modi-govt-which-can-benefit-your-personal-finances/1985671/ (accessed on 27 June 2021).
24. Poncela-Casasnovas, J., Gutiérrez-Roig, M., Gracia-Lázaro, C., Vicens, J., & Gómez-Gardeñes, J., (2016). *Humans Display a Reduced set of Consistent Behavioral Phenotypes in Dyadic Games*, 1–8.
25. Verelst, F., Willem, L., & Beutels, P., (2016). *Behavioral Change Models for Infectious Disease Transmission: A Systematic Review (2010–2015), 13*(125), 20160820. https://doi.org/https://doi.org/10.1098/rsif.2016.0820.
26. Touyz, S., Lacey, H., & Hay, P., (2020). Eating disorders in the time of COVID-19. *Journal of Eating Disorders, 8*(1), 8–10. https://doi.org/10.1186/s40337-020-00295-3.
27. DePietro, A., (2020). *Here's a Look at the Impact of Coronavirus (COVID-19) On Colleges and Universities in the U.S.* FORBES. https://www.forbes.com/sites/andrewdepietro/2020/04/30/impact-coronavirus-covid-19-colleges-universities/#dda6b6161a68 (accessed on 27 June 2021).
28. ILO, (2020). *Tackling the COVID-19 Youth Employment Crisis in Asia and the Pacific*. https://www.ilo.org/wcmsp5/groups/public/---ed_emp/documents/publication/wcms_753026.pdf (accessed on 27 June 2021).
29. Saraswathy, M., (2020). *10.8 Million and Counting: Take a Look at How Many Jobs COVID-19 has Wiped Out*. Money Control. https://www.moneycontrol.com/news/business/economy/10-8-million-and-counting-take-a-look-at-how-many-jobs-covid-19-has-wiped-out-5704851.html (accessed on 27 June 2021).
30. Power, K., (2020). The COVID-19 pandemic has increased the care burden of women and families. *Sustainability: Science, Practice, and Policy, 16*(1), 67–73. https://doi.org/10.1080/15487733.2020.1776561.
31. Asia Insurance Post, (2020). *Coronavirus: Keep a Check on Your Behavioral Changes During COVID-19 Pandemic*. Asia Insurance Post. https://www.asiainsurancepost.com/facts/coronavirus-keep-check-your-behavioural-changes-during-covid-19-pandemic (accessed on 27 June 2021).
32. Schoch-Spana, M., (2020). *COVID-19's Psychosocial Impacts*. https://blogs.scientificamerican.com/observations/covid-19s-psychosocial-impacts/ (accessed on 27 June 2021).
33. Roy, D., Tripathy, S., Kar, S. K., Sharma, N., Verma, S. K., & Kaushal, V., (2020). Study of knowledge, attitude, anxiety & perceived mental healthcare need in Indian population

during COVID-19 pandemic. *Asian Journal of Psychiatry, 51*, 102083. https://doi. org/10.1016/j.ajp.2020.102083.

34. Menon, P. C. S., (2020). *Spike in Self-Harm, Suicide Ideation Amid COVID Pandemic.* Times of India. https://timesofindia.indiatimes.com/india/spike-in-self-harm-suicide-ideation-amid-covid-19-pandemic/articleshow/77142884.cms (accessed on 27 June 2021).

35. Tribune India, (2020). *COVID-19 Triggering Panic Attacks, Depression and Suicides, Say Experts.* https://www.tribuneindia.com/news/nation/covid-19-triggering-panic-attacks-depression-and-suicides-say-experts-105222 (accessed on 27 June 2021).

36. Bavel, J. J. V., Baicker, K., Boggio, P. S., Capraro, V., Cichocka, A., Cikara, M., Crockett, M. J., et al., (2020). COVID-19 pandemic response. *Nature Human Behaviour, 4,* 460–471. https://doi.org/10.1038/s41562-020-0884-z.

37. Mohanbir, S., (2020). *The New Normal: 7 Behavioral Shifts that Will Persist Past the Pandemic.* LinkedIn. https://www.linkedin.com/pulse/new-normal-7-behavioral-shifts-persist-past-pandemic-mohanbir-sawhney (accessed on 27 June 2021).

38. Rohrich, R. J., Hamilton, K. L., Avashia, Y., & Savetsky, I. M., (2020). The COVID-19 pandemic: Changing lives and lessons learned. *Plastic and Reconstructive Surgery - Global Open, 8*(4), 2854. https://doi.org/10.1097/GOX.0000000000002854.

39. Post News Network, (2020). *Lockdown Transforms Software Engineer into Fish Farmer in Jagatsinghpur.* Orissa Post. https://www.orissapost.com/lockdown-transforms-software-engineer-into-fish-farmer-in-jagatsinghpur/ (accessed on 27 June 2021).

40. Sakshi, (2020). *Jobless Woman Software Engineer Sells Vegetables for Livelihood in Warangal.* https://english.sakshi.com/news/andhrapradesh/jobless-woman-sotware-engineer-selling-vegetables-livelihood-warangal-121914 (accessed on 27 June 2021).

41. Renee, C., (2020). *COVID-19's Long-Term Effects on Climate Change—For Better or Worse.* https://blogs.ei.columbia.edu/2020/06/25/covid-19-impacts-climate-change/ (accessed on 27 June 2021).

42. Lombrana, L. M., & Warren, H., (2020). *Oil Tankers Anchor Off the Coast of Southern California as Demand for Oil and Refined Products Plunge.* Source: U.S. coast guard video by Petty Officer third class Aidan Cooney: A pandemic that cleared skies and halted cities isn't slowing global warming. Bloomberg. https://www.bloomberg.com/graphics/2020-how-coronavirus-impacts-climate-change/ (accessed on 27 June 2021).

43. Vadlamudi, S., (2020). *Small Traders Diversify to Survive Pandemic Impact.* The Hindu. https://www.thehindu.com/news/cities/Hyderabad/small-traders-diversify-to-survive-pandemic-impact/article32311280.ece (accessed on 27 June 2021).

44. Falconer, T., (2020). *Shifting Focus: How COVID-19 is Encouraging Diversification.* IBIS World. https://www.ibisworld.com/industry-insider/coronavirus-insights/shifting-focus-how-covid-19-is-encouraging-diversification/ (accessed on 27 June 2021).

45. Cushion, I., (2020). *How Businesses are Diversifying Amid the COVID-19 Crisis.* WHITE OAK UK. https://www.whiteoakuk.com/blog/how-businesses-are-diversifying-amid-the-covid-19-crisis (accessed on 27 June 2021).

46. Thinking Hats Consumer Insights LLP, (2020). *Diversification - The Opportunity in Crisis.* Research Choices. https://researchchoices.org/covid19/findings/report/131/diversification-the-opportunity-in-crisis (accessed on 27 June 2021).

47. Ilyas, E. O., (2020). *A New Human Being Will Emerge in the Post-COVID-19 World.* https://www.orfonline.org/expert-speak/a-new-human-being-will-emege-in-the-post-covid-19-world-64275/ (accessed on 27 June 2021).

48. Namita, B., (2008). *Contradictions in the Indian Concept of Hygiene.* https://www.livemint.com/Politics/LAEvZVGuHxDtOT6WhRG9UP/Contradictions-in-the-Indian-concept-of-hygiene.html (accessed on 27 June 2021).

49. Suman, S., (2018). *The Paradox of Private Hygiene and Public Uncleanliness in India.* https://www.idealismprevails.at/en/the-paradox-of-private-hygiene-and-public-uncleanliness-in-india/ (accessed on 27 June 2021).

50. Hassaan, A., (n.d.). *Managing Your Relationship During COVID-19 Lockdown.* International Education Specialists. https://www.idp.com/global/blog/managing-relationships-COVID-story/ (accessed on 27 June 2021).

51. News 18, (n.d.). *Vulnerable Low-Income Groups, Racial Disparities: Lessons India Must Learn from US Healthcare System.* Retrieved from: https://www.news18.com/news/india/vulnerable-low-income-groups-racial-disparities-lessons-india-must-learn-from-us-healthcare-system-2567523.html (accessed on 27 June 2021).

52. WHO. (n.d.). *India further ramps up testing to curb the spread of COVID-19.* 2020. Retrieved August 10, 2020, from https://www.who.int/india/emergencies/coronavirus-disease-(covid-19)# (accessed on 24 July 2021).

53. Vijayaraghavan, P., & Singhal, D. (2020). *A Descriptive Study of Indian General Public's Psychological responses during COVID-19 Pandemic Lockdown Period in India.* 1–19. https://doi.org/10.31234/osf.io/jeksn (accessed on 24 July 2021).

54. Eenadu. (2020, August 9). *Say no to DoomScrolling.* 14. https://www.eenadu.net/sundaymagazine/article/320000692 (accessed on 24 July 2021).

55. Uma, S. (2020, April 29). *Migrant Workers Attack Employers, Cops At IIT-Hyderabad, Demand Wages.* https://www.ndtv.com/telangana-news/coronavirus-lockdown-migrant-workers-attack-cops-at-iit-hyderabad-demand-wages-passage-home-2220393 (accessed on 24 July 2021).

56. The Quint. (2020, March 30). *Surat: 93 Migrant Workers Held as They Defy Lockdown, Attack Cops.* https://www.thequint.com/news/india/covid-19-93-migrant-workers-held-for-violating-coronavirus-lockdown-attacking-cops (accessed on 24 July 2021).

PART IV
Role of Different Organizations and Professions

CHAPTER 13

Optimum Budget Allocation for Social Projects to Control the COVID-19 Pandemic: A Multi-Objective Nonlinear Integer Mathematical Model with a Novel Discrete Integer Gaining-Sharing Knowledge-Based Metaheuristic Algorithm

SAID ALI HASSAN,[1] PRACHI AGRAWAL,[2] TALARI GANESH,[2] and ALI WAGDY MOHAMED[3,4]

[1]*Department of Operations Research and Decision Support, Faculty of Computers and Artificial Intelligence, Cairo University, Egypt*

[2]*Department of Mathematics and Scientific Computing, National Institute of Technology Hamirpur, Himachal Pradesh – 177005, India*

[3]*Operations Research Department, Faculty of Graduate Studies for Statistical Research, Cairo University, Giza – 12613, Egypt*

[4]*Wireless Intelligent Networks Center (WINC), School of Engineering and Applied Sciences, Nile University, Giza, Egypt, E-mail: aliwagdy@gmail.com*

ABSTRACT

The resource allocation problem aims at achieving the best utilization of the available budget in governmental and non-governmental responsible parties for a proposed set of social control programs to fight against the COVID-19 pandemic. The best utilization is evaluated by determining a compromise solution to maximize the number of people who benefit from the intervention control programs and at the same to maximize the prioritized number of people relative to their category status of contact with the virus. The motivation to carry out this research comes from the extent of the seriousness of the coronavirus (COVID-19), which is currently spreading around the world, and the urgent need to implement a set of executive preventive social programs for different categories of people that help in preventing or treating the virus and helping families in which one of their relatives dies as a result of infection with the virus. The main objective of this chapter is to present a proposal for the optimum financial resource allocation (OFRA) for social intervention projects to control COVID-19 pandemic using a multi-objective nonlinear integer mathematical model.

The complete mathematical model for the problem is formulated, including the representation of the decision variables, the problem constraints, and the multi-objective functions. The proposed nonlinear integer mathematical model is applied to a real application case study in one district of Alexandria, Egypt (the second biggest city in Egypt). The case study is solved using a novel discrete integer gaining-sharing knowledge-based optimization algorithm (DIGSK). The detail procedure of the novel DIGSK is presented along with the complete steps for solving the case study.

13.1 INTRODUCTION

Currently, the entire world is suffering from a global epidemic of COVID-19 that has infected thousands of people in almost all countries [1]. In December last year, Wuhan in China, was the origin of pneumonia of unknown cause. By Jan in this year, assured cases were detected outside Wuhan [2].

Nowadays, the new coronavirus (COVID-19) put humans in all countries in front of the huge danger. The Centers for Decease Control and Prevention (CDC) declares the major signs of COVID-19 so that any individual can discover whether or not he has such symptoms [3]. The updated worldwide total cases and deaths of coronavirus are recorded daily [4]. The number of confirmed infected cases in all countries clarify that this is a vast evolving case, new situation changes may not be represented at once. Although the confirmed numbers in some countries is moderate till now, but numbers are expected to increase as new cases are discovered [5].

In light of this spread of this devastating pandemic, governmental, and non-governmental institutions are joining together to control the spread of the epidemic. This is done by proposing a set of social programs and activities to contribute to the awareness, treatment, and helping the economically and socially affected different people categories. Here, the role of allocating financial resources and distributing them to these proposed programs is highlighted, in order to achieve the highest desired benefit and aid reaching the largest number of people in the studied community.

The resource allocation may focus on specific types of resources, and budgetary allocation may be the most important type of these resources. The financial resource allocation to control COVID-19 pandemic is of great importance. This should be considered at the level of specialists and researchers for the optimal utilization of the available budget for both the governmental and non-governmental authorized parties.

This research is concerned with the optimal allocation of the available budget so that the optimal use of the budget is achieved, and the largest number of targeted people are effectively supported. At the same time, priority is given to people categories according to their conditions and infection by the virus, so that more weight is given to those who are in more dangerous status than others.

The structure of the chapter is as follows: Section 13.1 presents the introduction containing a concise point contents for each section in this chapter. Section 13.2 and its subsections explain the Epidemiological Model of COVID-19, Financial Resource Allocation Problem, Epidemic Social Control Programs, Mathematical Model for the Resource Allocation Problem, and A Real Application Case Study. proposes some social intervention control programs to help fighting against the COVID-19 epidemic. Nine different proposed control programs for both governmental and non-governmental parties to help all people categories: ordinary, contacts, infected, recovered, and deceased are suggested. The mathematical representation for the optimum financial resource allocation (OFRA) to control COVID-19 pandemic is designed, including all needed formulations. The proposed model is an Integer Nonlinear Constrained Multi-Objective formulation; the steps of the solution procedure are also explained. A Real Application Case Study in one district in Alexandria, the second big city in Egypt with all relative data is explained. In Section 13.3 the proposed solution methodology is introduced as a novel discrete integer version of a recently developed gaining-sharing knowledge-based technique (GSK) for solving the OFRA. GSK cannot solve the problem with discrete integer space; therefore, discrete Integer-GSK optimization algorithm (DIGSK) is proposed with two new discrete integer junior and senior stages. These stages allow DIGSK to inspect the problem search space efficiently. Section 4 gives the conclusions and the suggested points for future research.

13.2   METHODS AND MATERIALS

13.2.1   *EPIDEMIOLOGICAL MODEL OF COVID-19*

Suddenly, as a part of this world, we found ourselves face to face in front of a battle with COVID-19, the virus that necessitated tackling it, honing all medical efforts, and raising the level of preparedness in all sectors of health concerned.

Over the last few decades, mathematical models for the transmission of diseases were useful to gain information about the dynamics of transmission [6, 7]. Four commonly used phenomenological models are considered to mimic the initial exponential growth rate of an epidemic (Logistic, delayed logistic, Richards, and Exponential) in estimating initial epidemic growth rates [8].

The allocation of resources for epidemic control is not an easy task. A major source of complexity is that epidemics of infectious disease are dynamic and nonlinear. Figure 13.1 illustrates a typical S-shaped curve of epidemic growth.

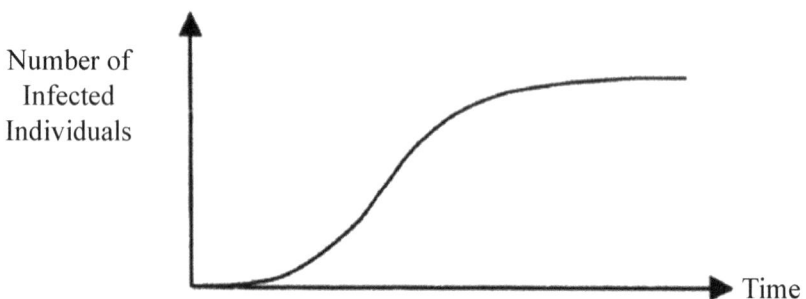

FIGURE 13.1   A typical S-shaped curve of epidemic growth.

The epidemiological model of COVID-19 is depicted in Figure 13.2; it is assumed that all people fall into one of five *categories*: Ordinary (O), Contacts (C), Infected (I), Recovered (R) or deceased (D). The "ordinary" category represents persons who have never catch the virus. The "contacts" are the individuals are those who are in contact with persons who are infected with the virus but who are not assured to become infected. The "infected" individuals are people who are infected with the virus and are contagious. The "recovered" are persons who are infected and survived. Finally, the "deceased" category represents the number of fatalities due to the virus. One should note that some persons may never leave the susceptible category (persons who do not contract the virus).

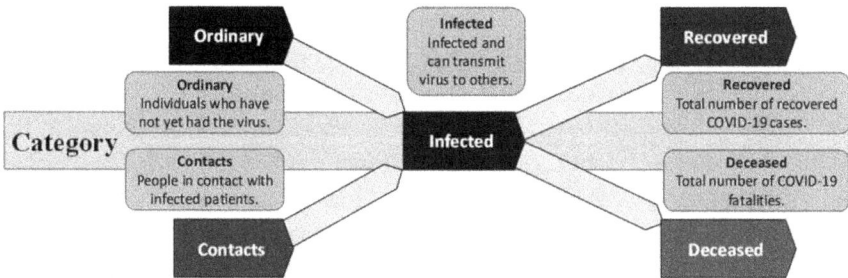

FIGURE 13.2   Scheme of the proposed epidemic model.

13.2.2   *FINANCIAL RESOURCE ALLOCATION PROBLEM TO CONTROL COVID-19 PANDEMIC*

Resource allocation is a critical part of managing any project(s), resources may include financial, technological, and human resources. When a task, project or program is to be accomplished, resources allocated is needed to the project to help get it done. Resource allocation is part of resource management or strategic management [9]. Budgetary allocations indicate the amount of money a community is allocating to a program.

The study may be focused on allocating monetary resources to specific purposes. As an example, Danneels's [10] study allocating financial, human, and technological resources to new entry to market. Souder and Shaver [11] studied the influence of managerial compensation on firms when put money into long-horizon payoffs capital projects; Maritan [12] compares the processes used to invest in new versus existing operational capabilities. Busenbark et al. [13] studied business capital allocation for reinforcement of the relation between capital allocation and business strategy. Ahuja and Novelli [14] focused on the allocation of financial resources to functional activities. Bardot et al. [15] observed that capital allocations to business units in a multi-business firm should not be done as independent but connected with evaluating all the possibilities. Vieregger et al. [16] challenged the idea of spreading the capital equally among an organization's business units.

A financial allocation model (RAM) is a methodology for determining where financial resources should be allocated within an organization. The problem is highly complex; the first complexity comes from the fact that distinct people categories generally have diverse risk of being infected, protecting a higher-risk one from being infected now may save other persons from infection later. However, the allocation of a large amount of protecting resources to high-risk persons may cause infection to other low-risk persons. Thus, the best allocation of resources may not engage the allocation of all the resources to high-risk persons. A second difficulty of allocating resources is the relation among expended resources and outcomes of a program; referred to as a "production function." For some situations, this production function can be linear in a manner that protecting one individual removes an individual from the infected category. For other cases, the production function may be nonlinear. A program may have a decreasing or increasing returns. A third complexity, epidemic social control programs may be correlated so that investing in one of them may influence other programs. As an example, an education program may raise the attention to the danger of an epidemic and then leverage the performance of other control programs. At last, the time span, whether it is long or short for the decision can influence the optimum decision [17].

13.2.3   COVID-19 EPIDEMIC SOCIAL CONTROL PROGRAMS

The most important governmental and non-governmental efforts and actions to confront the emerging coronavirus are based on the implementation of a group of national social projects at the state level and another group of projects at the level of governorates, cities, and villages. A list of those projects applied in a big city in Gharbia Governorate in Egypt is presented in Table 13.1 together with the relevant category and responsible party, where the symbols (O, C, I, R, and D) are for the Ordinary, Contacts, Infected, Recovered, and Deceased categories respectively; the symbols (G and N) denote the responsible party whether the Government or Nongovernment respectively.

TABLE 13.1   Proposed Epidemic Control Programs

Responsible Party	Category	SL. No.	Epidemic Social Control Programs
G	O	1.	Governmental specific assistance program.
	C	2.	Governmental home isolation protocol for contacts.
	I	3.	Hospital treatment protocol for infected persons.
	I	4.	Governmental home protocol for infected persons.
	R	5.	Treatment with convalescence plasma.
	D	6.	Dealing with dead cases due to COVID-19.
N	O	7.	Non-governmental assistance program.
	C	8.	Non-governmental assistance for home isolation.
	I	9.	Non-governmental home protocol for infected persons
	D	10.	Non-governmental assistance for families of dead cases.

A brief explanation of each of these control intervention programs for both the governmental and non-governmental parties is given in the following subsections.

13.2.3.1   *GOVERNMENTAL SOCIAL INTERVENTION PROGRAMS:*

i.   **Governmental Specific Assistance Program:** A series of strict preventive measures are being taken by the government, including the imposition of curfews in the evening; the suspension of air traffic; analyzing and tracking contacts; the closure of mosques and churches; the suspension of studies in schools and universities; the closure of cinemas, theaters, major malls, restaurants, parks, and beaches; and the analysis of quarantine for returnees from abroad. The preventive measures to raise the level of infection prevention and control is based on a number of pivots, foremost of which is raising awareness of people to social spacing and commitment to personnel protection measures. Other prevention activities include the advancement of the health sector, the provision of sterilization and disinfection tools and materials, raising the awareness of citizens about how to avoid infection with the virus, launching a national campaign for disinfection. All these measured are performed by the government at the national level for all citizens in all governorates of the country.

A complimentary special important program which is considered here is to provide virus protection materials and distribute them free of charge to people with low incomes, to distribute foods to poor families, to give cash grants to individuals who have lost their jobs, and distribute medicines that raise natural immunity to poor families, elderly people and those with chronic diseases and other financial and social aid for those in need.

ii. **Governmental Home Isolation Protocol for Contacts:** Home insulation is a separation carried out for those who are supposed to have had contact with an infected person or a foot on areas where the disease appeared. It is performed for a person who did not show clear symptoms of infection and his conditions do not require staying in the hospital according to the evaluation of the medical team. The person remains in his home for two weeks-the incubation period of the virus in the body until no injury is confirmed or negative test result.

The Ministry of Health has circulated to the health directorates in all governorates a list of medicines used in the treatment of the emerging coronavirus, according to the therapeutic guidelines.

COVID-19 home hygiene guidelines:

- Staying at home unless for medication;
- Do not use public transportation means as possible;
- Stay at home in a separate place with a special toilet if possible;
- Avoid mixing with animals;
- Wear a muzzle when out of the house for necessity or when around other people;
- Cover the nose and mouth when coughing and sneezing with a tissue and dispose it;
- Keep away from sharing personal household items with other people;
- Clean all frequently touched surfaces with sterilizers;
- Ensure that the common areas of the house are well ventilated;
- Wash hands with soap for more than least 20 seconds or with an antiseptic with at least 60% alcohol, especially after sneezing

and coughing, using the bathroom and before preparing food or eating. You should also avoid touching your mouth, nose, and eyes before washing hands;

- Monitor symptoms and when feeling a cough, high temperature or shortness of breath, a person should call the emergency phone and do not visit the hospital emergency directly to avoid transmitting the infection to others.

iii. **Hospital Treatment Protocol for Infected Persons:** The Ministry of Health and Population has published the latest protocol adopted by the Ministry's scientific committee to treat patients with the emerging coronavirus "COVID-19."

According to the WHO, the scientific committee added some new drugs to the protocol, such as "Lopinavir / Ritonavir" and an anti-HIV drug in the treatment of moderate and severe symptoms, to be inside hospitals and under direct medical supervision.

According to the protocol, giving AIDS medicine to patients will be another pathway with the drug "Hydroxychloroquine," which the committee has decided to keep in the treatment of some other cases.

There is an amendment to the treatment protocol for those affected with the virus, Tamiflu was removed, and alternatives to other antiviral drugs were added with Hydroxychloroquine, along with some medicines to strengthen immunity like vitamin C, zinc, and Antibiotics. The therapeutic protocol explains how to deal with the infected persons according to the clinical symptoms, whether for mild, moderate, or critical cases.

iv. **Governmental Home Treatment Protocol for Infected Persons:** The therapeutic protocol for the home isolation of people with coronavirus, which is determined by the Egyptian Ministry of Health and Population, affirmed that the infected cases that are allowed to be isolated at home are those that do not show symptoms at all, or the situation that shows minor symptoms and the doctor decides that they can receive treatment at home.

The ministry said that the aim of the therapeutic protocol is to follow up the improvement of the condition, follow up the appearance of signs of the severity of the disease, the non-transmission of infection to the rest of the family, and follow up with contacts.

The Ministry of Health added that the standard specifications for receiving Corona treatment include:

- Having a separate patient room;
- Having a private bathroom;
- There are no items in the patient's room that are not necessary for personal use.

The Ministry revealed the details of the drug doses that people get in-home isolation, and said that the patient gets Hydroxychloroquine 200 mg in the amount of 16 tablets for 6 days, Vitamin C 1 g in a total amount of 7 tablets for 7 days, Zinc 50 mg in a total amount of 7 tablets for 7 days, Lactoferrin sachets in a total amount of "14 sachets" for 7 days, Acetylcysteine 200 in the amount of "21 sachets" for 7 days, Paracetamol 500 mg with a total of 10 tablets obtained by the patient at high temperatures, and for children they receive Azithromycin syrup and Paracetamol syrup.

v. **Treatment with Convalescence Plasma:** Plasma treatment was one of the proposals that appeared last February to treat people infected with corona. China was the first country to announce testing of this technology with patients infected with COVID-19. This technology depends on the antibodies to the virus in the blood of recovered persons, the so-called "recovery plasma," which is derived from people who gradually restore their health after the disease and given to serious infected persons.

In April, American hospitals began using plasma to treat COVID-19 patients, and this came after the US Food and Drug Administration agreed to use this treatment. Egypt also began experimenting with plasma of recovering from the coronavirus, and the Ministry of Health withdrew samples from some of those recovered to use their plasma to treat the coronavirus patients.

National health authorities in many countries, called survivors of the coronavirus to donate blood in the hope of trying a promising plasma-based treatment for infected patients.

vi. **Governmental Assistance for Dead Cases Due to COVID-19:** The Ministry of Health and Population announced the procedures for dealing with deaths of corona's disease, confirming that the same precautions that were applied to the patient during his life should continue to be applied. To transfer of the body to the hospital refrigerator, the body is raised with the surrounding sheet and transported on a trolley that can be cleaned and disinfected taking into account the wearing of personal protection materials with the strict commitment to removing them in a correct manner and washing hands with the completion of removing the personal protection materials.

Procedures for transporting the body by ambulance:

- The body is transported after washing and shrouding inside a non-permeable bag, and the infection risk sign is marked on it.
- It should be noted that there are no people in the car other than ambulance personnel and only one of the relatives of the deceased.
- The body is placed in a closed box which can be cleaned and disinfected, taking into account not to open it except in the burial.
- Everyone in the car next to the corpse must commit to wearing the appropriate personal protective materials.
- While praying for the deceased, it should be noted that the box is not opened for any reason.

Burial procedures:

- When opening the box to transport the body inside the cemetery, the person in charge of the burial should wear the proper personal protective materials.
- Take into account the presence of the minimum number possible when entering the corpse to the cemetery.
- Complete commitment to washing hands or rubbing them with alcohol for everyone who deals with the deceased.
- Commitment to cleaning and disinfection of all work surfaces that have come into contact with the corpse starting from the deceased's bed, the dead-keeping refrigerator, the ambulance seats, and the dead transport box using disinfectants approved by the Ministry of Health such as liquid chlorine at a concentration of 5%.

13.2.3.2 *NON-GOVERNMENTAL SOCIAL INTERVENTION CONTROL PROGRAMS*

i.   **Non-Governmental Assistance Program:** The non-governmental sector with all constituents coordinates with each other with the aim of donating to the health and social care fund and providing all necessary means of support. The non-governmental sector is represented by major and small companies, social associations, religious institutions, popular institutions, charities, and a number of specialized unions. They provide protective materials, and all means of social and monetary support for elderly people with weak immunity, poor families, people who lost their jobs and for medical teams to alleviate the consequences of the negative consequences of the pandemic COVID-19.

iii. **Non-Governmental Assistance for Home Isolation:** Some civil societies and Non-governmental organizations launched initiatives to provide financial assistance for poor families to purchase food, medicine, disinfection materials, personal protection, and other necessary needs during the period of the home quarantine, especially those groups who lost their sources of income. The initiative is to enable poor families to receive weekly foodstuffs, and this was organized through a program that links the organization with a group of commercial stores. Some of these organizations not only work to provide aid, but also require that their beneficiaries receive training that enables them to start small projects themselves, ensuring their integration into social life.

iii. **Non-governmental Assistance for Home Treatment Protocol for Infected Persons:** Non-governmental organizations can assist in the therapeutic protocol for the home isolation of people with coronavirus, which is determined by the Egyptian Ministry of Health and Population. They help in providing treatment medicine necessary for infected persons; they can also help for providing protective materials, food, clothing, financial aid, and other needs.

iv. **Nongovernmental Assistance for Families of Dead Cases:** Non-governmental organizations and society societies can provide financial and moral assistance to the families of those who died as a result of the emerging coronavirus. Many of these families have lost their only breadwinner and need financial assistance to face life conditions. Also, these families are in urgent need of moral support to alleviate the shock of death due to the virus and the isolation imposed on them for fear of infection.

13.2.4   MATHEMATICAL MODEL FOR THE RESOURCE ALLOCATION PROBLEM

The model will be formulated as a multi-objective nonlinear problem as follows.

13.2.4.1   DECISION VARIABLES: LET

$x_{i,j}^k$ = The number of people (integer) to whom the epidemic control program No. i, for category of people j and responsible party k applies, $i = 1, 2, ..., n$.

$i \in I_j^k$ = Number of control projects in category j and for responsible party k.

$$j \in J = \{O, C, I, R, D\},$$

$$k \in K = \{G, N\}$$

where; O is the ordinary category; C is the contacts category; I is the infected category; R is the recovered category; D is the deceased category; G is the governmental responsibility; and N is the non-governmental responsibility.

13.2.4.2   CONSTRAINTS.

i   **Resource Constraints:** The amount of money spent for all control project by a responsible party should not exceed the available budget for that party:

$$\sum_{j \in J} \sum_{i \in I_j^k} f_{i,j}^k(x_{i,j}^k).x_{i,j}^k \leq B^k, \forall k \in K \tag{1}$$

where; $f_{i,j}^k(x_{i,j}^k)$ is a mathematical expression representing the cost of epidemic control project number with indices ($i, j,$ *and* k) as a function of the number of people $x_{i,j}^k$; B^k is the total budget available for responsible party k.

The mathematical expression of $f_{i,j}^k\left(x_{i,j}^k\right)$ as a function of $x_{i,j}^k$ can be a linear expression or a general nonlinear expression depending on the specific data relative to a considered case study.

ii. **Lower Bound for Each Program:** The minimum number of people who benefits from a specific program is not less than a lower bound. As requested by some donors, disbursements are made for this specific program.

$$x_{(i,j)}^k \geq L_{i,j}^k, i \in I_j^k, j \in J \text{ and } k \in K \tag{2}$$

where; $L_{i,j}^k$ is the lower bound for the number of people targeted by the program with indices i, j, and k.

iii. **Upper Bound for Each Program:** The number of people who benefits from a specific program should not exceed an upper bound limited by technical and administrative restrictions.

$$x_{i,j}^k \leq U_{i,j}^k, i \in I_j^k, j \in J \text{ and } k \in K \tag{3}$$

where; $U_{i,j}^k$ is the upper bound for the number of people targeted by the program with indices i, j, and k.

iv. **Maximum Number in Each Category:** The total number of people targeted by all programs for a specific category should not exceed the number of people in that category.

$$\sum_{j \in J} \sum_{k \in K} \sum_{i \in I_j^k} x_{i,j}^k \leq M_j, j \in J \tag{4}$$

where, M_j is the maximum number of people in category j.

Notes:

a. It is important to note that this constraint is redundant in case when the summation of the upper bounds for all control projects for a specific category is less or equal to the maximum number of people in that category:

$$\sum_{k \in K} \sum_{i \in I_j^k} U_{i,j}^k \leq M_j, j \in J$$

b. The maximum number of people in the infected category is equal to the sum of peoples in both the recovered and deceased categories:

$$M_I = M_R + M_D$$

v. **Integral Constraints:** All the decision variables are integers.

$$x_{i,j}^k = \text{Integers, } \forall i, j, \text{ and } k \tag{5}$$

vi. **Avoid the Trivial Solution:** In order to avoid the trivial solution that all intervention control projects can be implemented by the responsible parties, the following condition should hold:

The sum of the required amount of investments in all intervention control projects by all responsible parties should be greater than the total available budget of all the considered parties. This condition should be checked before writing the mathematical model and solving the problem.

In case of violation, then all intervention control projects can be implemented and no need to perform the optimization process of resource allocation.

vii. **The Objective Functions:** The COVID-19 crisis operation room decided on two main competing objectives, the first is to maximize the total number of people who benefited from the application of intervention control programs, and the second one is to maximize priorities depending on people conditions in terms of their track, category, and responsible party for each control program.

The problem is then a multi-objective one with two objectives. The multi-objective optimization (MOO) means searching the compromise (trade-off) solutions for problems with more than one contradictory objective functions.

The Weighted Sum or scalarization method is one of the classics (MOO) methods, it puts the considered objectives into one only by providing each one with a suitable relative weight. The method is simple, but it cannot find certain solutions in case of a nonconvex objective space [18]. The set of solutions represent the best trade-off between competing objectives [19]. The scalarization method deals with the multi-objective problem as composite objective function [20]. The composite objective function is expressed as follows:

$$Z = \text{Maximize } \sum_{i=1}^{q} w_i \cdot f_i(x)$$

where; w_i is the positive weight values; is one of the objective functions; and q is the number of objective functions. Maximizing Z will provide an enough condition for optimal multi-objective solution to be found. Since the objectives of this research is to provide a compromise between maximizing of total number of benefited people (NBP) and maximizing of prioritized category status (PCS), the following composite objective functions is considered:

$$Z = w_1 f_1(x) + w_2 f_2(x) \qquad (a)$$

$$\text{Maximize } f_1(x) = (NBP) = \sum_{i \in I} \sum_{j \in J} \sum_{k \in K} x_{i,j}^k \qquad (b)$$

$$\text{Maximize } f_2(x) = (PCS) = \sum_{i \in I} \sum_{j \in J} \sum_{k \in K} p_{i,j}^k \cdot x_{i,j}^k \qquad (c)$$

The weights w_1 and w_2 are related to each other as follows:

$$w_2 = 1 - w_1, \; w_1 \text{ is selected is in the range of } [0\text{--}1].$$

where; p_i is the relative importance of patient No i.

Considering that the available medical equipment of ambulance vehicles is different, then a variation of priorities in riding up ambulance vehicles will vary, and this will be considered by giving higher weights to better vehicles. From (a, b, and c), and the composite objective function will be:

$$\text{Maximize } Z = w_1 \left(\sum_{i \in I} \sum_{j \in J} \sum_{k \in K} x_{i,j}^k \right) + w_2 \left(\sum_{i \in I} \sum_{j \in J} \sum_{k \in K} p_{i,j}^k \cdot x_{i,j}^k \right) \qquad (6)$$

where; $p_{i,j}^k$ is the priority of people in program with indices i, j, and k.

The different weights in Eqn. (6) are obtained by choosing w_1 from 1 to 0 with a step of 0.1 [21].

13.2.5   A REAL APPLICATION CASE STUDY

The most important governmental and non-governmental projects to confront the emerging coronavirus are applied to one of the districts of Alexandria, the second-largest city in Egypt. These projects are presented in Table 13.2 together with the relevant category and responsible party, where $x_{i,j}^k$

represents the symbol for decision variables, the symbols (O, C, I, R, and D) are for the Ordinary, Contacts, Infected, Recovered, and Deceased categories respectively; the symbols (G and N) denote the responsible party whether the Government or Nongovernment respectively.

In this illustrative case study, the mentioned 10 epidemic social control programs are used by Governmental and Non-governmental responsible parties for a one-month planning horizon which can be repeated for other similar time periods. For simple accessibility of dealing with the decision variables, concise renaming is used as shown in Table 13.3 and Figure 13.3.

Constraint No. (1) will have the new forms:

$$\sum_{i=1}^{6} f_i\left(y_i\right) \cdot y_i \le B^G \text{ and } \sum_{i=1}^{4} f_i\left(z_i\right) \cdot z_i \le B^N,$$

The mathematical expression of $f_1(y_1)$ and $f_1(z_1)$ as a relation of the new decision variables y_1 and z_1 can be a linear expression or a general nonlinear expression depending on the specific data relative to the considered case study.

For the current planning month (June 2020) and after discussion with authorized persons in the corresponding Governmental and Non-governmental organizations, the relation between expended resources and outcomes of programs "production function" is linear for all decision variables except for the decision variable y_1 corresponding to "Governmental specific assistance program for ordinary persons." The unit cost is decreased by 20% as an economy of scale. The unit cost is 500 Egyptian pounds (L.E.) for a number of persons who benefit from the corresponding control project $= 3000$ to less than 5000, it is decreased to 400 L.E. when the number of persons is raised to 5,000 to 9,000, (1 US dollar $\cong 16.2$ L.E.).

The unit cost function $f_1(y_1)$ is obtained using a computer curve fitting program [22]. The function is a Nonlinear Symmetrical Sigmoidal one, a sigmoidal function refers to any function that retains the "S" shape [23].

A nonlinear symmetrical sigmoidal function is of the form $y = f(x)$:

$$y = d + \frac{a-d}{1+\left(\dfrac{x}{c}\right)^b}$$

where; a, b, c, and d are constants.

In this case and for the given data: $d = 400$, $a = 500$, $c = 4974.87$ and $b = 1392.443$, so:

$$f_1(y_1) = 400 + 100 / (1 + (y_1/4974.87)^{\wedge}1392.443).$$

The complete data for the case study is presented in Table 13.4.

The mathematical formulation for the given case is worked out by substituting in the previously described model for the given problem, the data for the maximum number of people in each category for this case results that constraint number 4 is redundant.

Fitting method and shape of the curve are shown in Figure 13.4. The complete steps of the solution procedure are presented in Figure 13.5.

TABLE 13.2 Proposed Social Epidemic Control Programs for the Case Study

SL. No.	Decision Variable	Epidemic Control Programs
1.	$x_{1,O}^{G}$	Governmental specific assistance program.
2.	$x_{1,O}^{N}$	Non-Governmental assistance program.
3.	$x_{1,C}^{G}$	Governmental quarantine protocol for contacts.
4.	$x_{1,C}^{N}$	Non-Governmental assistance for home isolation.
5.	$x_{1,I}^{G}$	Hospital treatment protocol for infected persons.
6.	$x_{2,I}^{G}$	Governmental Home treatment protocol for infected persons.
7.	$x_{1,I}^{N}$	Nongovernmental Home treatment protocol for infected persons.
8.	$x_{1,R}^{G}$	Treatment with convalescence plasma.
9.	$x_{1,D}^{G}$	Dealing with dead cases due to COVID-19.
10.	$x_{1,D}^{N}$	Non-governmental assistance for families of dead cases.

TABLE 13.3   Renaming of the Example Decision Variables

Decision Variables									
Math. Model Naming	$x_{1,O}^G$	$x_{1,C}^G$	$x_{1,I}^G$	$x_{2,I}^G$	$x_{1,R}^G$	$x_{1,D}^G$	$x_{1,O}^N$	$x_{1,C}^N$	$x_{1,I}^N$ $x_{1,D}^N$
New Naming	y_1	y_2	y_3	y_4	y_5	y_6	z_1	z_2	z_3 z_4

Responsible Party: - **Governmental Epidemic Control Programs (G)**
                       - **Nongovernmental Epidemic Control Programs (N)**

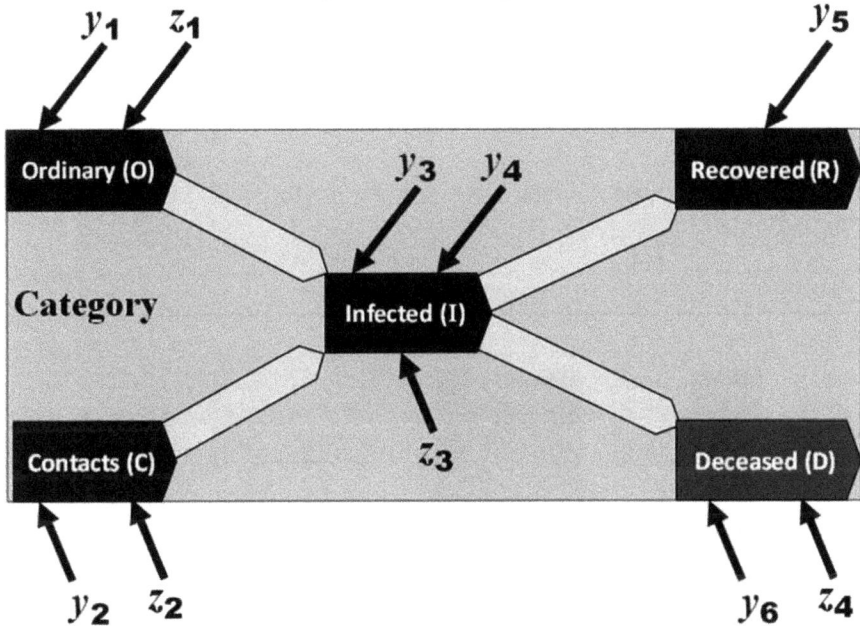

FIGURE 13.3   Scheme of the proposed epidemic control programs.

TABLE 13.4   The Data for the Case Study

Decision Variable		Upper Bound	Lower Bound	Cost Coefficient	Relative Priority	Available Budget
$x_{1,O}^G$	y_1	9,000	3,000	$f_1(y_1)$	3	
$x_{1,C}^G$	y_2	1,000	500	500	7	Governmental: 2.5 million pounds

TABLE 13.4   *(Continued)*

Decision Variable		Upper Bound	Lower Bound	Cost Coefficient	Relative Priority	Available Budget
$x_{1,I}^{G}$	y_3	200	50	1,000	10	
$x_{2,I}^{G}$	y_4	500	200	500	10	
$x_{1,R}^{G}$	y_5	2,000	50	1,000	9	
$x_{1,D}^{G}$	y_6	50	20	1,000	6	
$x_{1,O}^{N}$	z_1	15,000	4,000	500	3	
$x_{1,C}^{N}$	z_2	1,500	1,000	500	7	Non-governmental: 3.5 million pounds
$x_{1,I}^{N}$	z_3	1,000	300	500	10	
$x_{1,D}^{N}$	z_4	100	20	2,000	5	

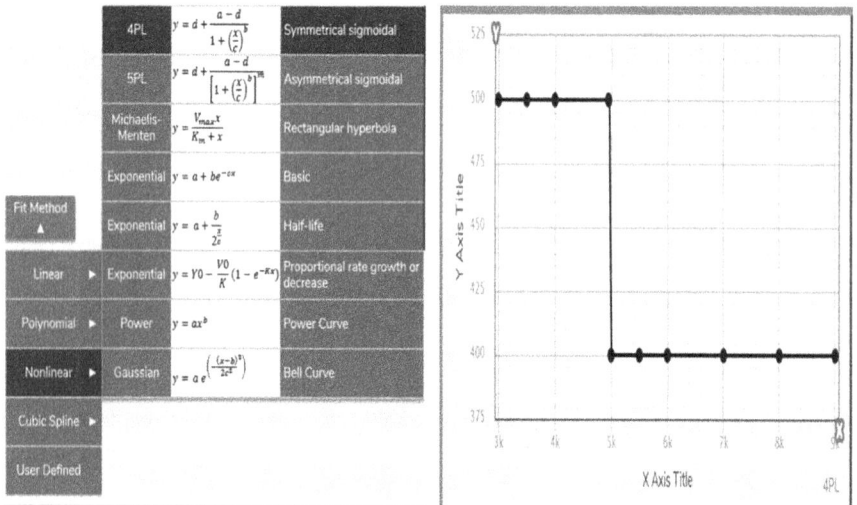

FIGURE 13.4   Fitting method and shape of the curve.

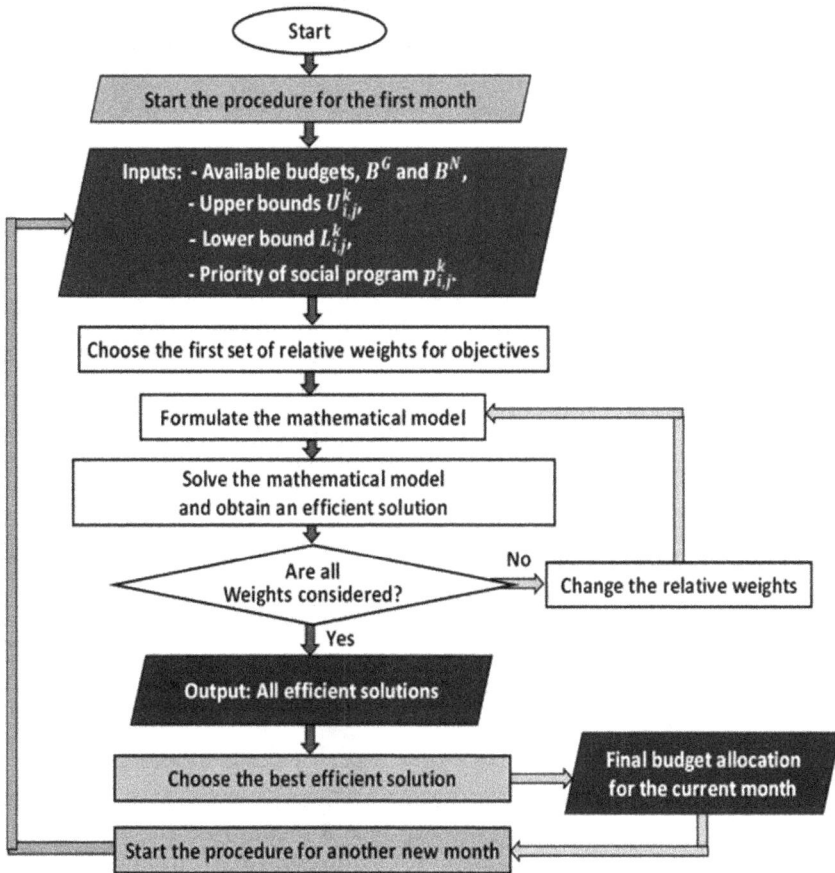

FIGURE 13.5 Steps of the solution procedure.

13.3 RESULTS AND DISCUSSION

13.3.1 PROPOSED SOLUTION METHODOLOGY

Metaheuristic approaches are developed for the complex optimization problems with continuous variables. Mohamed et al. [24] recently proposed a novel Gaining Sharing Knowledge-based optimization algorithm (GSK), setup on acquiring knowledge and share it with others throughout their lifetime. The original GSK solves optimization problems over continuous space, but it cannot solve the problem with integer space. So, a new variant of GSK is introduced to solve the proposed (OFRA). A novel discrete integer gaining sharing knowledge-based optimization algorithms (DIGSK) is proposed over discrete integer space with new integer junior and senior gaining and sharing stages. The proposed methodology is described in subsections.

13.3.1.1 DISCRETE INTEGER GAINING SHARING KNOWLEDGE-BASED OPTIMIZATION ALGORITHM (DIGSK)

DIGSK is proposed to handle the integer decision variables. The GSK algorithm is modified with an integer mutation leading to the development of a new integer gaining sharing knowledge (DIGSK) based optimization algorithm. Integer variables are handled with round operator, i.e., *round(a)*, which rounds the number *a*, to the nearest integer. The modifications are made in GSK to proposed DIGSK. The mathematical formulation of DIGSK is given in the following steps:

-   **Step 1:** Initially, the initial population is generated as:

$$x_{ij} = round\left(lb + rand * (ub - lb)\right);$$

where; *lb* and *ub* are lower and upper bounds of the optimization problem.

-   **Step 2:** At the beginning of the search for the solution, the dimensions for the junior, or senior phase must be set on. The number of dimensions that should be updated or changed during both phases should be computed by increasing and decreasing formula:

$$d_{junior} = d \times \left(1 - \frac{G}{Gen}\right)^k$$

$$d_{senior} = d - d_{junior}$$

where; *k* is the knowledge factor and a positive real number which controls the knowledge rate, *G* represents the generation number, and *Gen* is the maximum number of generations.

-   **Step 3: Integer Junior Gaining and Sharing Phase:** This phase considers at beginners' gain knowledge from their friends, family, etc., and share their views with other people who may or may not belong to their networks. This phase considers further two subphases as:

i.   The individuals are arranged in ascending order according to their objective function values as:

$$x_{best}, \ldots, x_{i-1}, x_i, x_{i+1}, \ldots, x_{worst}$$

ii. For each individual x_i, select two nearest best (x_{i-1}) and worst (x_{i+1}) individuals to gain knowledge and the select another individual randomly (x_r) to share their knowledge. Therefore, the individuals are updated in the following manner (Figure 13.6).

```
for i=1:NOP
    for j=1:d
        if rand≤ k_r (knowledge ratio)
            if f(x_i) > f(x_r)
                x_ij^new = round (x_i + k_f * ((x_{i-1} - x_{i+1}) + (x_r - x_i)))
            else
                x_ij^new = round (x_i + k_f * ((x_{i-1} - x_{i+1}) + (x_i - x_r)))
            end (if)
        else       x_ij^new = x_ij^old
        end (if)
    end (for j)
end (for i)
```

FIGURE 13.6   Pseudocode for integer junior gaining sharing knowledge phase.

– **Step 4: Integer Senior Gaining and Sharing Phase:** This phase concerns the impact and effect of others on an individual. Thus, each individual can be updated by arranging the individual on ascending order according to their objective function value. They are classified into three types of categories as best, middle, or worst individuals:

i.   **Best Individuals:** $100p\%$ (x_{pb}); middle individual: $d - 2 \times 100p\%$ (x_m);
ii. **Worst Individuals:** $100p\%$ (x_{pw});
     where; $p \in [0,1]$ is the percentage of best and worst classes.
After classification, select two random vectors from top and bottom $100p\%$ individuals to gain the knowledge part and to share the knowledge choose third vector from the middle individual $d - 2 \times 100p\%$.

The individuals are updated through the pseudo code (Figure 13.7) and the flow chart of DIGSK is shown in Figure 13.8.

```
for i=1:NOP
    for j=1:d
        if rand≤ k_r (knowledge ratio)
            if f(x_i) > f(x_m)
```
$$x_{ij}^{new} = round\left(x_i + k_f * \left((x_{pb} - x_{pw}) + (x_m - x_i)\right)\right)$$
```
            else
```
$$x_{ij}^{new} = round\left(x_i + k_f * \left((x_{pb} - x_{pw}) + (x_i - x_m)\right)\right)$$
```
            end (if)
            else        x_{ij}^{new} = x_{ij}^{old}
        end (if)
    end (for j)
end (for i)
```

FIGURE 13.7   Pseudocode for integer senior gaining sharing knowledge phase.

13.3.1.2   CONSTRAINT HANDLING APPROACH

To solve the constrained optimization problem, several techniques have been applied to metaheuristic algorithms [25–27]. Of these, penalty approach method is very popular and easy to implement to the constrained optimization problem. Bahreininejad [28] introduced augmented Lagrangian method (ALM) for the water cycle algorithm and solved the real-time problems. In this study, ALM is used, which is similar to the penalty approach method. In ALM, a constrained optimization problem is converted into an unconstrained optimization problem by adding a penalty to the original objective function with the Lagrange multiplier parameter. Suppose the constrained optimization problem is given as:

$Min = f(X)$
where; $(X) = (x_1, x_2,..., x_d)$
Subject to:
$g_i(X) \leq 0, i = 1, 2, ..., m$

When applying ALM method to the problem, it is converted into an unconstrained optimization problem as:

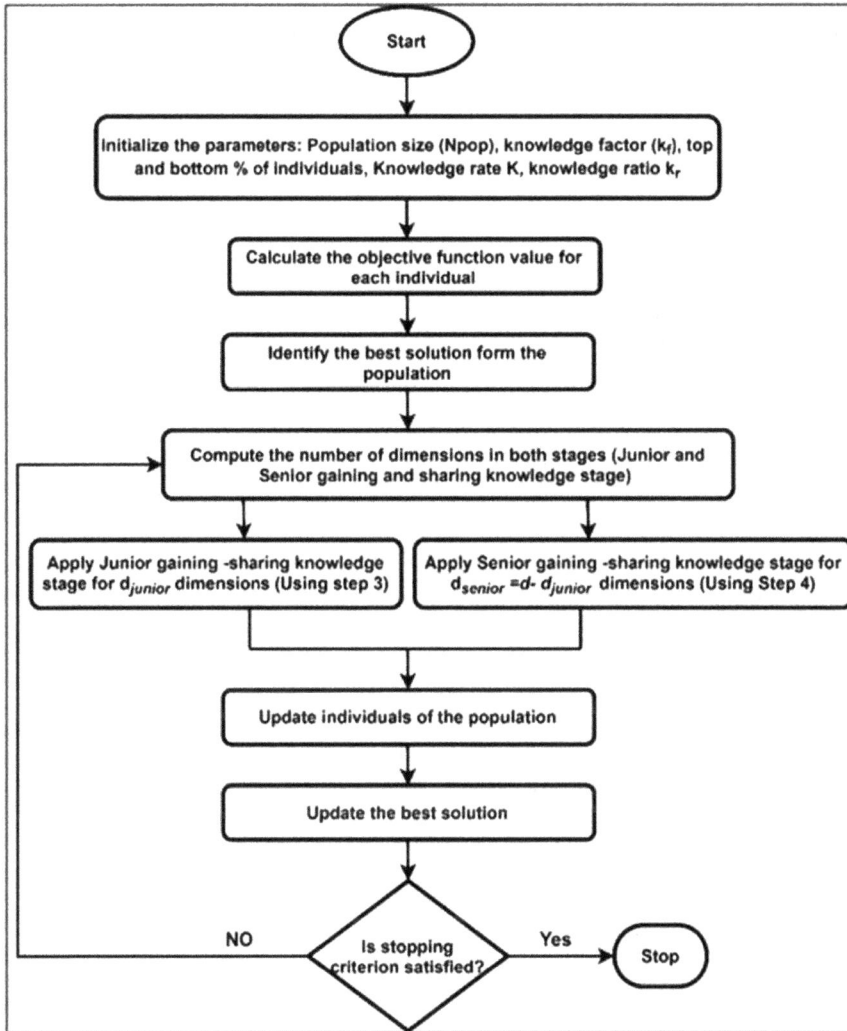

FIGURE 13.8   The flow chart of DIGSK.

$$Min = f(X) + \mu \sum_{i=1}^{m} (g_i(X))^2 - \lambda \sum_{i=1}^{m} (g_i(X))$$

where; μ is the penalty parameter, $\sum_{i=1}^{m} (g_i(X))^2$ is quadratic penalty and λ is the Lagrange multiplier. In the equation μ and λ are chosen in such a way that λ can remain small to maintain the strategic distance from ill condition. The advantage of ALM is that it reduces the possibility of ill-conditioning happening in the penalty approach method.

13.3.2   *EXPERIMENTAL RESULTS*

The (OFRA) is handled by using the proposed novel DIGSK algorithm, the used parameters are presented in Table 13.5. DIGSK runs over personal computer Intel ® CoreTM i5-7200U CPU @ 2.50 GHz and 4 GB RAM and coded on MATLAB R2015a. To get the compromise or effective solutions, 30 independent runs are complete, and the obtained statistics are provided in Table 13.6, including the best, median, average, worst solutions, and the standard deviations at the three groups of weights. Moreover, Figure 13.9 shows the convergence graph of the solutions of (OFRA) using the first group of the weights from the figure, it can be observed that after the 149th iteration, it converges to the global optimal solution (34460), which shows high convergence speed of DIGSK.

TABLE 13.5   Numerical Values of Parameters

Parameters of DIGSK	Considered Values
NoP	200
k	10
k_r	0.9
p	0.1
k_f	1
Max number of iterations	**400**

TABLE 13.6   Statistical Results of (OFRA) Using DIGSK

Weights	$f_1(x)$	Best	Median	Average	Worst	Standard Deviation
$w_1 = 1$	11819	11819	11819	11819	11819	0.00
$w_1 = 0.9$	11820	11820	11820	11820	11820	0.00
$w_1 = 0.8$	11819	11819	11789	11756	11700	87.00
$w_1 \in [0: 0.7]$	11690	11690	11690	11690	11690	0.00

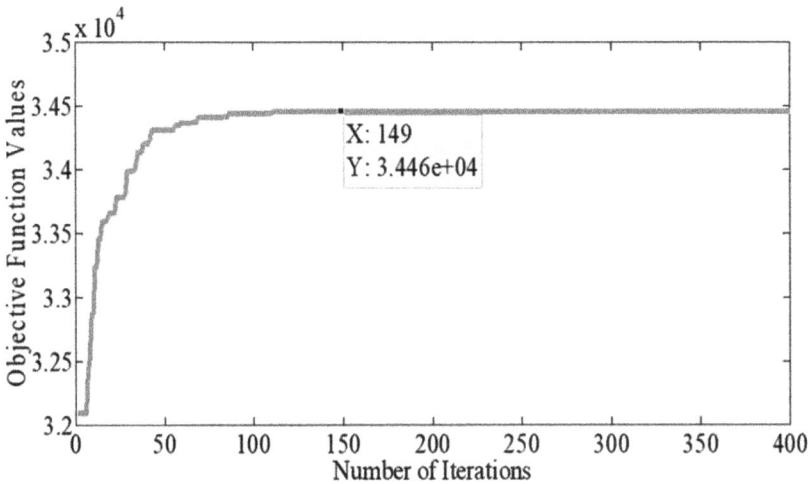

FIGURE 13.9   Convergence graph of DIGSK.

The efficient solutions for the problem for different weights of the two objective functions are presented in Table 13.7. From the table, it can be seen that there are multiple optimum solutions for $w_1 = 1$ and $w_2 = 0$. In this case, only the first objective is considered, and if the management is interested to consider only this first objective (maximizing the total NBP), then the second optimum solution will be chosen since it has the maximum value for the second objective function. There are also many efficient solutions for $w_1 = 0.8$ and $w_2 = 0.2$, any one of these efficient solutions can be used if management chooses these weights for the two objective functions.

When w1 is decreased in the range (0.9: 0.7) and w2 is increased in the range (0.1: 0.3), different efficient solutions are obtained for the multi-objective problem. When w1 is decreased in the range (0.6: 0) and w2 is increased in the range (0.4: 1), only one efficient solution is obtained for the multi-objective problem. In this case, there is no effect for the first objective function on the obtained efficient solutions and only the second objective function is significant. The number of beneficiaries and the allocated budget for each of the epidemic control programs for the solution with a weight of the second objective function w2 ≥ 0.4 are shown in Figure 13.10.

TABLE 13.7   Efficient Solutions for the Illustrated Case Study

w_1	w_2	Values of the Decision Variables										$f_1(x)$	$f_2(x)$
		y_1	y_2	y_3	y_4	y_5	y_6	z_1	z_2	z_3	z_4		
1	0	3386	899	50	474	50	20	5015	1223	682	20	11819	52787
		3632	671	50	455	50	21	4794	1358	768	20		52887
		3664	835	50	259	51	20	4841	1375	704	20		51794
0.9	0.1	3260	1000	50	500	50	20	4420	1500	1000	20	11820	56710
0.8	0.2	3020	1000	170	500	50	20	4420	1500	1000	20	11700	57190
		3032	1000	164	500	50	20	4420	1500	1000	20	11706	57166
		3198	1000	81	500	50	20	4420	1500	1000	20	11789	56834
		3258	1000	51	500	50	20	4420	1500	1000	20	11819	56714
0.7	0.3	3000	1000	180	500	50	20	4420	1500	1000	20	11690	57230
0.6	0.4												
0.5	0.5												
0.4	0.6												
0.3	0.7												
0.2	0.8												
0.1	0.9												
0	1												

	Governmental Epidemic Control Programs					
Decision Variable	y_1	y_2	y_3	y_4	y_5	y_6
No of Beneficiaries	3000	1000	180	500	50	20
Allocated Budget	1500000	500000	180000	250000	50000	20000
Total Budget	2.5 million Egyptian Pounds (L.E.)					

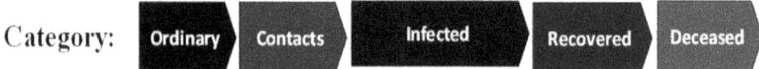

Category: Ordinary   Contacts   Infected   Recovered   Deceased

	Nongovernmental Epidemic Control Programs				
Decision Variable	z_1	z_2	z_3		z_4
No of Beneficiaries	4420	1500	1000		20
Allocated Budget	2210000	750000	500000		20000
Total Budget	3.5 million Egyptian Pounds (L.E.)				

FIGURE 13.10   Number of beneficiaries and the allocated budget.

13.4 CONCLUSIONS

The main conclusions for this chapter can be summarized as follows:

1. A financial resource allocation to control COVID-19 pandemic problem is presented. The resource allocation is aiming at achieving the best distribution of the available budget among several proposed social control projects for governmental and non-governmental responsible parties. The best distribution of the available budget is determined by two competing objectives. The first objective is to maximize the total number of people who benefit from the implementation of the proposed projects, the second objective will consider the relative priorities of people according to their category with respect to their relationship to the virus (Ordinary, Contacts, Infected, Recovered or Deceased).

2. A nonlinear integer constrained multi-objective mathematical model is formulated for the given problem. The integer decision variables represent the number of people who benefit from each of the proposed control programs. The obtained mathematical model and the solution method for obtaining efficient solutions are used to solve an illustrated case study in One district in Alexandria, Egypt.

3. The proposed problem is solved by a novel Discrete Integer Gaining Sharing Knowledge-based Optimization algorithm (DIGSK), which involves two main stages: Discrete Integer Junior and Senior gaining and sharing stages with a knowledge factor $kf = 1$. DIGSK is discrete integer variant of GSK, that solves the problem with integer decision variables.

4. DIGSK shows that it has the ability of finding the solutions of the problem, and the obtained results demonstrate the robustness and convergence of DIGSK towards the efficient solutions.

The points for future researches can be stated in the following points:

1. To propose other mathematical models' formulation for the same problem comprising designing the objective function, decision variables and constraints, and then to compare the effectiveness of computations for each model.

2. To continue applying the problem to other months and to other districts, cities, and the whole country.

3. To build an online decision support system that can handle instantaneous situations with timely updated data, and in turn, update the resource allocation for such an important problem.

4. To check the performance of the DIGSK approach in solving different complex optimization problems, and further works can be investigated by the extension of DIGSK with different kinds of constraint handling methods.

KEYWORDS

- **control COVID-19 pandemic**
- **gaining-sharing knowledge**
- **integer gaining sharing knowledge-based metaheuristic algorithm**
- **multi-objective nonlinear integer problem**
- **resource allocation**
- **social programs**

REFERENCES

1. Sara, C., Wim, D., Vagner, F., Wasim, A. K., Marta, G., Luiz, C. A., Koen, D., & Tulio De, O., (2020). Genome Detective Coronavirus Typing Tool for rapid identification and characterization of novel coronavirus genomes. *Bioinformatics*, btaa145. Retrieved at: https://doi.org/10.1093/bioinformatics/btaa145.

2. THE LANCET website, (2020). *A Novel Coronavirus Outbreak of Global Health Concern.* Retrieved from: https://www.thelancet.com/journals/lancet/article/PIIS0140-6736(20)30185-9/fulltext (accessed on 27 June 2021).

3. World Health Organization (WHO) Website, (2020a), *Novel Coronavirus (2019-nCoV) Situation Report-7.* Data as reported by 27 January 2020.

4. Worldometer website, (2020a). *COVID-19 Coronavirus Pandemic.* Retrieved from: https://www.worldometers.info/coronavirus/#ref-13 (accessed on 27 June 2021).

5. Wikimedia Commons Website, (2020). retrieved from: https://commons.wikimedia.org/wiki/File:COVID-19_Outbreak_World_Map.svg (accessed on 27 June 2021).

6. Heesterbeek, H., Anderson, R. M., Andreasen, V., Bansal, S., De Angelis, D., Dye, C., Eames, K. T., et al., (2015). Modeling infectious disease dynamics in the complex landscape of global health. *Science, 347*(6227).

7. Ross, R., (1911). *The Prevention of Malaria.* John Murray.

8. Ma, J., Dushoff, J., Bolker, B. M., & Earn, D. J., (2014). Estimating initial epidemic growth rates. *Bulletin of Mathematical Biology, 76*(1), 245–260.

9. Bower, J. L., (2017). Managing resource allocation: Personal reflections from a managerial perspective. *Journal of Management, 43*(8), 2421–2429.

10. Danneels, E., (2007). The process of technological competence leveraging. *Strategic Management Journal, 28*(5), 511–533.
11. Souder, D., & Shaver, J. M., (2010). Constraints and incentives for making long horizon corporate investments. *Strategic Management Journal, 31*(12), 1316–1336.
12. Maritan, C. A., (2001). Capital investment as investing in organizational capabilities: An empirically grounded process model. *Academy of Management Journal, 44*(3), 513–531.
13. Busenbark, J. R., Wiseman, R. M., Arrfelt, M., & Woo, H. S., (2017). A review of the internal capital allocation literature: Piecing together the capital allocation puzzle. *Journal of Management, 43*(8), 2430–2455.
14. Ahuja, G., & Novelli, E., (2017). Activity overinvestment: The case of R&D. *Journal of Management, 43*(8), 2456–2468.
15. Bardolet, D., Brown, A., & Lovallo, D., (2017). The effects of relative size, profitability, and growth on corporate capital allocations. *Journal of Management, 43*(8), 2469–2496.
16. Vieregger, C., Larson, E. C., & Anderson, P. C., (2017). Top management team structure and resource reallocation within the multi business firm. *Journal of Management, 43*(8), 2497–2525.
17. Eastman, B., Meaney, C., Przedborski, M., & Kohandel, M., (2020). *Mathematical Modeling of COVID-19 Containment Strategies with Considerations for Limited Medical Resources.* medRxiv.
18. Marler, R. T., & Arora, J. S. (2004). Survey of multi-objective optimization methods. *Structural and Multidisciplinary Optimization, 26*, 369–395.
19. Gunantara, N., (2018). A review of multi-objective optimization: Methods and its applications. *Cogent Engineering, 5*(1), 1502242.
20. Hemamalini, S., & Simon, S. P., (2009). *Economic/Emission Load Dispatch Using Artificial Bee Colony Algorithm.* iPi, 1, 2.
21. Naidu, K., Mokhlis, H., & Bakar, A. A., (2014). Multi-objective optimization using weighted sum artificial bee colony algorithm for load frequency control. *International Journal of Electrical Power & Energy Systems, 55*, 657–667.
22. MyCurveFit website, (2020). *Online Curve Fitting.* Retrieved from: https://mycurvefit.com/ (accessed on 27 June 2021).
23. Spiess, A. N., Feig, C., & Ritz, C., (2008). Highly accurate sigmoidal fitting of real-time PCR data by introducing a parameter for asymmetry. *BMC Bioinformatics, 9*(1), 221.
24. Mohamed, A. W., Hadi, A. A., & Mohamed, A. K., (2019). Gaining-sharing knowledge based algorithm for solving optimization problems: A novel nature-inspired algorithm. *International Journal of Machine Learning and Cybernetics*, 1–29.
25. Deb, K., (2000). An efficient constraint handling method for genetic algorithms. *Computer Methods in Applied Mechanics and Engineering, 186*(2–4), 311–338.
26. Coello, C. A. C., (2002). Theoretical and numerical constraint-handling techniques used with evolutionary algorithms: A survey of the state of the art. *Computer Methods in Applied Mechanics and Engineering, 191*(11, 12), 1245–1287.
27. Muangkote, N., Photong, L., & Sukprasert, A., (2019). Effectiveness of constrained handling techniques of improved constrained differential evolution algorithm applied to constrained optimization problems in mechanical engineering. *ITMSOC Transactions on Innovation & Business Engineering, 04*(2019), 1–21.
28. Bahreininejad, A., (2019). Improving the performance of water cycle algorithm using augmented Lagrangian method. *Advances in Engineering Software, 132*, 55–64.

CHAPTER 14

Solace in Social Media: Women Unite Under COVID-19

JYOTI AHLAWAT

Post-Doctoral Fellow, University of Victoria, Canada,
E-mail: jyotiahlawat@icloud.com

ABSTRACT

The chapter is an attempt to bring forth the power of technology in bringing life-enhancing changes and opportunities for women and girls, especially the disenfranchised community of women. The objective of the chapter is to highlight the significance of social media during the COVID-19 pandemic in uniting women across the globe from recreation to support and inclusivity. The chapter focuses on three diverse perspectives of how social media turned into a boon for women and helped them cope up with the adversities of the global pandemic. The chapter analyzes social media posts, and feeds collectively over a period of three months to conclude how social media has played a crucial role in forming a virtual global community of sisterhood for women and further how it can be made more inclusive for the digitally deprived communities of women to empower and support themselves.

"The world will no longer be the same," a statement that has sprung up in everyday conversations, with an uncertain future facing us. The world has undergone tremendous change in terms of working, living, and socializing. The pandemic has certainly morphed into a global socio-economic crisis, posing a threat to women's safety and livelihoods. This chapter is a research inquiry to investigates how social media in the current COVID-19 crisis has the capacity to turn into a significant digital space for women to connect, share, and bond for support or to seek help. The research brings forth three different perspectives on how social media can bring life-enhancing changes for women. Gauging the impact of social media on the female communities around the world from articles, stories, and data available online. Keeping the three diverse aspects of recreation, support, and inclusivity as the foundation for the argument.

COVID-19 crisis has highlighted how social media can be used for community and emotional support suggests Associate Professor Kristine de Valck in her article, 'What is the role of social media during the COVID-19 crisis? [1]. If and how social media turned into a site for recreation for active women users during the COVID-19 crisis? How has social media turns into a viable platform for many who might be in need of immediate help? How can the disenfranchised community of women and girls benefit from being brought within the folds of social media? Are the questions the enquiry intends to seek answers to using secondary data of social media websites, posts, and news articles.

The broad objective is to analyze if social media has brought any significant changes for better into the lives of women and how women as active users of social media capitalized it for their wellbeing and support. For this, the review enquiry takes into account the various social media posts from popular social media sites-Facebook and Twitter, websites displaying content where women can virtually participate for recreation as well as find support in cases of emergencies due to the uptick in the number of cases of domestic violence, third, the chapter brings forth data to support the fact that online media has the capacity to bring enhancement in the lives of women and girls who remain offline. The research shall keep a time period of three months from March 2020 till end of May 2020. Since the focus is on social media hence there is no specific country being the target of study.

The idea put forward in the chapter is to base the objectives within the framework of social participatory media and digital feminism. Does there exist any alignment between digital-social media of participation, based on core values of openness, networking, and collaboration with feminism, based on access, cooperation, and inclusion questions Kate Ott in her research article social media and feminist values? [2]. The attempt in this chapter is to understand the current situation through the gendered lens that does social media has the capacity to metamorphosize into an anchor for women, thereby connecting themselves with the virtual community of global solidarity of women. Josiane Jouet in her working research paper, 'Digital Feminism: Questioning the Renewal of Activism,' brings forth the idea of digital feminism as the new source of feminist activism. How feminist collectives use digital media to promote their cause of justice for women and inequities they suffer. Digital connectivity has the capacity to widen its audience base and further leading to the building of virtual communities [3]. Amy Lacount in her article, 'Digital Feminism: A New Frontier,' clearly states that a new digital environment makes the dream possible of organizing online and creation of cohesive feminist communities [4].

Hence digital feminism creates a virtual movement which may translate into an on-ground movement but certainly helps take the cause on a higher level with its global participation, results which manifest in the forms of the better and more secure environment with stronger legal frameworks put into place [5, 42] The rise of feminist campaigns #MeToo, #BeenRapedNever-Reported, #EverydaySexism reflect the growing trend of digital resistances to sexism, patriarchy, and other forms of oppression [43].

Social Participatory Media is media where the audience can play an active role in creating content, disseminating information in the form of blogging, via personal accounts on social media sites [5]. Thus, social participatory media has made allowances for people to create new content and share. This democratic flow of communication helps the audience to take active participation in shaping the flow of new ideas across different formats of media [6]. A free virtual space which gives more power to control and create content as one pleases, availing the affordances of social media, to simply share their stories with those who matter and make a difference to this community worldwide. The structure of social networks and social media spaces facilitate in accessing the expertise available as well as there is a greater amount of exposure to the levels of conflicts which in turn the willingness for participation leading to the endogeneity of network formations [7].

Within this framework of digital networked technologies and communicative practices, the chapter presents the core idea that social media has brought solace and element of recreation and relaxation amidst fear and uncertainty for women who are tech-savvy or digitally active users. Second, women create a community of unity and solidarity in the virtual space with the use of social media. Third, women who are isolated and remain offline can benefit and have life-enhancing opportunities if they are included within the fold of online media. The review enquiry in the chapter explores these three diverse strands of the impact of technology upon women, especially during the COVID-19 crisis.

14.1   WOMEN CREATE A NETWORKED COMMUNITY

The first aspect of how social media kept the women connected and brought in the solace into their lives amidst confusion and stress the pandemic created. The research takes into account two popular social media sites Facebook and Twitter, as well as some women-focused websites to curate the posts and content, which brings forth the urgency of their use and support offered on the accounts on these sites for women looking for recreation, help, and support. Prior to that, it is important to understand that women are active users of popular social media sites by analyzing the data about the percentage of women users around the world. Facebook has 2.5 billion users worldwide, out of which 56% are women and 46% men till February 2020 [8]. This establishes the fact that women have been a proactive user and content consumers of social media Facebook. Twitter, on the other hand, has more male users than female as per the data shared by Omnicore, a data processing company [9], popular blog website-Blog-Hootsuite shares the statistics on the gender demographics as 62% male and 38% female users of Twitter [10]. This clearly reflects those women are tech-savvy and keep themselves connected with social media in order either obtain information, exchange, and share content.

A global digital report compiled a data-sharing website-We Are Social confabulates that during the COVID-19 crisis that the world's digital behaviors have been impacted during the pandemic with people getting connected online to cope with life and to work under the lockdown [11]. The data further reflects that more women have increased their social media engagements as compared to men during the pandemic in the month of April 2020 and the trend will continue [11, 12].

The enquiry in this chapter brings forth the websites operated by women, for women which have brought special events in the form of webinar series which focus on handling and coping up with the COVID-19 crisis in multiple manners; domestically, socially, and economically. The website Empower Women is one such website that stand for women empowerment and women's rights. The platform has been endorsed by United Nations (UN) women. Empower women have been organizing regular webinars for members, non-members as well as organizations connected with them focusing on domestic violence, economic empowerment and opportunities, gender equality, and COVID-19 crisis response and recovery, and many more based on sharing information and support [13]. The possibility of these webinars was created by companies like Zoom.us, a web-based format by

Zoom video communications, an American company, has become exceedingly popular and in use for webinars, teleconferencing, and videotelephony, especially during the COVID-19 crisis. Zoom.us is not alone, there certainly is more competition in the market with the likes of Skype and most recently with the addition of Meet-Google. Women and non-governmental organizations (NGOs) like Empower Women are using this platform to connect women and share vital information with members and non-members or those participating. It is important to bring the relevance of an earlier survey shared by a media researcher Johanna Blakely in her TED Women talk brings out the new change in the offing about social media and the end of gender, basing the essence of her talk on the new data and understanding of social media user demographics [14]. It is the emotional and psychological support that women find from one another that creates solidarity and support building new virtual communities. These virtual spaces of social media like Facebook, Twitter, etc., are locations where women build communities with multiple goals from safe spaces for entertainment to relaxation as well as garnering support when needed as well as relatability [15].

Another popular website for women and queer community; women on a roll has been organizing social engagement events. The operators of this website have created a special feature of free events: for women to connect in the current times of social distancing, offering free online social experiences of variety, from celebrities connecting and sharing stories virtually to women musicians and DJs or disc jockeys belting out music to entertain, for all who connect from any and everywhere across the globe. The virtual list of events laid out for women to choose from, participate, and enjoy irrespective of any differences as long as one is interested in the essence of the event, which is to meet, greet virtually and enjoy a new sense of merriment. Endless choice of live sessions on humor to salon chat to specific themes, a respite for women, to divert stressed minds [16]. A recent article by website Connect Americas reiterates the fact that women are driving the social media revolution [17]. The increasing active participation of women and teenage girls on social media is due to the emotional component that prevails in their action in the form of likes, sharing, and resharing on social media sites. This could mean that gender stereotypes are being dismantled in the online platforms leading to the end of gender divisions in the virtual world.

As Roxanne Brown states in her article published post-COVID-19 lockdown, in a news and updates website Daily Commercial, titled aptly, "Local ladies bringing people together virtually amid social distancing." She highlights the way women have been playing a key role in creating new groups and virtual hangouts for friends as well as strangers who wish to share the same camaraderie, with uncertainty looming large [18] This reflects how much time women might be spending on the internet, simply surfing, and searching for nothing in particular yet finding what suits their interests or becoming a part of an activity which has gone viral. These examples establish the fact that women like to connect and find solace in especially in the current pandemic, in order to pacify the growing concerns and rising stress levels. As a recent Leger poll conducted by the Association of Canadian Studies reveal that during the COVID-19 crisis, women of all ages and specifically the young women between the age group of 18–24 was more stressed as compared to men [19]. The digital connectivity has brought in relief to the anxious minds of women. A study published in the Journal of Computer-Mediated Communication in the July 2016 issue suggests that when we receive communication from people, we have strong ties with-in the form of a direct message, a photo share or a comment, the wellbeing tends to improve, though the effect may be less when the communication is from one with whom we have weaker ties [41]. To take the point further post-Doctoral fellow Izabella Pena, at the Department of Biology, Whitehead Institute for Biomedical Research, Cambridge, Massachusetts, USA, suggests how she uses social media to combat misinformation about COVID-19 pandemic and utilizes the power of social media via videos to connect and dispel false information [20].

14.2   FINDING SUPPORT IN SOCIAL MEDIA

How has social media affected a change in the wake of the pandemic with cases of domestic violence rising or appear to be rising? The second part of the enquiry reviews the creation of #Hashtag posts, on social media sites: Facebook and Twitter and how women are using them in the current time. At the same time how some government agencies as well as government officials taking advantage of social media to reach out to women in need of immediate or urgent support. Since obtaining reliable data on IPV-Intimate Partner Violence as the very nature of the phenomenon, therefore the chapter tries to use the new reports published and data shared by websites during the period of March 2020 till May 2020, which showcase the rise in IPV worldwide. According to the research paper-Methodological issues in the study of violence against women, published in the Journal of Epidemiology and public health, IPV can be defined as "any behavior within an intimate relationship that causes physical, psychological or sexual harm to those in the relationship" [21].

An article written by Melissa Godin for Times, USA, titled, "As Cities Around the World go on Lockdown, Victims of Domestic Violence Look for a Way Out," states how the National Domestic Violence Hotline has been buzzing with calls from the victims of IPV since the lockdown began. Melissa further highlights an important fact in her article that the current pandemic is expected to push the economy into recession, therefore making it even more difficult for victims to leave abusive relations [25, 44].

In Canada, the situation is no different as reported in the web-based newspaper National Observer, in an article written by Alastair Sharp, dated 28th April 2020 titled, "An uptick in domestic violence happening in Toronto due to COVID-19 experts say," states the spike in such cases and rise in the number of calls by four times, received per day reported by Assaulted Women's Helpline, a 24/7 crisis counseling service [22].

Amanda Taub, in her article written for The New York Times dated 14th April 2020 titled, "A New COVID-19 Crisis: Domestic Violence Rises Worldwide," brings out important facts about on intimate partner violence cases during the lockdown as reported in different countries. From China where Equality, a Beijing-based NGO-non-government organization dedicated to combating domestic violence, has seen a surge in the calls to their helpline ever since the lockdown. She further reports a similar situation prevailing in Spain, France, and Italy, where the domestic violence cases have risen many folds with an equal increase in distress calls seeking support by the victims of intimate violence [23].

A leading newspaper in India-Times of India, published an article on its website "Domestic violence cases in India on the rise during the lockdown, report says," brings forth data shared by National Legal Service Authority-NALSA, on the rapid rise of domestic violence cases across the states in the country [28]. The number of reporting cases of domestic across the globe clear state the rise in IPV during the COVID-19 pandemic.

The rising reports and updates by new agencies across the world on domestic violence have seen a surge during the COVID-19, whether they are authenticated completely is a matter of speculation. The idea is to map the use of social media via #Hashtags to combat IPV world over in order to extend support and bring vulnerable women and girls under protection from this abuse. It is interesting to note how government and non-government agencies and celebrities have used the social media platform to curb the rise of IPV. The United Kingdom (UK), France, and Italy have set fine examples of using social media #Hashtags-#EndVAW-end to violence against women, #YouAreNotAlone, #DomesticAbuse, #WhenHomeNotSafe, #WhyIGive-ToWin, #TogetherForHer are some of the many #Hashtags campaigns started to rescue women facing domestic abuse in this pandemic. For instance, #YouAreNotAlone campaign launched by the Home Secretary, Government of the UK-Ms. Priti Patel, on Twitter [24], a new public awareness campaign to help domestic abuse sufferers, received more than 400 posts every day.

The posts range from those who are the victims sharing pictures of their assault injuries to posts from the agencies extending support to anyone who might be in a situation needing urgent help from domestic violence. Government officials are #Hastagging their messages in the form of video messages and sharing contact number details to reach out to. For instance, the Ministry of Justice, Government of the UK, has repetition of video messages to reach anyone needing help and the video explains in detail how to access help (@ MoJGovUK [25]. Another tweet by a friend of a victim shares photos of her friend and her abusive partner [26]. The same #Hashtag has been used the world over-as in India as well where a lady police officer holding a senior position as Additional Commissioner of Police, Hyderabad city has tweeted a message using #YouAreNotAlone as well as #DomesticViolence to say that one is not alone and can reach out to the police with phone numbers being shared in the form of a picture-poster also a part of the message [27].

On the other popular social media site Facebook, there has been similar use of #Hashtag-#domesticviolenceawareness, #domesticviolencesurvivors are some of the many #Hashtags created by groups and people as well as agencies working towards stopping domestic abuse. For example, a popular Facebook group: 'Stand Up Survivor-Domestic Violence Awareness [28] has more than 60,000 members, are creating content to help those needing it however there were not many messages confirming that they needed help, this could be due to the inhibitions women face when reporting abuse on a public platform. As Bianca Fileborn and Rachel Loney-Howes in their introductory chapter in their edited book, "#MeToo and the Politics of Social Change," clearly state that the survivors who speak out about their sexual abuse routinely face scrutiny from public, police, and even friends or family [29]. Rosemary Clark in her research article, 'Hope in a hashtag: the discursive activism of #WhyIStayed,' states that hashtag feminism has become a powerful tactic for fighting gender inequalities around the world with potential and limitations. She further argues that hashtag activism has the ability and the potential to connect individual stories with collective action but with certain underlying conditions as how much of online activation leads to on-ground mobilization as well as women coming forward to share their abuse [30]. The use of technology in eliminating violence against women is certainly the way forward with greater inclusivity of those offline.

14.3   GENDER DIGITAL DIVIDE WIDE OPEN

The third part of this chapter brings into the discussion the status of those women and girls who remain offline or digitally disconnected. COVID-19 has emphatically revealed a plethora of problems especially for disenfranchised, displaced, homeless/stateless women and girls. Amidst plunging economies, financial strains, and uncertain future, trouble seems to be aggravating for the women. A report published by United Nations Population Fund (UNFPA) reiterates the fact that the pandemic has led to a rise in threats and vulnerabilities, apart from the risk of infection especially for women and girls [31]. The crisis precipitated by COVID-19 exposes not only the gender gap and inequities for women but also the digital divide it brings along [32]. The challenge does not end here, the food scarcity, loss of jobs, and unemployment make matters worse. Digital exclusion leaves women and girls out of life-enhancing and lucrative opportunities. Despite the progress the world has made in terms of digitization, increased accessibility of web applications, affordable handsets, the challenges of digital illiteracy, and exclusion of women and girls in transforming towards a digital-enabled society, remains [38].

A recent survey conducted by GSMA, the mobile gender report 2018, which reveals the vast difference region-wise gender gap in mobile usage and the gender gap in mobile ownership. The challenge is evident that women and girls who are disconnected from the digital environment need accessibility as well as the knowledge to use the technology in order to be able to assert their rights wherever required. Smitha in her research paper, 'Empowerment of women through digital literacy strategies-new challenges,' brings forth the urgency for digital literacy in isolated communities of women, to be able to support themselves, to live in a violence-free domestic environment apart from the other benefits that digital literacy can bring to them. She brings out a significant aspect of gadget availability and network connectivity in the context of India, where there are 1 billion mobile subscriptions until 2016–2017, but this is indicative of the SIM cards sold [33].

14.4   THE WAY FORWARD WITH TECHNOLOGY-SHORT- AND LONG-TERM MEASURES

Digital education program needs to begin at the grassroots level. Using technology for the creation of a database, region-wise, of the vulnerable population of women and girls. Who needs what in terms of financial help, food availability and shelter, and protection from abuse. It is an apt time for the telecom sector to step in to iron out the hurdles of communications, by creating viable internet ecosystems. A fine example of this from the initiative taken in Indonesia with regards to women's digital literacy, where women have now started creating and sharing content on social media as well as equipped themselves with technology in day-to-day necessities of online banking to using online trade markets [36].

The women leader's virtual roundtable hosted by the UN WOMEN on COVID-19 had the agenda of women and girl's safety and inclusion, as a top priority, agreeing that gender equality and women's rights are essential to get past this pandemic, with faster recovery, towards building better safer future [34]. The leaders have asked the governments and stakeholders, especially private sector telecom companies for creating innovative solutions for stronger advocacy and awareness about VAWG, violence against women and girls. To put women and girls at the center of their efforts with vigilant staff responding to helpline calls and proper shelters in place.

The long term, measures will be created on the foundations of those steps taken currently. Measures of inclusivity of women and girls, with special focus on advancing digital fluency, capacity building, upskilling of the underrepresented women's population. All the stakeholders, which include governments, the private sector, academia, and civil societies should revisit and reframe strategies for gender digital inclusion with an assessment of barriers that create digital exclusion [38]. An integrated and cohesive action plan for gender spells out hope and progress.

14.5 CONCLUSIONS

With the accessibility and knowledge of the use of social media, there can be improved advocacy and awareness of women's legal rights. Safe future with seeking out help via #Hashtags and online messages. Social media can bridge the gap between those women and girls in need of help and those agencies and individuals extending help. Social media has the potential to help create connected virtual communities of women worldwide, in order to safeguard their interests and rights.

Amidst confinement, quarantine, and lockdown, the challenges are plenty, from intimate partner violence to online harassment and an uncertain future. COVID-19 brings in its set of new problems amidst the old existing gender inequities. However, women fight back, create space for themselves, connect with the likeminded via social media and online platforms to vent out their fears and anguish, share their pleasure and moments of merriment.

Social media serves as a platform to connect with women and girls who in the current lockdown conditions want to secure relief from abuse. Yet, there are many who harbor their own inhibitions to open up, especially in the online environments due to cyber violence. Social media has turned as an inexpensive tool for women and girls against abuse. Social media has the potential to curb further deprivation of women and girl's rights. However, cohesive efforts of individuals, civil societies, governments, and private sector to collectively widen their reach for the displaced, anxious, and fearful women and girls who do not have access of any kind to media. Social media and online platforms to be made more accessible with stricter legal frameworks to curb cybercrime. Use of technology wherever possible to ensure faster response to emergencies faced by thereby ensuring safety for women of the world. Revival is the new normal way henceforth.

Picking up the pieces of their pandemic struck life, women forge ahead and fight back with their renewed resilience. Social media has brought motivation in forms of creating, connecting, and sharing posts, articles of simple affirmations, and camaraderie. It has helped women shed their inhibitions and open about themselves and their experiences, dreams, or doubts and found support from each other, building virtual strands of solidarity. Social media platforms for women are those rays of hope in the gloom, joyful virtual locales to rush back to, loose oneself and let go of the pain. Women have found solace in social media where they create life-changing moments, attaching themselves to their golden clasp of gaiety.

KEYWORDS

- **demographics**
- **digital behaviors**
- **global digital report**
- **organizations**
- **social media**
- **teleconferencing**

REFERENCES

1. Valck, K. D., (2020). *What is the Role of Social Media During the COVID-19 Crisis.* Retrieved from: https://www.hec.edu/en/knowledge/instants/what-role-social-media-during-covid-19-crisis-0 (accessed on 26 June 2021).

2. Ott, K., (2018). Social media and feminist values- aligned or maligned? *Frontiers: A Journal of Women Studies, 39*(1), 93–111.

3. Jouet, J., (2017). *Digital Feminism: Questioning the Renewal of Activism.* Retrieved from: http://www.lse.ac.uk/media-and-communications/assets/documents/research/working-paper-series/WP48.pdf (accessed on 28 June 2021).

4. Lacount, A., (n.d.). *Digital Feminism: A New Frontier.* Retrieved from: https://bust.com/feminism/9982-digital-feminism-a-new-frontier.html (accessed on 28 June 2021).

5. Carpentier, N., (2009). Participation is not enough: The conditions of mediated participatory practices. *European Journal of Communication*, 407–419. https://doi.org/10.1177%2F0267323109345682.

6. Benkler, Y., (2006). *The Wealth of Networks: How Social Production Transforms Markets and Freedom.* Connecticut: Yale University Press.

7. Siegel, D. A., (2009). Social networks and collective action. *American Journal of Political Science*, 122–138. Retrieved from: https://www.jstor.org/stable/25193871 (accessed on 28 June 2021).

8. Clement, J., (2020). *Gender distribution of social media audiences worldwide as of January 2020.* Retrieved from: https://www.statista.com/statistics/274828/gender-distribution-of-active-social-media-users-worldwide-by-platform/ (accessed on 28 June 2021).

9. Aslam, S., (2020). *Twitter by the Numbers: Stats, Demographics and Fun Facts*. Retrieved https://www.omnicoreagency.com/twitter-statistics/ (accessed on 28 June 2021).

10. Sehl, K., (2020). *Top Twitter Demographics That Matter to Social Media Marketers.* Retrieved from: https://blog.hootsuite.com/twitter-demographics/ (accessed on 28 June 2021).

11. Kemp, S., (2020). *Digital Around the World in April 2020.* Retrieved from: https://wearesocial.com/blog/2020/04/digital-around-the-world-in-april-2020 (accessed on 28 June 2021).

12. Rana, U., & Singh, R., (2020). Emotion analysis of Indians using google trends during COVID-19 pandemic. *Diabetes & Metabolic Syndrome, 14*(6), 1849–1850.

13. EmpowerWomen, (2020). *Events and Opportunities.* Retrieved from: https://www.empowerwomen.org/en/community/events-opportunities (accessed on 28 June 2021).

14. Blakely, J., (2010). *Social Media and the End of Gender.* Retrieved from: https://www.ted.com/talks/johanna_blakley_social_media_and_the_end_of_gender#t-179926 (accessed on 28 June 2021).

15. Ahlawat, J., (2020). *How Social Media Has Become a Site for Sisterhood in the COVID-19 Pandemic*. Retrieved from: Feminism in India: https://feminisminindia.com/2020/07/01/social-media-safe-space-for-women-sisterhood-covid-19/ (accessed on 28 June 2021).

16. Meyerson, A., (2020). *Women on a Roll.* Retrieved, from https://womenonaroll.com (accessed on 28 June 2021).

17. Connect Americas, (2015). *Women Are Driving Social Media Revolution.* Retrieved from: https://connectamericas.com/content/women-are-driving-social-media-revolution (accessed on 28 June 2021).

18. Brown, R., (2020). *Local Ladies Bringing People Together Virtually Amid Social Distancing.* Retrieved from: https://www.dailycommercial.com/news/20200328/local-ladies-bringing-people-together-virtually-amid-social-distancing (accessed on 28 June 2021).

19. Scott, M., (2020). *Coronavirus: Stress Hitting the Young Women Most: Poll.* Retrieved from: https://montrealgazette.com/news/local-news/coronavirus-stress-hitting-young-women-the-most-poll (accessed on 28 June 2021).

20. Ferriera, F., (2020). *Myth-busting on Youtube.* Retrieved from: http://news.mit.edu/2020/myth-busting-youtube-izabella-pena-0503 (accessed on 28 June 2021).

21. Ruiz-Pérez, I., Plazaola-Castano, J., & Vives-Cases, C., (2007). Methodological issues in the study of violence against women. *Journal of Epidemiology & Community Health, 26*–31.

22. Sharp, A., (2020). *A Spike in the Domestic Violence Happening Due to COVID-19 Experts Say.* Retrieved from: https://www.nationalobserver.com/2020/04/28/news/spike-domestic-violence-happening-toronto-due-covid-19-experts-say (accessed on 28 June 2021).

23. Taub, A., (2020). *A New COVID-19 Crisis: Domestic Abuse Rises Worldwide.* Retrieved from: https://www.nytimes.com/2020/04/06/world/coronavirus-domestic-violence.html (accessed on 26 June 2021).

24. Murphy, N., (2020). *YouAreNotAlone Campaign to Tackle Domestic Abuse During Lockdown Launched by Priti Patel.* Retrieved from: https://www.mirror.co.uk/news/uk-news/government-launches-youarenotalone-campaign-tackle-21851363 (accessed on 28 June 2021).

25. @MoJGovUK, (2020). *If You are a Victim of Crime, or You've Experienced Domestic Abuse or Sexual Violence, #YouAreNotAlone.* Support services are open & available to you. Retrieved from: https://twitter.com/hashtag/YouAreNotAlone?src=hash&ref_src=twsrc%5Etfw%7Ctwcamp%5Etweetembed%7Ctwterm%5E1248995977538809859&ref_url=https%3A%2F%2Fwww.mirror.co.uk%2Fnews%2Fuk-news%2Fgovernment-launches-youarenotalone-campaign-tackle-21851363 (accessed on 28 June 2021).

26. @TaylorBlack2014, (2020). *One of My Best Friends Outed Her Abuser Today and I Am So Proud of this Strong Woman! #Domesticviolence.* Retrieved from: https://twitter.com/taylorblack2014/status/1269809454704459776 (accessed on 28 June 2021).

27. @AddlCPCrimesHyd, (2020). *#YouAreNotAlone #EnoughisEnough.* Say no to #domesticviolence reach us at Bharosa. Retrieved from: https://twitter.com/hashtag/domesticviolence?ref_src=twsrc%5Egoogle%7Ctwcamp%5Eserp%7Ctwgr%5Ehashtag (accessed on 28 June 2021).

28. Survivor, S. U., (2020). *Stand up Survivor- Domestic Violence Awareness.* Retrieved from: https://www.facebook.com/standupsurvivor/?epa=SEARCH_BOX (accessed on 26 June 2021).

29. Bianca, F., & Loney-Howes, R. (2019). Introduction: Mapping the emergence of #MeToo. In: Bianca, F., & R. L. H., (eds.), *#MeToo and the Politics of Social Change* (pp. 37, 38). Switzerland: Palgrave Macmillan.

30. Clark, R., (2016). Hope in a hashtag: The discursive activism of #WhyIStayed. *Feminist Media Studies, 788*–804. https://doi.org/10.1080/14680777.2016.1138235.

31. News, (2020). *As Pandemic Rages, Women and Girls Face Intensified Risks.* Retrieved from: https://www.unfpa.org/news/pandemic-rages-women-and-girls-face-intensified-risks; www.unfpa.org (accessed on 28 June 2021).

32. McGill, M. H., (2020). *Coronavirus Exposes the Digital Divide's Toll.* Retrieved from: https://www.axios.com/coronavirus-exposes-the-digital-divides-toll-7c270aab-82e4-4719-840f-fc06e2b9083c.html; www.axios.com (accessed on 28 June 2021).

33. Smitha, H., (2017). Empowerment of women through digital literacy strategies- new challenges. *IOSR Journal of Humanities and Social Sciences, 21*–23. Retrieved from: http://iosrjournals.org/iosr-jhss/papers/Conf.17036/Volume-3/7.%2021-23.pdf (accessed on 26 June 2021).

34. OECD, (2020). *Women Leaders Virtual Roundtable on COVID-19 & the Future Issues Call to Put Women and Girls at the Centre of Response Efforts.* Retrieved from: http://www.oecd.org/newsroom/women-leaders-virtual-roundtable-on-covid-19-and-the-future-issues-call-to-put-women-and-girls-at-the-centre-of-response-efforts.htm (accessed on 28 June 2021).

35. Lyons C. Angela, Zucchetti Alessia, Kass-Hanna Josephine, & Cobo Cristobal, (2019). Bridging the Gap Between Digital Skills and Employability for Vulnerable Populations. *T-20 JAPAN.* https://t20japan.org/policy-brief-bridging-gap-between-digital-skills-employability/ (accessed on 28 June 2021).

36. Robertson, Danielle, Ayazi, Mina, (2019). How Women are Using Technology to Advance Gender, Equality and Peace. United States Institute of Peace, July 15 2019. https://www.usip.org/publications/2019/07/how-women-are-using-technology-advance-gender-equality-and-peace (accessed on 28 June 2021).

37. India, T. O., (2020). *Domestic Violence Cases in India on the Rise During the Lockdown.* Retrieved from: https://timesofindia.indiatimes.com/life-style/relationships/love-sex/domestic-violence-cases-in-india-on-the-rise-during-lockdown-says-report/articleshow/75801752.cms (accessed on 28 June 2021).

38. Judith, M. G. M., (2019). Bridging the gender digital gap. *Economics.* The open access. *Open-Assessment E-Journal 13,* 1–12. http://dx.doi.org/10.5018/economics-ejournal.ja.2019-9 (accessed on 28 June 2021).

39. Kaitylnn, M. J. R., (2019). *Digital Feminist Activism: Girls and Women Fight Back Against Rape Culture.* London: Oxford Scholarship Online. https://oxford.universitypressscholarship.com/view/10.1093/oso/9780190697846.001.0001/oso-9780190697846 (accessed on 28 June 2021).

40. Meco, L. D., (2019). *A Woman's Place in a Digital World.* Retrieved from: https://thehill.com/opinion/technology/432029-a-womans-place-in-a-digital-world (accessed on 28 June 2021).

41. Burke Moira, & Kraut E. Robert, (2016). The relationship between Facebook use and well-being depends on communication type and tie strength. *Journal of Computer-Mediated Communication,* 265–281. https://onlinelibrary.wiley.com/doi/full/10.1111/jcc4.12162 (accessed on 28 June 2021).

42. Mariscal Judith, Mayne Gloria, Aneja Urvashi, & Sorgner Alina, (2019). Bridging the Gender Digital Gap. *Economics E-Journal 13, 1.* https://www.degruyter.com/document/doi/10.5018/economics-ejournal.ja.2019-9/html (accessed on 28 June 2021).

43. Mendes Kaitlynn, Ringrose Jessica, & Keller Jessalynn, (2019). Hashtag Feminism. *Digital Feminist Activism: Girls and Women Fight Back Against Rape Culture.* Oxford University Press. https://oxford.universitypressscholarship.com/view/10.1093/oso/9780190697846.001.0001/oso-9780190697846 (accessed on 28 June 2021).

44. Godin, Melissa, (2020). "As Cities Around the World Go on Lockdown, Victims of Domestic Violence Look for a Way Out." *TIME Magazine.* https://time.com/5803887/coronavirus-domestic-violence-victims/ (accessed on 28 June 2021).

45. Times of India, (2020). Domestic violence cases on the rise during the lockdown, says report. *Times of India.* 2020 May 18. https://timesofindia.indiatimes.com/life-style/relationships/love-sex/domestic-violence-cases-in-india-on-the-rise-during-lockdown-says-report/articleshow/75801752.cms (accessed on 28 June 2021).

CHAPTER 15

The South African Police and the Challenges They Are Encountering During COVID-19

VANNIE NAIDOO

School of Management, Information Technology, and Governance, University of KwaZulu-Natal, Durban, Westville Campus, Durban, South Africa, E-mail: naidoova@ukzn.ac.za

ABSTRACT

In whatever country in the world, the police or our "men in blue," as they are often referred to, are the first responders, called upon by members of the community whether it is a crime, disturbance, disaster, or health hazard. They are the ones who serve and protect the public during times of uncertainty, disasters, or conflicts. These men and women have a duty and have pledged to serve their countrymen. This is not an easy job, as the emergence of COVID-19 has put a strain on our society, and now more than ever, worldwide the police officers are needed to prevent chaos and retain the peace during these difficult and uncertain times. The motivation for this research was to explore and discuss the challenges faced by the members of the South African police, during the COVID-19 outbreak. The key objectives in this chapter will highlight themes on the police and their duty to members in society, reflections on how COVID-19 impacts on the policy will be discussed with specific inference to South African police. The challenges faced by police and stress and how it affects the police during the pandemic will also be brought to light. Lastly, the theme on how the police can manage their stress during the pandemic and maintain quality of life for themselves and the nation they serve will be discussed.

15.1 INTRODUCTION

The police are unique members of society who are sworn to serve and protect the community and broader society they serve. There are no racial, political, elite lines for the police, they protect all people in the country under their jurisdiction. The police are the first responders. On the 15 March 2020, due to the outbreak of COVID-19, a National State of Disaster was declared by the South African government. On the 23 March 2020, Lockdown came into effect in South Africa. This was a national 21-day Lockdown. This LockDown was further imposed after three weeks as the country's infection rate was on the rise, till 30 April. Lockdown at stage 5, was where all citizens of South Africa, who were not essential workers were asked to stay home. During stage 5, Lockdown, there were certain special circumstances, namely buying food or medical supplies and seeking medical assistance that permitted South Africans to leave their homes. The different stages of Lockdown have followed in the preceding months from March, 23. At present in July-August, the country is on Lockdown stage 3. In this stage, there is a curfew, where people must have a permit to move around after 10 pm. The curfew was at 9 pm at night but moved to 10 pm so that people would be allowed to frequent restaurants and have ample time to take their dinner and return home before curfew. Curfew can only be broken if a person needs medical attention. The police during Lockdown were asked to ensure that the public follow the rules and regulations of Lockdown, put forward by the government. In this chapter, the following key areas will be discussed in detail. They are as follows:

- The police and their duty to members of the public during COVID-19.
- Reflections on how COVID-19 impacts on the police with specific reference to South African police.
- The challenges faced by the police.
- Stress and how it affects the police during the pandemic.
- How can the police manage their stress during the pandemic and maintain quality of life for themselves and the nation they serve?

The discussion will begin by outlining the police and their duty to the community they serve.

15.2   THE POLICE AND THEIR DUTY TO MEMBERS OF THE PUBLIC DURING COVID-19

The police have a pivotal responsibility and duty towards the public. The discussion that follows reflects these important duties members of the police are tasked with to serve the nation in South Africa.

The various duties allocated to police officers vary, depending on their rank. The main duty and responsibility of a police officer is to support and defend the law and maintain law and order. Some of their main duties and responsibilities are as follows:

- The police officers maintain law, order, and peace;
- They investigate crime;
- They are responsible for prisoners detained in the jail where necessary;
- They make arrests on people who are guilty of criminal negligence or guilty of breaking the (South African) law;
- They are responsible to be called on the scene of traffic and roadblocks;
- They are responsible to attend a scene of an accident where applicable;
- They are responsible for promoting community policing;
- They guard prisoners in hospital;
- They are responsible for visiting prisoners in hospital where necessary;
- They are responsible to guard prisoners in court;
- They act as community liaison officers where applicable;
- They act as community spokesperson where applicable;
- They can sign and endorse affidavits provided original documents are presented;
- They secure crime scenes and collect evidence where applicable;
- They engage in workshops and police forums and studying towards a Diploma in Policing in order for them to acquire a higher rank;
- They are called on to assist the Department of Health, in investigating in the tracking down of COVID cases;
- They are called on to assist in investigating possible threats during COVID. For example, if there are too many people at a mall during a sale, they must investigate to check that social distancing is maintained;
- They are called on to protect Government politicians;
- They are called on to escort the ambulance into rural communities or informal sectors since the ambulance service can be assaulted on the scene if they enter without police protection;

- They are called on to help assist the firemen where applicable to ensure road closures and evacuations to prevent loss of life in certain circumstance;
- The police are tasked during COVID-19 to do patrols and investigate members of the public who are in a gathering and not respecting social distancing etiquette. They also have to investigate if complaints are made of funerals, weddings, religious services, and other gatherings and ensure that social distancing etiquette is followed accordingly.

Some of the police members' duties have been briefly outlined above, and from this, it can be clearly seen that the police members are in direct and close contact with the public. This in itself makes them vulnerable to infection, especially during COVID-19. The police are the first call the public makes, whether it is a crime, a disturbance, or a health pandemic. The police have a job that requires them to continuously interact with members of the public at all times. The researcher would like to highlight the European Union and the United Nations (UN) Office on Drugs and Crime recommended behavior to be followed [1]. Important areas focused on will be maintaining social distancing while working at stations, managing public order situations, contact tracing of infected members of public, arresting protocols during COVID-19. They will now be discussed.

15.2.1 WORKPLACE SOCIAL DISTANCING AT POLICE STATIONS

While performing duties when working in police stations, officers should follow the recommended behavior below [1]:

- At a police station unnecessary contact with visitors should be limited [1];
- At the police station, exposed office surfaces and office equipment should be regularly sanitized [1];
- When police officers handle documents, there is a possibility that they may be contaminated. Avoid unnecessary contact with documents. The use of gloves in such circumstance is necessary, or police officers have to immediately wash their hands after handling a document [1];
- To avoid unnecessary contact with the public, consider suspending the enforcement of minor offenses and traffic violations [1];

• The police should maintain strict compliance with existing national legislation to prevent overcrowding in specific locations, namely taverns, clubs or sports stadiums, beaches, which are considered hotspots in the transmission of the COVID-19 virus [1].

15.2.2   MANAGING PUBLIC ORDER SITUATIONS

When police are managing public order situations, the following recommended behavior is put forth [1]:

• A police officer must have on personal protective equipment (PPE). These should include gloves, eye protection goggles, and a disposable face mask before coming in close contact with a crowd [1].
• Stay calm.
• The crowd should be briefed on the regulation for COVID-19 prevention measures and then explained that it is in the interest of their own safety, that they disperse [1].
• Force should only be used on members of the public only when absolutely necessary to achieve order in accordance with existing national legislation [1].
• Clean and disinfect all equipment before and after the use.

15.2.3   CONTACT TRACING

While contact tracing, police should embark on the following recommended behavior [1]:

• You may be called upon to assist public health officials and related entities in tracing members of the public who are possible carrier of the virus [1];
• Duties need be performed in strict compliance with national legislation, in liaison with relevant agencies where necessary, whilst respecting the individual's legal rights [1];
• When interacting with members of the public who are possible carrier of the virus wear PPE and exercise an abundance of caution [1];
• Police officers must wash or sanitize their hands, and any other surfaces that may have come into contact with the infection at the earliest opportunity [1].

15.2.4   *MAKING ARRESTS*

When making arrest the police should engage in the following recommended behavior [1]:

- It is crucial to limit the number of individuals detained in jail to prevent infection;
- During the current pandemic detaining a potential suspect should be a last resort, to be used only in relation to serious offenses [1];
- Only, when necessary, should a potential suspect be searched. The police officer should ask the potential suspect to display any items of interest on their person, or amongst their personal possessions. Police should only physically touch a potential suspect of it is absolutely required, and under safe conditions using PPE [1];
- Of the law permits, release detainees on bail;
- If the suspect is detained, the police officer must consider how and where the detainee can be held safely and for what duration; and also, who is going to interact with the detainee whilst they are in custody. Enforce social distancing measures at all times [1];
- The detention facilities should be regularly and thoroughly cleaned. The staff doing the cleaning need to use proper PPE's [1].

After discussing the duties of police officers during COVID-19, the discussion that follows will be on how COVID-19 impacts on South African police members.

15.3   REFLECTION ON HOW COVID-19 IMPACTS ON THE POLICE- WITH SPECIFIC REFERENCE TO SOUTH AFRICA

The pandemic has affected people across the globe in all facets of their everyday lives. Under National Disaster, South Africa had different stages of Lockdown. Level 5 being complete shutdown of business and only allowing essential services like police, army, medical practitioners, petrol stations, food, and grocery shops, firemen, navy, and limited bus and taxi transport to continue services. Anyone who was not an essential worker had to stay at home during this stage of Lockdown. The police were called upon to enforce the Lockdown. During all stages of Lockdown, the police are a vital force that has to serve and protect people during this time of national crisis brought on by the pandemic. Many rules and regulations governing how civilians should behave, were instated by the South African government, and the police were called upon to ensure public compliance to the new, Lockdown policies, rules, regulations, and laws. During Lockdown, stage 5, in South Africa, police had to ensure limited movement of people be enforced during this stage. Roadblocks were put up to catch illegal people from moving around or crossing provincial and foreign borders. Essential workers had to carry on them a work permit at all times. People who were traveling between provinces also had to have necessary documentation and permits to travel. Trucks and other vehicles crossing the South African border had to have the necessary documentation to enter or leave the country. At all times, the South African police, together with Metro Police and the South African army were at the forefront to protect the South African nation. During Stage 3 of Lockdown, brought on in July/August 2020, there is a curfew in place and the police must ensure there is no illegal movement from 10 pm, as this is the time everyone in the county must be at home, unless the person has a permit to move around. The police also had to use their discretion as people who require immediate medical treatment must be allowed to travel.

The police had to ensure civilians maintain social distancing, wear masks and are not engaged in large gatherings. Wearing of masks in public was mandatory from May 2020 when the government took this decision for all citizens of South Africa to wear masks in public. This was an added function to the police officers' daily job which was brought on during COVID. If people did not comply with government regulations pertain to COVID, they had to be fined by the police. This in turn, is putting a strain on the police, as the police stations jails become overcrowded and the court being overrun with cases being brought forward because of negligent people who are not upholding the Lockdown rules and are breaking the law. In South Africa, some people refuse to abide by the rules and wear mask. In many shops and malls in South Africa, you cannot enter without a mask. Yet, still certain South Africans' refuse to follow the rule of law during COVID-19 times.

The major challenges to police officers has been their ability to enforce social distancing and voluntary quarantine in communities and restricting civilians to their own neighborhoods [2]. It is often problematic for police officers to enforce social distancing, since civilians need access to shop for food and obtain medical care. In spite of South Africans' being educated on the norms of social distancing and how it promotes health and safety, there are those members of the public who just do not follow rules in society. The police also picked up the homeless during COVID-19 who were roaming the streets of South Africa, destitute, and hungry and took them to homeless shelters and places of safety.

The army was brought in to work with the South African police to bring about compliance of Lockdown during stage 5, as many people, especially from the locations, certain African townships and informal settlements refused to abide by the rules and stay home during National Lockdown. Since the police community numbers are so limited in South Africa, to actively police these areas during stage 5, Lockdown, the army was effectively brought in, and they ensured that these members of South African society stayed in their homes and not roam the streets freely. Some South African's have argued against such harsh measures being brought into action by the government and see South Africa as being governed as a "police state." Ordinary South African's have ganged up on social media to speak poorly about the brute force shown by the police against members of the public, who had not following Lockdown regulations. The big picture, emerging is that the strong arm of the police and other armed forces like the army is essential during COVID-19 to protect ordinary South Africans.' For this, the South African police are becoming the most feared and hated in the country because they are trying to prevent the infection rate, by ensuring that people in South Africa follow the rules and regulations stipulated in Lockdown.

Another important job the South African police was tasked with was to cease and arrest members of the public who were transporting illegal goods, especially cigarettes and alcohol that was banned during Lockdown stage 5. During COVID-19, the South African police controlled unnecessary movements during Lockdown. Numerous roadblocks were set up, and the police were on the lookout for vehicles transporting illegal substances. Drugs, alcohol, and cigarettes were confiscated during these roadblocks, and many members of the public were arrested for transporting these illegal goods.

A high police and army presence had to be present at borders as South Africa closed its borders during National Lockdown. A large movement to cross the border into their own home countries occurred. Mozambican and Zimbabweans were assisted safely across the border to their own countries that neighbor South Africa's border. SA during their nationwide lockdown, closed off their ports and borders with their neighboring countries. A few days before SA national lockdown, around 23,000 mineworkers from Mozambique were estimated to have embarked on the border crossing successfully. Around 13,500 Zimbabwean nationals had also made border crossings back to their home country. They were asked to self-isolate, once they reached their homes. Dr Aaron Motsoaledi, the SA Home Affairs

Minister, visited the Beitbridge border post into Zimbabwe and was greeted by queues stretching for up miles who had not made the border crossing before lockdown commenced [3]. They were allowed safe passage across the SA border posts and return home.

During COVID-19, police conducted raids and illegal drugs and counterfeit cigarettes were confiscated. Many people who were illegally selling cigarettes and alcohol during Lockdown stage 5 were arrested, as they were breaking the law in terms of COVID-19 Lockdown regulations put forth by the South African government.

Another duty police were tasked with during COVID-19, were to close down illegal shebeen and taverns and arrest the owners and the people who were frequenting them during Lockdown, stage 5. After the ban on alcohol was removed, police had the daunting task to control threats coming from the public, about drunk men who were driving while intoxicated or meeting accidents while intoxicated. Police were also called in on domestic violence incidences because the spouse got drunk and was verballing and physically assaulting the women and children in the home. Once the SA government removed the ban on alcohol, violence in South Africa, specifically within the locations and rural townships increased drastically. These drunk and unruly South Africans were rushed to hospitals by the police and ambulance service. These hospitals were operating beyond capacity and overburdened with treating COVID-19 patients, and were now forced to also treat these drunk and unruly criminals. During Lockdown, stage 3, in South Africa, the ban on alcohol had to be reinstated. This was due to many people being unable to control their liquor, or listen or abide by the rules while intoxicated. They often became violent and harmful to other members of society, more often than not even their own family.

Police have to be fair in upholding the law to protect members of the public during the pandemic. Theorists define procedural justice along the line of the public placing their trust and faith in the police officers and their institution of law and order. The public in return, should be treated in a fair and equitable manner, and the police should maintain a good rapport amongst its' officers and civilians that they are tasked with protecting [4]. The police force was not provided with restrictions for Lockdown as timeously as possible in South Africa. This could be because the government themselves were overwhelmed with the COVID-19 pandemic reaching South Africa and had to battle to make quick decisions to save the lives of their nation. In South Africa, not all stations are following similar protocols. For example, Station A will be fining members of the public if they do not use masks and Station B would not follow the same protocols. It stands to reason that; in SA, such behavior should change, and all police officers should utilize a procedurally just approach that commits to enforcing the law accordingly irrespective of circumstance and situation. This would ensure that the public views the police as exercising their authority in a fair and just manner towards all people who live within our countries borders [5].

Gender violence is prevalent in high levels in South African society. This has not changed during COVID-19. Women police officers in South Africa have been victims of abuse or violence from members of the public while conducting their regular jobs. During COVID-19 women police officers had to be especially careful that they were not caught off guard by criminals. Members of the South African public do not respect female officers as they would their male counterpart's. In African culture, the common sentiment is that "men rule and women are subservient." This perception by members of African society can perpetuate this sort of unequal respect and impact on why these members disrespect the authority of a female officer as opposed to a male police officer.

During COVID-19 a threat that police had to constantly monitor was crowd control, during strikes and illegal strikes that took place in South Africa. It is near impossible to maintain social distancing during a strike when there are huge crowds of people gathering. Police officers had to make sure illegal strikes were disbanded and strikes that were legal had to conform to Lockdown regulation of wearing masks and maintaining social distancing.

To ensure proper law enforcement, the police need constant updated information to do their duties effectively. In South Africa, where there is often load-shedding and power-cuts, this makes it difficult for members to be briefed timeously on new mandates pertaining to COVID-19 and Lockdown procedure and rules of engagement with the public. The argument raised is that police officers require factual and timely information to fulfill their duties successfully. This entails police officers being properly briefed as to why they are carrying out these specific tasks. Apart from information sharing, police officers also require the support of their senior officials, which would encourage them to serve the public with equality, freedom, and justice [6].

PPEs were needed for the police to stay safe as they worked directly with the public. The Police Executive Research Forum Washington, together with the Bureau of Justice in Assistance (USA) [2] indicate that a crucial step in protecting police offices and their administration staff is the mandatory use of PPE's during the disease outbreak. When responding to a contaminated scene, PPE's must be used at all times to promote the officers' safety. Police personnel must have PPE well in advance before an outbreak occurs. Law enforcement use the following three main classes of PPE namely; hand sanitizers, gloves to protect against blood and body fluids, and masks for respiratory protection [2].

In South Africa, the country was in the middle of the Lockdown, stage 5, and the government was trying to acquire PPEs for the police and other essential service workers. The police had to buy their own PPE's and only when stock of PPE's was later sent to them did, they have access to it. Some police stations only had gloves, and police members had to take their own initiative to safeguard their lives and that of the public, by buying their own masks until they became available at their station. It is important to note that [8] despite police officers being first-line responders during the pandemic, they are not regularly tested for the virus. In South Africa, the health care system was over-taxed, and at certain times there were no test kits available to test for COVID-19, and the lack of testing first-line responders during COVID-19 like the police is unacceptable and the South African government failed dismally in protecting their police force. There are ongoing stories of corruption and stealing of PPE's and unaccounted PPEs to date. If the government cannot protect its members in the police force, how can they expect them to be motivated to do their jobs properly? This is the question often raised by the public and policy communities in South Africa.

Especially during the COVID-19 pandemic, it is clearly reflected and seen that the roles of the police have changed, as they now we're tasked with the mammoth task of maintaining the peace and calm amongst the general public. They are the first call that vulnerable women and children make when they feel threatened, scared, or confused. The South African police especially during COVID-19 went to great lengths to safeguard the rights of vulnerable people. Children and women, the most vulnerable in the South African society, were under attack by men on a daily basis. During Lockdown, abused women and children who were involved in domestic violence incidents with family members, placed their hope in the police community, who were the first responders to assist them in taking them to a place of safety. The identity of the police force has changed. Police officers are now content with their social identity that symbolizes them as 'peacekeepers' rather than 'crime-fighters' [9].

15.4   CHALLENGES FACED BY THE POLICE

Research have alluded to many challenges faced by police during COVID-19 pandemic. They are outlined below:

- There is a shortage of police officers on duty at a station. Added to this is the police not being able to cope with the public during the pandemic due to many officers being sick or booked off due to having underlining conditions that they make susceptible to contracting the virus. Arguments indicate that while there are only a handful of accounts of the police role during a flu pandemic, personal accounts allude to the many deaths resulting and the overwhelming destruction that comes with it. This is a clear indicator that the repercussions of a 21st-Century flu pandemic could result in the police services being stretched to its' limits [2].
- Members of the police are close to retirement age and have underlying health conditions that make them unfit to work during the pandemic. In India, for example, officers aged 55 years and older were asked to not report for duty as many of them lost their lives in serving the public during the pandemic. This is not the case in South Africa, although many policemen have lost their lives, the government has done nothing to safeguard members of the police community that is close to retirement age.
- The police officers do not have the necessary PPEs to do their job, even though they in direct contact with the public during the pandemic.
- The policemen and women are human, and the pandemic and the uncertainty and death it brings with it can cause members of the police to have doubts, fears, and anxiety that can contribute to their high stress levels, which can lead to poor health or depression in police members.
- In South Africa, there are too few police members' available to control the low-income sectors living in a huge number of informal settlements.
- People do not respect the law and hate or fear the police. This can be a great challenge as these citizens will break the law and cause chaos or malicious acts of violence during the pandemic.
- The occupation of a police officer involves close cooperation with the public, this can put them in a high risk and vulnerable situation and they can become infected whilst carrying out their duties to uphold law and order;
- Police officers have to enforce Lockdown procedures and rules especially pertaining to the general public. If the members of the public refuse to abide by these rules, the police can issue them a fine. A good example where police can find members of the public if they do not

wear a mask in public. Another example is where people are crossing provinces with fake permission documents.

15.5   STRESS AND HOW IT AFFECTS THE POLICE DURING THE PANDEMIC

The discussion that follows will address stress and how it affects the police during the pandemic. The pandemic has placed undue stress on the lives of police officers. In the line of duty, officers can experience post-traumatic stress. This can lead to ill-health and many mental disorders like depression and anxiety. In August 2020, South Africa was registered as having the 5th largest infection rates in the world. The death toll is also on the rise, and this coupled with communities being sick and dying at the hand of the pandemic can take its' toll on the mental psyche of members in the SAP. They would circum in the ongoing months to post-traumatic stress, which can severely impair their health. Police officers must have regular counseling, especially during COVID-19 as their mental capacity can be overwhelmed during the pandemic and can lead to impaired concentration levels and inability to perform their tasks at optimum. Current research suggests that counseling can be an effective tool for managing these wellness issues, especially those associated with post-traumatic stress [11].

The diverse roles of police officers make them very highly stressed as their job entails enforcing the law and order in society and maintaining the peace. Since police officers' roles are very broad, there is no clear picture on specifying "what they can do," but infringes on "what they are called on to do" to maintain order and peace within South African society. Dating back to the early 1990s, the role of a police officer includes various tasks namely; anti-terrorism, relief, and assistance services, arresting criminals, crime control and crime prevention [12]. In South Africa, especially during COVID-19, the police were called on to maintain the peace and disband crowds during illegal strike action. When dealing with crowds, there is always the uncertainty and volatility of something going wrong. Police officers many a times in South Africa have been privy to stoning, petrol bombs being hurled at them, and violent confrontations with members of a rioting mob. Again, this behavior can traumatic a police officer who can experience post-traumatic stress due to the trauma and violence he/she was exposed to during this incident.

Police are also fearing infecting their loved ones and family as they constantly in contact with the public and can at any time become infected, in spite of wearing PPE's. This causes great mental strain in their family unit and can lead to the police officer being angry or agitated or constantly worrying over the safety of their family because of their job environment and circumstances. Some police officers are living apart from their families to keep them safe, or they are practicing social distancing even in the same household that they share with their loved ones, thus adding to their anxiety and stress levels.

Many white police officers can feel threatened while enforcing the law because the perceptions of many black South Africans are steeped in racial beliefs due to the past Apartheid laws. The Black people in South Africa would have a tough time taking instructions from a white police office during an ethnic confrontation as they would want an African officer present who understands their culture and would understand the ethnic conflict better. Although culture and diversity are taught to police officers, the perceptions of the majority of the public have not changed. In fact, it has gone worst during strikes where police officers are violently assaulted irrespective of their color as well. The lack of racial tolerance and acceptance as a rainbow nation has never been properly articulated to all levels of South African society. Some, many a time choose to live in anger based on racial, ethnic or gender tensions. With respect to, women police officers who are not given the due respect as male officers purely based on gender. This is a sad reality as oppression and violence against women in South Africa continues unabated till today. Gender and racial tension can also cause stress and anxiety to be experienced by police members. Especially during COVID, such negative attitude portrayed by the public towards police members based on gender and racism can impede police in their duties. The stress of dealing with members of the public during COVID-19 can be especially difficult due to the disrespect shown by members of the public towards South African law enforcement officials. Stress can add up, if members feel disrespected as it can poorly affect their morale.

Community policing is an important aspect of an evolving role within the police departments in South Africa. The ongoing budgetary cuts made in the sectors of health, social care, and mental health services and policing has changed the dynamics of police officers' duties. Police officers are now also tasked with an increasing range of non-crime related activities. In SA, the College of Policing estimates that around 83% of all calls that come through to a police stations' call center staff are non-crime-related [13]. During COVID-19 the police were inundated with calls requesting assistance in illegal gatherings of people during the pandemic. Police were also requested in the CSC charge office to assist in getting ambulances through to assist sick people during the pandemic. When university students unlawfully during Lockdown, stage 5, lived at residences that were not vacated, police had to go in when these students complained of needing medical attention. These students had to be delivered by the police to the necessary quarantine centers, for example, in order for them to receive medical assistance. This again can expose the police to contracting the virus. It can also cause worry and stress after the incident, as many police officers battle to manage their doubts about COVID and becoming infected.

In the discussion that follows how the police manage their stress during the pandemic whilst maintaining quality of life for themselves, and the nation they serve will be outlined and discussed.

15.6   HOW CAN THE POLICE MANAGE THEIR STRESS DURING THE PANDEMIC AND MAINTAIN QUALITY OF LIFE FOR THEMSELVES AND THE NATION THEY SERVE?

During this global pandemic, the police force will be one of the sectors of essential service workers hardest hit in a country. South Africa will be no different. In protecting the public and maintaining the peace during COVID-19, many officers will be exposed to the virus. This can lead to compromising their quality of life in the long term or in certain severe circumstances, even loss of life. In the line of duty, many police officers during COVID-19 will lose their lives. These are the unsung heroes, who often are not appreciated by members of the community in spite of their hard work and sacrifice in protecting the community they police.

Another clearly challenging aspect that COVID-19 would have world-wide on the police community is the stress and trauma that goes with the job during the pandemic. As more and more police officers in South Africa get infected while in contact with infected members of the public, this would have a devastating impact on the morale of police officers and can lead to heightened stress and anxiety on the job. COVID-19 is the silent killer stalking the public and it is an unseeing violent predator that makes it all the more dangerous. The reality of the situation at present, makes the police officers more paranoid and anxious to have such a violent threat like COVID-19 on the loose, that can attack silently, any member of society, police included, or "brothers in Blue" like they often referred to.

Police officers experience high levels of stress due to the complexity of their job. Although mental fitness is important for a police officer, these individuals are also human, and if continuously surrounded by traumatic events, these can trigger mental anguish and stress. Stress is an unseeing killer that can affect the lives of police officers. Stress can be a contributing factor to heart disease. This is one possible reason why police officer has a shorter lifespan compared to normal civilians [10]. Job related stress can cause police officers to over-indulge in food, alcohol or smoking or having affairs as a form of escapism from their stressful jobs. Many police officers also experience severe mental conditions, most common are depression, anxiety, and paranoia, fear of dying on the job, or panic attacks. Police officers also commit suicide as the world around them and their stressful jobs becomes too much to deal with, that death is the only way out. Within the policing context members who display distancing and avoidance behavior due to stress and trauma may become unstable [15]. Avoidance behavior by police officers can lead to them having psychosomatic symptoms and dysfunctional work/family relationships [16], psychological distress that triggers mental health issues like depression [17, 18], post-traumatic stress disorder (PTSD) [19, 20], mental fatigue and exhaustion [21], and suicidal tendencies [22].

Mental anguish is often experienced by police officers. Since the idea taught by society in South Africa is that "grown men don't cry," there is a lot of stigma attached to seek medical and professional attention for stress by police officers. This perception has to change, as human beings, anyone at a given time can be exposed to stress or a traumatic experience that can bring on mental anguish and stress that has to be treated through counseling and medicine prescribed by a psychiatrist. If South Africans' can see that there is no shame in this, then maybe stress a silent killer can be combated, as more police officers seek medical and professional counseling for stress and trauma. Avoidance coping strategies practiced by police officers as a way of dealing with stress, and traumatic experiences, registered in these members having high levels of cynicism. They were often exhausted. They registered feeling low in terms of their accomplishment and professional efficacy at work [14].

COVID-19 will constantly heighten stress levels of the police community worldwide. As more members in their community die around them and more officers test positive and circum to the pandemic, this rising death toll will place undue pressure on the lives of South Africa police officers. The trauma and death that goes with COVID-19 will result in police officers' experiencing devastating stress levels that can hinder their job performance. High levels of absenteeism will increase as more members of the police force in South Africa test positive for COVID or have mental distress and related medical issues associated with stress. A proactive way forward is to ensure that police members are provided adequate counseling and support during the pandemic and post-pandemic. Research suggests that counseling can be an effective tool for managing these wellness issues [10]. Pienaar and Rothmann indicate that problem-focused coping is the most practices therapy administered to people coping with emotional shock, grief, and stress [7]. In the discussion that follows, future research areas aligned to the chapter topic will be outlined.

15.7   FUTURE RESEARCH AREAS

Research should be carried out to ascertain police perceptions, on how to manage unruly gatherings and mobs during COVID-19. Another area that requires further research is how the police officers are coping with post-traumatic stress during COVID-19. Research is also required on police roadblocks and how police officers maintain COVID-19 regulations with members of the public who are transporting illegal goods like cigarettes and alcohol. The focus of such research should look at arresting people who transport illegal products during Lockdown. Research on how police officer's family's lives are disrupted and how they cope during COVID-19 should be explored in further research. The studies for future research can be South African based or internationally based.

15.8   CONCLUDING REMARKS

COVID-19 is a silent killer, it sees no race, ethnicity, age, or gender. It attacks people in society and, more often than not, has devastating consequences on society. The only way to keep the South African nation safe is to force the nation to practice the use of masks, self-isolation, and maintaining social distancing protocols at all times, so that COVID-19 can be curtailed. For now, especially in COVID-19 times, the time for talking and negotiating is over. To stop the infection rate, the police had to take drastic measures to ensure the protection of the nation during the pandemic. If South Africans are not in agreement, their opinion should be benched, as this is "not normal times," this is a pandemic, and it kills humans. To protect and preserve the safety of human life, the police have to be strict and defend ordinary South Africans against the pandemic, even if it means being members of South

African society that are the most feared and hated during COVID. The police members need to be respected during COVID-19 as they are the fearless warriors defending the nation and maintain order in communities during COVID. This makes the police vulnerable to the virus. As more members lose their lives during COVID-19, let the government ensure that the police community is also provided with proper counseling and medical services during these sad, traumatic, and tragic times brought on in the wake of the pandemic.

KEYWORDS

- **civil society**
- **COVID-19**
- **law**
- **order**
- **police**
- **stress**

REFERENCES

1. European Union and the United Nations Office on Drugs and Crime, (2020). *Nigeria Police Force Guidelines for Policing During the COVID-19 Emergency*. European Union and the United Nations Office on Drugs and Crime, Nigeria.
2. Luna, A. M., Solé, B. C., & Sanberg, E. A., (2007). *Police Planning for an Influenza Pandemic: Case Studies and Recommendations from the Field*. Police Executive Research Forum, Washington.
3. Institute for Security Studies, (2020). *Peace & Security Council Report* (Issue 123). Institute for Security Studies, Kenya.
4. Quinton, P., Myhill, A., Bradford, B., Fildes, A., & Porter, G., (2015). *Fair Cop 2: Organizational Justice, Behavior and Ethical Policing*. College of Policing, Ryton.
5. Tyler, T. R., (2004). Enhancing police legitimacy. *The Annals of the American Academy of Political and Social Science, 593*, 84–99.
6. Bradford, B., & Quinton, P., (2014). Self-legitimacy, police culture and support for democratic policing in an English constabulary. *The British Journal of Criminology, 54*, 1023–1046.
7. Pienaar, J., & Rothmann, S., (2003). Coping strategies in the South African police service. *SA Journal of Industrial Psychology, 29*, 81–90.
8. Express & Star, (2020). *"Significant Confusion" in Role of Police in Enforcing Coronavirus Legislation*. https://www.expressandstar.com/news/uk-news/2020/03/23/

significant-confusion-in-role-of-police-in-enforcing-coronavirus-restrictions/ (accessed on 28 June 2021).

9.   Charman, S., (2018). *From Crime Fighting to Public Protection: The Shaping of Police Officers' Sense of Role.* The police Foundation: London. www.police-foundation.org.uk (accessed on 28 June 2021).

10. Tanigoshi, H., Kontos, A., & Remley, T., (2008). The effectiveness of individual wellness counselling on the wellness of law enforcement officers. *Journal of Counselling and Development, 86,* 64–74.

11. Patterson, G., Chung, I., & Swan, P., (2012). The effects of stress management interventions among police officers and recruits. *Campbell Systematic Reviews, 8,* 1–54.

12. Millie, A., (2013). The policing task and the expansion (and Contraction) of British policing. *Criminology and Criminal Justice, 13,* 143–160.

13. College of Policing, (2015). *College of Policing Analysis: Estimating Demand on the Police Service.* http://www.college.police.uk/documents/demand_report_21_1_15.pdf (accessed on 28 June 2021).

14. Klopper, J., (2003). *Stress and coping in the South African Police Service in the Free State.* http://univofpretoria.worldcat.org/title/burnout-stress-and-coping-in-the-south-african-police-servicein-the-free-state/oclc/55954828&referer=brief_results (accessed on 28 June 2021).

15. Violanti, J. M., (1993). What does high stress police training teach recruits? An analysis of coping. *Journal of Criminal Justice, 21,* 411–417.

16. Burke, R., (1998). Work and non-work stressors and well-being among police officers: The role of coping. *Anxiety, Stress and Coping, 11,* 345–362.

17. Aaron, J., (2000). Stress and coping in police officers. *Police Quarterly, 3,* 438–450.

18. Moller, A., (2008). *The Relationship Between Coping Behavior, Personality Characteristics and Psychological Distress in South African Police Trainees.* http://univofpretoria.worldcat.org/title/relationship-between-coping-behaviour-personality-characteristics-and-psychological-distressin-south-african-police-trainees/oclc/284988693&referer=brief_results (accessed on 28 June 2021).

19. LeBlanc, V. R., Regehr, C., Jelley, R. B., & Barath, I., (2008). The relationship between coping styles, performance, and responses to stressful scenarios in police recruits. *International Journal of Stress Management, 15,* 76–93.

20. Menard, K. S., & Arter, M. L., (2013). Police officer alcohol use and trauma symptoms: Associations with critical incidents, coping, and social stressors. *American Psychological Association, 20,* 37–56.

21. Naud'e, J. L. P., (2003). Occupational stress, coping, burnout and work engagement of emergency workers in Gauteng. Unpublished doctoral thesis/dissertation.

22. Pienaar, J., Rothmann, S., & Van De, V. F. J. R., (2007). Occupational stress, personality traits, coping, and suicide ideation in the South African Police Service. *Criminal Justice and Behavior, 34,* 246–258.

CHAPTER 16

Role of Journalism and Media During the Crisis of the Coronavirus Pandemic in India: A Review

PALLAV MUKHOPADHYAY

Assistant Professor, Department of Journalism and Mass Communication, West Bengal State University, West Bengal, India, E-mail: journalist430@gmail.com

ABSTRACT

The COVID-19, alias coronavirus, has spread to the majority of the countries, areas, and territories in the world. Coronavirus has become a worldwide phenomenon. World Health Organization (WHO) announced this outbreak as a pandemic on 11th March, 2020. The outbreak of coronavirus has created havoc across the world. It has caused severe damage ranging from several lakhs of deaths to economic devastation and leading lockdowns in many countries that have a significant impact on our lifestyles. The rate of infection has increased, but safety and precautionary measures have been taken to fight against this infectious disease to spread across the globe. It includes social distancing, wearing masks and sanitization. The unrest, pessimism, and frustration are spreading day by day. In this time of crisis, the media have to face an examination. The society expects that the coverage of media should be responsible and responsive. While a large section of the media, especially corporate-owned has showed deviation from the role of social responsibility, a small section is maintaining the expected ethics of journalism, which shows its courage. In this prevailing situation, journalists, and media have crucial roles in democratic structure. However, corporate media rely on commercialization and profit. Lack of adequate public health infrastructure, dillydallying in treatment has been ventilated by the media coverage. These issues claim serious investigation and review, but the large section of the mainstream media excepting some has forgotten its role. The central government and various state governments emphasized on social distancing, wearing of masks and usage of sanitizers to fight against the infection. Critics are of opinion that the self-quarantine and isolation have caused a negative impact in the psychology of the common mass. Since we have not adequate information about the novel coronavirus, it is important and significant to cater true news and information collected from trusted and reliable sources. It is not easy to gather the latest and updated information and statistics of the spread of the dangerous Virus during the unprecedented situation caused by the Corona pandemic. Various media have been and are used to aware the common public to obey the rules of quarantine and to decrease the tension among the common mass. The COVID-19 pandemic can be considered as a unique case as far as the role of journalism and media sector in India is concerned. The medical misinformation has continuously spread over mass media platforms at a breakneck speed. The quantum of fake news and misinformation had so negative impact on the mind of individual and the society that its harmful impact has been agreed from all corners of the society. The fake news, false information, gossip have created hindrance in the entire process of news and communication and have increased tension and anxiety among the mass.

Due to the fast dissemination of information through social networking sites, the major drawback of it is that it has been applied to cater false news and information. After the appearance of various social networking sites such as Twitter, Facebook, and YouTube, the dissemination of information in this prevailing time of crisis has enhanced worldwide. These social networking sites provide a domain for exchanging reactions and feedbacks which may have a negative impact during an emergency situation like the existing Corona pandemic. Fake News and false information on the Corona pandemic are spreading with an accelerating pace through the online and new media, creating a change in the behavior of the common people during this emergency situation. These fake news and false information urgently need serious attention and introspection for ensuring community awareness, quick response and prompt decision making. This chapter has examined whether the autonomy of journalism has been maintained in this crisis situation. Within this framework, what was the role of different mass media on the individual and social life as far as the effective health communication is concerned. What were their role for taking preventive measures and combating the spread of false information, maintaining physical distancing, reduction of prejudice, discrimination, and inequalities caused due to fake news or misinformation? Do media provide a way for misinformation and how it affects the private domain of individuals? How fake news impact the largest democracy in the world? Does fake news put forward acute problem on the psychology of people? If so, how? It is essential to look into how the media have catered every minute updates to crores of citizens during this situation of pandemic. This chapter has followed the observational and analytical method to investigate the role of journalism and media during the crisis of the coronavirus pandemic in India. The country has seen significant growth and development in the domain of media during the last three decades, and the indigenous media market has considered one of the biggest in the world. Globalization and neo-liberalization have also shaped it.

Maximization of profit, commercialization, and commoditization has appeared as its main characters. What will be the role of mass media and the journalists during this prevailing crisis situation? The role of capitalism, the market, and the media has to be assessed. Will this pandemic radically change the role of the media and the journalists? Will the country see the increased efforts of building social responsibility among the temptation of finance capital and profit maximization?

Indian media and the journalists need to introspect their respective stands in the context of these significant and serious questions and issues. Media have vital influence over people during the present coronavirus pandemic, so all information should be more transparent and authentic, which is of paramount importance in this crisis. Fake news and misinformation can fill in the void if genuine and trusted information fail to appear in time to the target audience of the mass media. As a consequence, it can lead to hazardous effects. The news and information catered by various media have an influence on the mind of the prospective target audience, so it should be presented with utmost care and sincerity after repeated rechecking and cross-checking because single misinformation that gain attention can negate the importance of correct information and can pose a serious challenge about the credibility and trustworthiness of the media. It is vital to consider that in such a time of crisis, the news media should respond with responsibility and social accountability. The media should disseminate reliable information to the mass during this existing pandemic situation. The mass and social media have been flooded with news, data, statistics, and information during the pandemic situation. A considerable amount of information is catered to aware the general public regarding the nature of the COVID-19. On the other hand, false information about the COVID-19 and its medical treatment are increasing anxiety, tension, and common people's fear psychosis. Media should introspect that whether it have been able in teaching and increasing awareness among the people and reducing anxiety, tension, fear, and panic.

16.1 INTRODUCTION

The COVID-19 alias coronavirus has affected the majority of the countries of the world and has spread to the vast areas and territories across the globe. Coronavirus has become a worldwide phenomenon. The World Health Organization (WHO) announced the outbreak as a pandemic on 11th March, 2020. The outbreak of coronavirus has caused havoc across the world such as causing several lakhs of deaths, economic disintegration leading lockdowns in many countries. This pandemic situation has a negative impact in the life style of the common people belong to almost all the countries.

The style of its spread and pace of infection has increased, but safety measures have been taken to combat the spread of this virus across the world. It includes social distancing, wearing masks and sanitization. The unrest, pessimism, and frustration have spread day by day. In this time of crisis, the media have to face an examination. The society expects that the coverage of media should be responsible and responsive. While a large section of the media, especially corporate-owned has showed deviation from the role of social responsibility, a small section is maintaining the expected ethics of journalism, which shows its courage. In this prevailing situation, journalists, and media have crucial roles in democratic structure. However, corporate media rely on commercialization and profit.

Lack of adequate public health infrastructure, dillydallying in treatment has been ventilated by the media coverage. These issues claim serious investigation and review, but the large section of the mainstream media, except some has forgotten its role. On 30th January, 2020, the first case was identified in Thrissur District of Kerala. It was regarded as the first case in the country. Under the Epidemic Diseases Act (1897, https://legislative.gov.in/sites/default/files/A1897-03.pdf), COVID-19 was announced as an epidemic in more than a dozen states in the country. The country observed 14-hour public curfew on 22nd March, which was followed by a 21-day lockdown of the entire country.

The central government and various state governments emphasized on social distancing, wearing of masks and usage of sanitizers to fight against the infection. Critics are of opinion that the self-quarantine and isolation have caused a negative impact in the psychology of the common mass.

Since we have not adequate information about the novel coronavirus, it is important and significant to cater true news and information collected from trusted and reliable sources. It is not easy to gather the latest and updated information and statistics of the spread of the dangerous Virus during the unprecedented situation caused by the Corona pandemic. Various media have been and are used to aware the common public to obey the rules of quarantine and to decrease the tension among the common mass.

The COVID-19 pandemic can be considered as a unique case as far as the role of journalism and media sector in India is concerned. The false information about the treatment of the dangerous Virus has constantly expanded through various channels of the mass media at an accelerating pace. The quantum of false information was so irritating on the sphere ranging from individual to social that its impact has been felt and agreed from all corners of the society.

The false information, lack of knowledge and gossip can create damage in the process of communication and increase anxiety and tension amongst the common mass. Social media have the scope to spread the information within a couple of minutes, therefore, the major drawback of it is that it has been purposefully applied as a tool to disseminate false information. After the appearance of various social networking sites such as Twitter, Facebook, and YouTube, the dissemination of information in this prevailing time of crisis has enhanced worldwide. These social networking sites provide a domain for exchanging reactions and feedbacks which may have a negative impact during an emergency situation like the existing Corona pandemic. False information on COVID-19 is expanding quickly through media and the internet, which alters the behavior of the public during the epidemic. This misinformation needs serious monitoring and evaluation for enhancement of the awareness, development of quick responses and in cooperation in the process of decision making.

16.2   AIMS AND OBJECTIVES

The nature and standard of journalism and mass media in a democratic structure can be examined in this prevailing crisis situation. This chapter has examined whether the autonomy of journalism has been maintained in this crisis situation. The boom in media consumption in this time of crisis is seen. Within this framework, what were the roles of different mass media on the individual and social life as far as the effective health communication is concerned and dealing with physical distancing, reduction of prejudice, discrimination, and inequalities caused due to fake news or misinformation? Do media provide a way for misinformation and how it affects the private domain of individuals? How fake news impact the largest democracy in the world? Does fake news put forward acute problem on the psychology of people? If so, how? It is essential to look into how the media have helped in reaching out to millions of citizens with minute-to-minute updates in this situation of pandemic.

16.3   METHODOLOGY

This chapter has followed the observational and analytical method to investigate the role of journalism and media during the crisis of coronavirus pandemic in India.

16.4   RESEARCH QUESTIONS

The chapter has tried to investigate and get the answer of the following research questions:

1. Have the media houses having business interests investigate the real state of affairs? Have they covered the disaster with empathy?
2. Have the global online and new media on the internet and small, indigenous, domestic media performed its due role in catering true and objective information though they do not possess the reach and penetration that large media moguls enjoy?
3. Have most media forced to cover the worker's penury to satisfy the sensationalism? Have the media become a tool of sensationalism during the pandemic?
4. Can the trusted media sources just ignore misinformation? How fake news impact Democracy during coronavirus pandemic? Are there attempts by the media to counter it because this infodemic is undermining the democratic function of the media in a country? What are the effects of infodemic during coronavirus pandemic? What are laws and regulations to curb fake news in India?
5. What is the economic situation of the media sector in India during the COVID-19 situation? How have the media served to shape prospects of the sector of 4th estate in India during the prevailing situation of crisis?

6. Have the journalists use the proper terminology prescribed by the Guidelines of Disaster Reporting? Have the reporters taken the risk of crossing the line from journalism to activism where the situation demands?
7. Have the vast audience of the web-enabled media participated actively in the interactions in the context of media reports?
8. Has the nation witnessed cyberchondria and information overload of the citizens?

16.5   STARK REALITY OF MEDIA DURING PANDEMIC IN INDIA

In a democratic structural framework, journalism is considered to be a business of public service. But instances have shown that the autonomy of the profession and the freedom of the press have been time to time violated in the hands of corporate ownership. This conflict of interest has appeared as a trait of Journalism in the country. Though a lion's share of Indian media is under the control of corporate ownership, there are presences of several exceptions. Thus, the indigenous media sector has appeared as a battleground of ideologies and values. In this prevailing crisis, alternative media have upheld issues with public interest during this crisis. The global online and new media on the internet and small indigenous domestic media have performed its due role in catering true and objective information though they do not possess the reach and penetration that large media moguls enjoy. A section of the indigenous mainstream media has not performed its expected role during this crisis through a portion of the newspapers has upheld some relevant issues.

A section of critics has argued that the declaration of the lockdown created a tension and the migrant laborers are the worst affected. A few media have covered the stories of the migrant laborers from their sense of deep feeling while other's representations have directed to the affluent class. A section of the middle class labels the migrant workers' behavior during this pandemic situation as irresponsible and blames them [1, 2]. Besides, another section of the media covers the issue of migrant laborers because of its sensational value. Serious journalism still exists because of some committed journalists. A few English newspapers were seen with their investigative journalism to cover the pandemic with more empathy.

16.6   NEED FOR GREATER RESPONSIBILITY AND COMMITMENT

The period of lockdown witnessed a growth of consumption of media. People were and are dependent on various media for corona virus related information. The problem sighted in many cases is that what information has been provided is far from factuality and reality. A section of critics is of opinion that in several cases, the media have become a tool of sensationalism. In several cases, the real picture has not been reflected properly. Thanks to a handful of committed, dedicated journalists of whose presence things did not turn ugly further. It was seen in the coverage of almost all television channels that a considerable section of the people was clapping, banging utensils, blowing conch shells on the streets, forgetting the social distancing, when the Janata curfew was announced.

A section of the Economists is of opinion that the pandemic is also threatening the deteriorating economy of the country. The media, however, are worried due to its own economic condition. Media, especially Print, are facing a resource crunch. The decay of advertisements, reduction in circulation and readership has made this segment of media worried. A large section of journalists, correspondents, reporters, and media persons has covered the COVID-19 situation day after day taking risks. Cutting wages have seen in some media organizations, some journalists even have lost their jobs. The Corona pandemic has created a new crisis in Indian Journalism.

The country has seen significant growth and development in the domain of media during the last three decades, and the indigenous media market has considered one of the biggest in the world. The role of capitalism, the market, and the media has to be assessed. The country has witnessed the increased efforts of building social responsibility among the temptation of finance capital and profit maximization.

During the pandemic, news media are the fundamental origin of information, insights, and exploration that needs to be crosschecked. The pandemic has made the job of the Journalists tough. Journalists now have to protect themselves against not just the virus but misinformation too. A journalist's responsibility is to verify and counter check the news and information gathered from various sources. Journalists and correspondents are advised by the guidelines of how to report disaster for usage of accurate nomenclature. They have also been advised not to lose their power of critical analysis.

According to Mr. Summer Lopez, a Senior Director of PEN America, truth-tellers have an essential role in maintaining freedom of speech and expression in free societies [6].

Various media ranging from print to audio to audio-visual disseminate accurate news and information to fight against false news. Timely monitoring over the interactions through social networking sites for the sake of public interest will foster the awareness of stakeholders and will facilitate in framing the policies essential for subsidence of risk effectively and thus ensuring efficient management of events at a time of crisis. In reality, the common masses apply various sources of news and social networking sites for exchange of information mutually. It is important to maintain fruitful communication between the government/authorities regarding public health. In this process, the mass media and social networking sites may play a vital role in successful pandemic responses.

16.7 ROLE OF MEDIA DURING SPREAD OF MISINFORMATION DURING THE PANDEMIC

The role of media in today's world is of paramount importance. Media are often described as the silent revolution in the 21st century. Media help in shaping public opinion, raise crucial issues related to public interest, make the common people aware of various news and information happening across the world, its genesis in this country initiated from the decade of 1940s when the concept of development communication commenced.

The world has turned upside down after outbreak of coronavirus pandemic and it has become a global phenomenon. The news and information disseminated through various media have made the people conscious about the circumstances and its subversive effects. Many scientists, virologists, researchers, medical practitioners appealed to the common people to take everything seriously about COVID-19 and obey all preventive steps for ensuring health care through the mass media, including a variety of social media.

But today media are facing a serious problem of the expansion of fake news and false information. The expansion of the false information on coronavirus that it was made in the laboratory as an agent of bioterrorism, 3 in addition thousands of listings of promoting fake COVID-19 cures have been reported and the price of some sanitizers and face makers have increased by over 2000%. During the pandemic circumstances caused by COVID-19, a scarcity of transparent communication can increase confusion and even tension and anxiety among the common mass. So, it is very important that credible media should not just afford to ignore misinformation but should attempt to counter it because this type of infodemic not only undermines the democratic function of the media as well as questions its credibility and trustworthiness. During a pandemic, without credible Journalists and Media for checking the facts, rumors would become the only information available that will increase fear psychosis.

Since we have not adequate information about the novel coronavirus, it is important and significant to cater true news and information collected from trusted and reliable sources. It is not easy to gather the latest and updated information and statistics of the spread of the dangerous Virus during the unprecedented situation caused by the Corona pandemic since there are possibilities of risk for the reporters and journalists. Besides, social networking sites can be applied to motivate people to obey the guidelines prescribed by the appropriate authority concerned and to reduce panic among people.

16.8   MASS AND SOCIAL MEDIA AS SOURCE OF INFORMATION DURING CRISIS

Now, social media is a vital source of information. The constantly developing social media have appeared as a crucial domain for communication during this prevailing crisis. Popular social networking sites like Twitter, Facebook and YouTube have made the people aware of the steps to combat against the false information during the existing coronavirus pandemic. However, questions have arisen regarding their roles.

16.9   EFFECTS OF INFODEMIC DURING CORONAVIRUS PANDEMIC

Media have radically changed the way of communication with each other. The news and information catered by the various types of media regarding precautionary steps and pace of infection has helped people in identifying its harmful effects. At the same time, misinformation and fake news have put life at risk prompting some unproven remedies that create a ray of hope in the minds of the common mass that it will facilitate them for cure from coronavirus which directly restrains them to disclose information regarding their health conditions. As a consequence, it will lead virus to widespread.

A report of a survey conducted on 8,914 adult people during March 10th to 16th 2020 in the USA has been published. According to the report, four-fifth of respondents have been witnessed to some false news and information regarding the COVID-19 such as the figure of death tolls exaggerating the seriousness of the virus that several lakhs of people could succumb due to the Virus and some respondents demanded that the media undersold the gravity of the virus as they are equalizing the virus with flu and 10% reported about concocted stories [12]. An E.U. Monitoring Team found 80 instances of disinformation between January and March in this year [9]. Misinformation about remedies from virus includes sipping water and more dangerous one drinking bleach, etc. This has led to devastating effect in Iran, where many citizens died by consuming methanol in the belief that it will protect them against COVID-19.

16.10   LAWS, RULES, AND REGULATIONS TO CURB FAKE NEWS IN INDIA

Section 66 of The Information Technology Act [3] states that a person dishonestly doing any act referred in Section 43 will be punished for 3 years or fine [3]. Civil or criminal defamation is another area for fake news. Indian Penal Code has specific sections which check fake news.

Section 54 of The Disaster Management Act [4] explains about deceitful warning about pandemic leading to fear among the mass [4].

On the other hand, Section 3 of The Epidemic Disease Act [5] says penalty for a person violating any regulation under this Act deemed to have committed crime u/s188 of IPC [5].

The Ministry of Home Affairs' Cyber Crime Portal Guidelines tell how Media should function during the COVID-19 pandemic [10] and also have listed some provisions under which steps can be taken against anybody who transgresses the law.

16.11   CYBERCHONDRIA AND INFORMATION OVERLOAD

Cyberchondria and information overload have been observed in many cases from excessive internet usage and application during COVID-19 pandemic situation. Cyberchondria is characterized as an obsession for online enquiry for health (in general and specific symptoms in particular) related news and information. Overload of Information is a situation where all communications and information inputs cannot be processed. It has resulted in the collapse of the information collecting network. It has also made the entire process ineffective.

The excessive and random usage of social networking sites as a source of news and information has created both cyberchondria and overload of information.

A considerable section of the critics is of opinion that the news and information exchanged through social networking sites are more impressionable to the slant of individual. These news and information have the deficiency of the balanced, objective, and extensive direction dissimilar with the news of reporters, correspondents, and journalists of the various news media.

The developers of social networking sites and various search engines should take measures for ensuring true, reliable, and transparent news and information to the users to combat the ill effects of overload of information and cyberchondria.

It is essential to aware people for the safe application of social media. It will help to decrease the negative impact of the social media.

16.12   ARE TWITTERING, FACEBOOKING JOURNALISM?

A section of journalists, columnists has raised this question-are twittering, face booking journalism at all? No. Journalism has appeared in various cases as the contraposition of the phrase, 'Here Comes Everybody' proposed by Clay Shirky. It has indicated inundation of raw material that new social media disseminate [11] journalism is distillation. It is an option of material upholding the truest, pure, and most detailed manifestation of a circumstance. It appears by means of an intelligence and sensibility. It depends on form without which significance is lost to chaos [13]. As Aristotle suggested more than two millennia earlier, form necessitates a beginning, middle, and end. It claims unity of theme. Journalism cuts through the atwitter phase to coherence of theme [14].

Presence is essential. Because a portion of the choice lies in something inexpressible that cannot be devoured or rendered at a distance [15].

Technology has expanded the medium and the raw material on which the profession is based and thus enriched journalism. But it has also cut down the incentive and the revenue. Martha Gellhorn's view 'from the ground' remains absent. Nature hates emptiness, journalism does so and so it fills absence with windiness [18].

16.13   FINDINGS AND OBSERVATIONS

By a careful critical analysis of the contents of various mass media during the prevailing pandemic situation, this chapter has observed that in few cases, the media have provided more in-depth news and analysis of the events. Sometimes, they have turned their attention to nursing their local neighborhoods and have taken up issues that are of immediate concern for their prospective target audience. Sometimes, they have also widened their circuit of target audience to include the concerns of the marginalized sections of the society like small peasants, workers, agricultural laborers, and other backward classes as well as the coverage of environmental and human rights issues. They have interpreted and analyzed news, events, trends, and happenings in important fields like politics, economics, social issues, etc. They have shown features of interest to the target audience or through an interactive mode.

16.14 DISTORTION

Distortion of news occurs when wrong or facts full of errors substitute genuine facts or when a biased explanation is blended into the news report. In this present situation of pandemic, distortion of news has happened. News content, analysis, and presentation have been influenced by the editorial policy. Some of the Indian media which has by and large accepted the role of social responsibility has earned the reputation of a mature media and has shown the way to others in this situation of crisis.

16.15 CRISIS JOURNALISM

Crisis journalism has created disturbances sometimes on the rationality and peace of a society. Sometimes, people have felt uneasiness, become nervous, etc. No good media can afford to forget its social responsibilities even in a competitive market situation. They should keep in mind the interests of all sections of the society including the deprived, the underprivileged and the inarticulate.

16.16 ROLE AND IMPACT OF THE MEDIA

The media as a mass communicator, representative of the society, regular, and constant spokesperson of the citizen, can discuss and propose essential steps regarding various policies, schemes, and projects. A section of it has succumbed to sensationalism, obscenity, and vulgarism. A large section has followed commercialization.

The role of mass media in social change is without doubt. The mass and the newcomer social media have to play their due ranging from the public to private sector. This chapter suggests some recommendations that the Indian mass media and the social media platforms of the country need to follow in this time of crisis:

- Media should cater authentic information.
- It should welcome the positive and constructive changes that are going to happen around the people and should tell them about its utilities in their life.
- The media can help the people to accept the challenges in time of crisis.
- It can educate the people about the policies, practices, and mechanisms of public health and hygiene.
- During the present pandemic condition, media should cover the incident with pace to enable authorities and voluntary organizations and the people to undertake quick rescue, relief, and rehabilitation steps and medical treatment. It can also cater courage to the people to cope with the challenge.

The media have the strength to do its due especially in the time of crisis but it should have the will to do it. It is expected that media will awaken the collective conscience of the society at the time of crisis, disasters, sufferings, and emergency.

If the mass media are to achieve the required trust from the people, it has to introspect seriously. This chapter has earmarked some weaknesses and shortcomings that need to be addressed if the media are to discharge its social responsibilities. It is essential, especially in this time of acute crisis is to stress the need for a social audit of the media to see that it remains on the right track, to check deviations and to take remedial action.

1. Catering to the Elitist, Neglecting the Problems of the Less Privileged: The majority of the urban and metropolitan media have not focused its attention sufficiently on the problems of the have-nots and the deprived sections of the society.

   The growing population of the country has presented many challenges and has reflected the inequities present in the society in terms of rich-poor divide, urban concentration, imbalance in health care facilities, and in terms of those that are educated and those are not.

Some big media have sometimes focused the people's attention on some selective problems of the poor and the rural areas including the deprived and the displaced.

2. Ignoring or Suppressing News of People's Concern: It has also been observed that some media have no place for the real issues before the nation and for problems facing the people. They have been hardly ever discussed and even reported. They have made no appeal to the target audience. On the other hand, celebrity journalism has found a prominent place.

3. Misinformation: and disinformation are not unknown. When such misleading information has touched socially sensitive matters, they have often led to panic and crisis.

   It has been observed that there have been some media which sensing the crisis promptly present the requisite true, authentic information to defuse the anxiety and panic and to warn people against fake news and misinformation.

4. Crass Commercialism-Market Oriented, Not Mass Oriented: A large section of today's media owners and controllers are more concerned with the commodification of their respective medium by treating news, views, events, advertisements, programs, and publicity as saleable commodities with scant regard for journalistic ethics and integrity. Social responsibility and morality are essential human needs. No doubt, media must sell but not by ignoring the socio-economic aspirations and agonies, cultural decency, ethos, and developmental imperatives of the people. There is an entire area of knowledge that is denied to people by a section of media that is more concerned with profit than proper dissemination and promotion of meaningful information among the people.

5. Trivialism: Giving undue space to unimportant and insignificant issues is on the increase. This is not a little on account of market orientation of the media.

6. Sensationalism: It indicates the usage of emotional issue or extreme style of drama, language or artistic expression desired to bang, flash, vibrate or arouse the readers, listeners, and viewers, etc., [16]. A section of the media has always been suffering from this ailment which has to be curbed.

7. Intruding into Personal Grief at Times of Crisis: Some in the media have intruded through photography and visual clippings into moments of personal grief which can be a cause of further distress to

the aggrieved family and friends. Although this section of the media has often claimed that the photography and visual clippings of victims have been done in larger public interest, still such photography and visual clippings have to respect the privacy of the individuals, which is often forgotten.

8. Superficialism: It has been observed that there is no in-depth analysis of issues and their implications for the benefit of the common people. Even some events have not been interpreted to bring home their significance. Sometimes, a section of the media has depended on shallowness and mere gossiping. Impressions and not knowledge has been conveyed to the audience who are made no benefitted by such coverage.

Marshall McLuhan, the author of 'The Medium is the Message,' said that the medium unknowingly creeps inside the media person and makes him or her do things differently [17].

Mass media have impact over public opinion. Advertising influences it openly. Film and theater remain powerful tools in the question of public influence. And journalism is regarded as the 4th estate of democracy because it is supposed to influence public opinion by true, objective, and just information [18].

Democracy offers an array of informed alternatives. News media showing objectivity, unbiased, and authenticity make it possible. Various lobbies and interest groups have always tried to apply this power of media to fulfill their own interests. Corporate houses and ownerships have been influencing journalists to influence the policymakers and the people for the sake of their own interest [19].

In this prevailing situation of pandemic, the ethics of journalism needs to introspect. Objectivity has to be maintained at any cost. If journalism loses credibility, it will not act anymore as a trusted source of authentic news and information [20].

McLuhan was an advocator in favor of media as a 'make happen agent' rather 'a make aware agent.' If media want to retain its credibility and somewhat lost glory, the recast and reshape of it is needed. The sincere, dedicated journalists and public-spirited media need to go back to the basic values of the business of public service and insist that it should be abide by all [21].

Besides, indicating some weaknesses and shortcomings of the media that need to be addressed, this chapter also recommends the following proposals for the smooth and proper functioning of a responsible and responsive media during the period of pandemic situation:

1. Insurance Coverage for Journalists/Editors: Journalists, correspondents, reporters, newspersons, editors, editorial staffs and others related with news and information organizations across the domain of mass and social media should be provided adequate insurance cover through special schemes to protect them during the period of crisis situation.
2. Social Audit of Mass and Social Media: Initiative of Social Audit at regular interval should be taken by the mass and social media to examine their respective roles. It will also help to earmark the problems and issues of the society, especially of its underprivileged sections. Besides, it will also help to point out the needs for the development of the country.
3. Media Watch Groups: Initiatives of establishment of Media Watch Groups at local, state, regional, and national level should be taken to evaluate the contents of the mass and social media at regular intervals focusing on the suppression, distortion, manipulation, planting of news along with any deviations of ethics of journalism, etc.

16.17 CONCLUSION

The country has seen significant growth and development in the domain of media during the last three decades, and the indigenous media market has considered one of the biggest in the world. Globalization and neo-liberalization have also shaped it. Maximization of profit, commercialization, and commoditization has appeared as its main characters.

What will be the role of mass media and the journalists during this prevailing crisis situation? The roles of capitalism, the market, and the media have to be evaluated. Will this pandemic radically change the role of the media and the journalists? The country has witnessed the increased efforts of building social responsibility among the temptation of finance capital and profit maximization. Indian media and the journalists need to introspect their respective stands in the context of these significant and serious questions and issues.

Media have vital influence over people during the present coronavirus pandemic, so all information should be more transparent and authentic, which is of paramount importance in this crisis. Fake news and misinformation can fill in the void if genuine and trusted information fail to appear in time to the target audience of the mass and social media. As a consequence, it can lead to hazardous effects.

All the news disseminated by media has an important influence on the mind of the prospective target audience, so it should be presented with utmost care and sincerity after repeated rechecking and cross-checking because single misinformation that gain attention can negate the importance of correct information and can pose a serious challenge about the credibility and trustworthiness of the media.

It is vital to consider that in such a time of crisis, media must respond collectively and intelligently. The media should disseminate reliable information and daily updates to keep the people informed during the crucial time of this prevailing crisis.

The various media have been inundated with news, data, statistics, and information during the pandemic situation. There is information which helps to aware people regarding the nature of COVID-19. On the other hand, the medical misinformation has continuously spread over mass media platforms at a breakneck speed. The quantum of fake news and misinformation had so negative impact on the mind of individual and the society that its harmful impact has been agreed from all corners of the society. The fake news, false information, gossip have created hindrance in the entire process of news and communication and have increased tension and anxiety among the mass. The media should introspect that whether it have been able in teaching and increasing awareness among the people and decreasing anxiety, tension, fear, and panic among them.

16.18   FUTURE SCOPE

This chapter has tried to assess the role of journalism and media during the crisis of the corona virus pandemic in India and to make a prognosis of its future, especially in the time of any crisis, disaster, and emergency. The chapter has tried to fulfill its aims and objectives of analyzing at least the issues and problems with which the Indian media deal while performing its functions. Besides, the chapter has tried to recommend some measures for the smooth and proper functioning of a responsible and responsive media during the period of pandemic situation in the future. It will help the media to meet the forthcoming challenges. The conclusions drawn and the recommendations made at the chapter are designed to serve as the possible signposts of the way of the exploration of the subject further. The issues dealt with in this chapter are indeed vast and interconnected, and their widths and depths are ever-increasing day by day.

KEYWORDS

- **corona**
- **crisis**
- **India**
- **journalism**
- **pandemic**
- **virus**

REFERENCES

1. Abi-Habib, M., & Sameer, Y., (2020). *For India's Laborers, Coronavirus Lockdown is an Order to Starve*. New York Times. https://www.nytimes.com/2020/03/30/world/asia/coronavirus-india-lockdown.html (accessed on 28 June 2021).
2. Ellis-Petersen, Hanna, & Chaurasia, M., (2020). *India Racked by Greatest Exodus Since Partition Due to Coronavirus*. Guardian. https://www.theguardian.com/world/2020/mar/30/india-wracked-by-greatest-exodus-since-partition-due-to-coronavirus (accessed on 28 June 2021).
3. The Information Technology Act, (2000). https://www.indiacode.nic.in/bitstream/123456789/13116/1/it_act_2000_updated.pdf.
4. Disaster Management Act, (2005). https://indiankanoon.org/doc/640589/.
5. Epidemic Disease Act, (1897). https://legislative.gov.in/sites/default/files/A1897-03.pdf.
6. Ram, A., (2020). *Journalism in the time of COVID-19 Pandemic*. The Times of India.
7. http://www.vox.com/policy-and-politics/2020/4/15/21222458/study-people-coronavirus-fake-news (accessed on 28 June 2021).
8. Ibid.
9. http://mediawatchjournal.in/fake-news-and-social-media-indian-perspective/ (accessed on 28 June 2021).
10. http://www.thehindubusinessline.com/opinion/fighting-fake-news-during-covid-19/article31233348.ece (accessed on 28 June 2021).
11. Cohen, R., (2009). *Twittering is no Journalism*. The Asian Age.
12. Ibid.
13. Ibid.
14. Ibid.
15. Ibid.
16. Press Council of India, (2001). *Future of Print Media: A Report* (pp. 184, 185). New Delhi.

17. Dev, S. A., (2010). *Fall of the Fourth Estate?* The Asian Age.
18. Ibid.
19. Ibid.
20. Ibid.
21. Ibid.

PART V

Closure of Schools and Colleges During COVID-19: Remote Learning Challenges

CHAPTER 17

Information Curation, Psychosocial Response, and Hygienic Practices in the Context of the COVID-19 Pandemic: A Case Study of Indian Students of Higher Education

MRINAL MUKHERJEE,[1] CHANCHAL MAITY,[2] and
SOMDUTTA CHATTERJEE[1]

[1]*Department of Teacher Education, The West Bengal University
of Teachers' Training, Education Planning and Administration
(WBUTTEPA), Kolkata, West Bengal, India,
E-mail: dr.mmrinal@gmail.com (M. Mukherjee)*

[2]*Bankura University, Bankura, West Bengal, India*

ABSTRACT

The COVID-19 pandemic has influenced a wide spectrum of life triggering psychological and other problems in almost all countries. In consonance with the advocacy of the World Health Organization (WHO), the national and regional administrative authorities in India have imposed lockdown and have propagated general hygienic advocacies through Government and Non-government agencies. The degree of effectiveness of such mitigation strategies largely depends on cooperative response and compliance of the public in general and youth in particular. How Indian students pursuing undergraduate (UG) and Post Graduate studies are reacting to the present pandemic context is of paramount importance as this educated section is supposed to influence and shape the future architecture and practice of the society. Hence the present study is trying to investigate how UG and postgraduate (PG) level students are curating information, responding to psychosocial issues, and maintaining an elementary hygienic practice in the context of the COVID-19 outbreak. An online survey was employed to collect data from Indian students pursuing UG and PG courses. The data was collected through a validated questionnaire by snowball sampling method. Responses of all 470 participants were valid and considered for analysis. Apart from percentage analysis of demographic data, Chi-square analysis was also employed to observe the influence of the demographic category on psychosocial response and hygienic practices. It has been found that Television and Newspaper are still enjoying dependency from educated youth along with social media. Though they are agreed on the tendency of information amplification but still believe that media can play an instrumental role. The UG and PG students reacted in a positive manner showing pro-social attitude in the context of the COVID-19. The study also has thrown a ray of hope as the majority of respondents are ready to adapt hygienic practices in this current situation in order to restore post-COVID new normalcy.

17.1   INTRODUCTION

The COVID-19 pandemic has tremendously influenced a wide spectrum of life triggering psychological and other problems [1–3] everywhere around the world. In such a scale of paralysis of normalcy and uncertainty, the COVID-19 is continuously posing new kinds of challenges to our societal practices and designs. The academia as a community needs to respond to the gravity of this crisis. While every section of society is affected by the COVID-19 in one way or another, we need to respond in two ways to study the ongoing societal impacts. Apart from general approach towards the impact of the COVID-19, we also need to approach the crisis from cross-section study. Every section of society has been affected in a unique manner. The crisis caused by the COVID-19 is really unprecedented and in forced lockdown while we are trying to adapt to compulsive virtual engagement, people are craving for social intimacy and association. The society which is inherently unequal still has shown tons of positive examples of empathy, humanity, and care not only extended by acquaintances but also by the strangers. Every experience of such pandemic might be instrumental in strengthening our community, society, and nation to thrive in post-pandemic era. Thus, every aspect of human response needs to be analyzed and documented. It is a fact that we are not only a part of the local web of supply system of commodities but also an integral part of the flow of network of our experience, knowledge, attitudes, and insight. Therefore, a critical approach is an urgency to adopt in documenting and analyzing the ongoing events in social dynamics.

Despite having international instruments like the Universal Declaration of Human Rights [4], where education has been considered as a human right, in reality in a globalized market economy the higher education has been treated not as a right of individual for greater societal perspective; rather higher education has become a vehicle to supply the needs of the economic design. So, we are at the juncture of the unsolved debate of the nature of higher education-whether this would be completely a public good discharged by the government or it should be private in nature where education is completely a commodity and the learners in higher education are customers. This pandemic has shown us a gloomy picture of the sufferings of the student community in higher education in the global scale. In India, undergraduate (UG) and postgraduate students are going through rough sailing. They are the unique section of the population. It is of utter importance how the Indian UG and postgraduate (PG) students of higher education are reacting and responding to the situation, because this is an entirely educated section that is supposed to influence and shape the future architecture and practice of society.

The policy paralysis at global scale caused by the COVID-19 induced pandemic has revealed the fragility and inadequacy of the policies and practices in different countries. The crisis has hinted at the need of reconnection between 'humanity and planet' to ensure food, health, and education for all (EFA) to build a more resilient supply chain. The World Bank [5] in its recent article 'Building a Balanced Future' decisively asserted 'how the world responds to this tragedy will either amplify global threats or mitigate them, so countries need to choose wisely.' The innovative solution of the existing challenges needs a lot of insight, and it is time for wise decision-making where youths might have the most crucial role to play. In another report of World Bank Group, Education [6] revealed that youth in global scale exhibited immense creativity and innovation in mitigating the challenges in ensuring food health and job, and thus they showed the ray of hope and resilience. For instance, from South-East Asia, SM Anamul Arefin, a graduate in the Sher-e-Bangla Agricultural University, took recourse to his 3D printer to develop 'face shields' that protect doctors and nurses [7], which are cost and medically effective. Students of Instrumentation Engendering Department of Jadavpur University, Kolkata, India, innovated such an electronic mask which can denature the COVID-19 virus coming in contact with the mask instantly. So, youths are major facilitators for future design of normalcy we are heading to. Hence studying the behavioral aspect of UG and PG students should be a priority in social sciences research.

It has been revealed from researches of previous episodic epidemic outbreaks of contagious diseases and also the experience of the COVID-19 pandemic reconfirms that media in all its forms have played instrumental roles in not only shaping the perception of risk of the common people including youth but also influenced the behavioral pattern of the individuals in such times of crisis. Propagation of misinformation and deliberate amplification of the gravity of crisis through all sorts of media shape up the risk perception of the people and specific populations are showing high degrees of the COVID-19-related wide spectrum of psychological distress [1, 8–10]. Apart from mainstream media, social media due to their global virtual presence [11] became the platform for public dialog and debate on the COVID-19 related pandemic and has been contributing to opinion formation in public and in particular among UG and PG level students of tertiary education [12–14]. It is therefore essential to pay attention to the psychological states of the public in the context of the COVID-19 [15] as people are becoming much worried about the extreme uncertainty. Hence in this study researchers felt the need to focus on the nature of media engagement of university students and tried to assess how this particular educated group of the general population curate information among the vast field of media and whether there is at all any influence of gender, level of education or nature of course they are pursuing on their information curation pattern.

The pandemic caused by the COVID-19 has been negatively impacting in creating panic and fear and leading to a wide range of psychological stress [16]. Students of tertiary education most often experience compounded negative emotions while their institutions remain closed due to this pandemic and apart from education, they are denied from their campus life [17]. Many of them are suffering from a crisis of loneliness and isolation and craving for socialization while they are forced to remain disconnected from partners and friends. UG and PG students are passing through severe distress due to abrupt disruption and long-term paralysis of their education. The majority of higher education institutions are compulsorily switching over to virtual learning teaching with high-end digital gadgets, all students are not comfortable with such modalities primarily because many of them do not have appropriate access to digital gadgets and are deprived of required internet connectivity and secondly lot of them are in further stress in this digital climate which leads to deterioration of mental health [18]. They might also be fearful that they could be potential sources of infection and transmission of the COVID-19 to others and specially their family members [19]. Despite such a worrisome situation, the Indian higher education student being youths have created precedents of positive leadership roles. In this context, the present study has tried to assess how UG and PG students are reacting and responding to the psychosocial issues in respect to their gender, level of education, and nature of course they are pursuing.

The outbreak of COVID-19 influenced hygienic practices to the maximum extent among different aspects of life, and therefore the study of hygienic behavior analysis is relevant [3]. Even after the repeated advocacy, a majority has not paid enough attention to the guidelines and ignored the suggestive hygienic practices [20]. The COVID-19 related hygienic practices are supposed to play an instrumental role in determining the overall readiness of society to accept new norms of pro-hygienic social behavior [21]. Educated youths are the potential future leaders, and considering the age, it is expected they might provide leadership in carrying forward such positive behavior as "new normal" than other sections of the population. Adaptation of such non-pharmaceutical protective hygienic practices may vary in terms of gender, grades of study and might be related to the nature of the courses the students are pursuing. The present study analyzes the hygienic practice of Indian College and University students both who are studying at UG and PG level at different institutions.

17.2 METHODOLOGY

17.2.1 STUDY DESIGN

An online survey was employed during lockdown to collect data from Indian students pursuing UG and PG courses (either directly belonging to central and state-aided university departments, affiliated, and autonomous colleges; private universities and general degree colleges; private law and medical colleges; and central institutions like Indian Institute of Technology and Jawaharlal Institute of Post Graduate Medical Education and Research). The data was collected from 5th to 20th June 2020. The survey was made available in the public domain by social media platforms to reach the potential target respondents. After providing the consent, the student participants were directed to self-administered questionnaire. The data was collected through a validated questionnaire by Snowball sampling method. All 470 samples were valid and considered for analysis.

17.2.2 RECRUITMENT PROCEDURE

A convenient snowball sampling was applied in which the university students were invited to take part in the study through social media, mainly Facebook and WhatsApp. The response schedule was prepared in the Google form and survey link was uploaded in the social media. By accessing the link, the respondent got auto-directed to the information about the study and informed consent. Thereafter, the participants had responded to a set of items in the survey schedule which appeared sequentially. The participants were also requested to share and forward the link in their own/other UG and PG student groups so that the survey schedule could be distributed apart from the first point of contact. All subjects were informed of the survey purpose, and the aim and objectives were clearly explained before recording any response. There was also a provision that they may withdraw from the study at any point of time during the survey. Thus, the participants voluntarily participated in the study. The inclusion criterion was that the participants must be UG or PG pursuing students, having attained the age of 18 years, and should be able to understand the English language.

17.2.3 STUDY INSTRUMENT

A structured questionnaire was designed by the researchers to meet the objectives of the study, and it was validated by four academicians who have noted expertise in the related research work. The questionnaire consisted of two major parts. The first part comprises the socio-demographic characteristics, including age, gender, level of education, name of the course along with its nature (weather general or professional), name, and address of the institute. The second part of the survey instrument has three sections designed in the context of the COVID-19 pandemic. The first section was meant to document the trends of information curation of the respondent, having six items (Items 1–6). As each item in this section is unique in nature hence instead of any common pattern, each of the items has its own kind of alternative options for response. The second section has been designed with five items (Items 7–11) to collect data for documenting the respondent's reaction on psychosocial issues (where every item is provided with Yes/No options). The third section is framed with five items (Items 12–16) in Likert type design with three alternative options-completely, partially, or not at all-to collect data on the hygienic practices of the respondents.

17.2.4   STATISTICAL ANALYSIS

All 470 responses were found valid and thus has been considered for analysis. For this study, the collected data has been analyzed through SPSS, version 16 (IBM Corporation). For assessing the pattern of response, descriptive analysis focused on frequencies and percentages while chi-square tests were employed, where necessary, to determine the differences between groups for selected demographic variables. The threshold level for statistical significance was set at $p < 0.05$ where applicable.

17.3   FINDINGS

17.3.1   DEMOGRAPHIC CHARACTERISTICS

A total of 470 participants responded to the study. Among the total respondents, 45.3% were male, and 54.7% were female. The students pursuing UG study were 65.3%, and those studying PG were 34.7%. And it is also worth mentioning that 49.1% and 50.9% of students were from general and professional courses who participated in the study. The demographic characteristics of respondents are shown in Table 17.1.

TABLE 17.1   Sample Demographics (N = 470)

Variables		Sample	Percentage (%)
Gender	Male (M)	213	45.3
	Female (F)	257	54.7
Education	Undergraduate (UG)	307	65.3
	Postgraduate (PG)	163	34.7
Course type	General (Gen)	231	49.1
	Professional (Prof)	239	50.9

17.3.2   ASSESSMENT OF INFORMATION CURATION PATTERN

A total of six questions were used to assess the information curation pattern of the university-level students in the context of the COVID-19 pandemic. The percentage analysis of the respondents' information curation trends for each of the items was done to estimate total respondents as well as demographic category.

TABLE 17.2　Percentage Analysis of Overall and Category-Wise Response with Respect to Information Curation

Item	Category	Response Pattern Against Each Item (N, %)	Gender		Education		Nature of Course	
			M	F	UG	PG	Gen	Prof
1. Where from you first came to know about the outbreak of novel coronavirus in the Wuhan Province of China?	Television (TV)	185, 39.4	62, 29.1	123, 47.9	128, 41.7	57, 35.0	87, 37.7	98, 41.0
	Social Media	149, 31.7	73, 34.3	76, 29.6	87, 28.3	62, 38.0	78, 33.8	71, 29.7
	Newspaper	67, 14.3	34, 16.0	33, 12.8	47, 15.3	20, 12.3	28, 12.1	31, 13.0
	Digital Media Outlets	69, 14.7	44, 20.7	25, 9.7	45, 14.7	24, 14.7	38, 16.5	39, 16.3
2. Where from you first informed about the serious outbreak of the COVID-19 virus in India?	Government notification on websites and TV	174, 37.0	77, 36.2	97, 37.7	120, 39.1	54, 33.1	75, 32.5	99, 41.4
	Social media	202, 43.0	83, 39.0	119, 46.3	126, 41.0	76, 46.6	110, 47.6	92, 38.5
	Newspaper	44, 9.4	22, 10.3	22, 8.6	28, 9.1	16, 9.8	18, 7.8	26, 10.9
	Digital media outlets	50, 10.6	31, 14.6	19, 7.4	33, 10.7	17, 10.4	28, 12.1	22, 9.2
3. Which source you are exploring for regional/state level every day update for COVID-19 related information?	Government notification on websites and TV	280, 59.6	113, 53.1	167, 65.0	189, 61.6	91, 55.8	136, 58.9	144, 60.3
	Social media	60, 12.8	27, 12.7	33, 12.8	33, 10.7	27, 16.6	32, 13.9	28, 11.7
	Newspaper	60, 12.8	39, 18.3	21, 8.2	36, 11.7	24, 14.7	30, 13.0	30, 12.6
	Digital media outlets	70, 14.9	34, 16.0	36, 14.0	49, 16.0	21, 12.9	33, 14.3	37, 15.5

TABLE 17.2 (Continued)

Item	Category	Response Pattern Against Each Item (N, %)	Gender		Education		Nature of Course	
			M	F	UG	PG	Gen	Prof
4. Are you navigating in a regular manner the website of WHO, ICMR, AYUSH for non-pharmaceutical self-care advocacy related to the COVID-19?	Yes	363, 78.2	163, 76.5	200, 77.8	241, 78.5	122, 74.8	178, 77.1	185, 77.4
	No	107, 22.8	50, 23.5	57, 22.2	66, 21.5	41, 25.2	53, 22.9	54, 22.6
5. Are you searching for specific detail at the global and national level of developments about the COVID-19 situation?	At least once in a day	220, 46.8	100, 47.0	120, 46.7	143, 46.6	77, 47.2	110, 47.6	110, 46.0
	Occasionally	92, 19.6	48, 22.5	44, 17.1	60, 19.5	32, 19.6	44, 19.0	48, 20.1
	Usually	158, 33.6	65, 30.5	93, 36.2	104, 33.9	54, 33.1	77, 33.3	81, 33.9
6. Are you searching for latest updates about local specific development regarding the COVID-19 situation?	At least once in a day	219, 46.6	103, 48.4	116, 45.1	143, 46.6	76, 46.6	100, 43.3	119, 49.8
	Occasionally	82, 17.4	42, 19.7	40, 15.6	51, 16.6	31, 19.0	41, 17.7	41, 17.2
	Usually	158, 33.6	68, 31.9	101, 39.3	113, 36.8	56, 34.4	90, 39.0	79, 33.1

As far Item No. 1 is concerned, the respondents have come to know the first global outbreak of Novel coronavirus in Wuhan, China, from different sources. Among all (N=470), the percentage of students were reported from television, newspaper, social media, and digital media outlets as 39.4%, 14.3%, 31.7%, and 14.7%, respectively (refer to Table 17.2). So, among the four types of media, the University level students in India preferred the television most till the time for getting information relevant in global context.

Female respondents obtained the first information about the COVID-19 from television was higher (47.9%) than male respondents (29.1%). On contrary, male students showed higher dependency on social media, digital media outlets and newspaper than their female counterparts, respectively, for *Item No. 1*, as reported in Table 17.2 and Figure 17.1(A). The UG respondent showed little higher dependency on television (41.7%) and newspaper (15.3%) than Post Graduate students (35% and 12.3%) for similar purposes. The majority of PG students had come to know the first COVID-19 outbreak report through social media. The information obtained from digital media outlets were similar in percentage for both the UG and PG students (refer to Table 17.2 and Figure 17.1(B)). A higher percentage of students pursuing professional courses got the first news of COVID-19 from Television and newspaper than students pursuing general course. While students of general course access social media a little bit more than students of professional course. Again the information obtained from digital media outlets were almost similar in percentage for students of the general and professional course (refer to Table 17.2 and Figure 17.1(C)).

In response to *Item No. 2*, as far as the first serious COVID-19 outbreak in India is concerned, the majority of Indian students were primarily informed by social media and Government notification in comparison to the other two sources mentioned in the items (refer Table 17.2). The result shows that female respondents had greater dependency on social media (46.3%) and Government notification (37.7%) than male respondents (39% and 36.2%). On the other hand, the male respondents were greater exposed to newspaper and digital media outlets than the female respondents (see Table 17.2 and Figure 17.2(A)). The Under Graduate students showed little higher dependency on government notification than PG students; on the contrary, Post Graduate students exhibited higher affinity for social media than its UG counterparts; but very little difference was there between UG and PG respondents in terms of newspaper and digital media outlets (see Table 17.2 and Figure 17.2(B)). Students belonging to general course showed greater dependency on social media (47.6%) and digital media outlets (12.1%) than student of professional courses (38.5% and 9.2); but the respondents of professional course had greater dependency on government notification and newspaper than general course students (see Table 17.2 and Figure 17.2(C)).

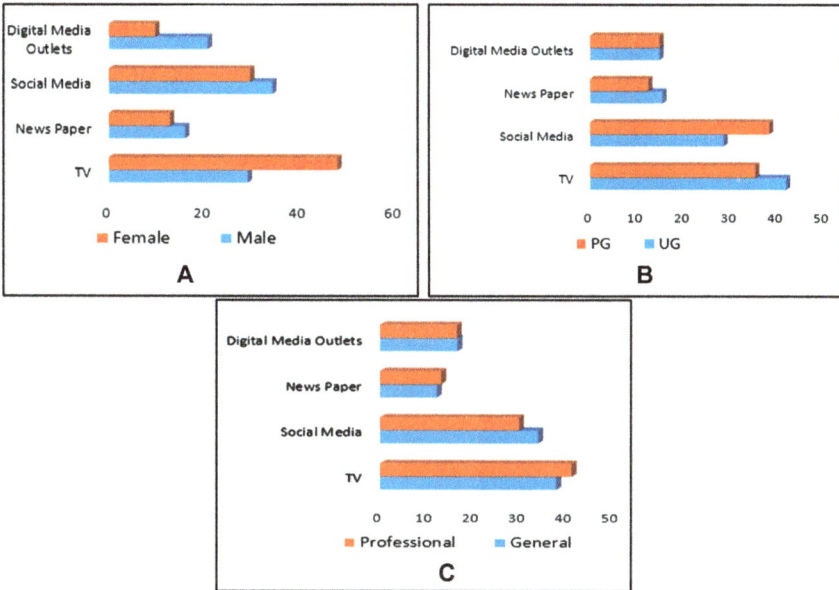

FIGURE 17.1 Chart showing the distribution of percentage of different media use patterns for curating information of first case of novel corona outbreak in China (A-gender, B-level of education, C-nature of the course).

Being anxious about the COVID-19 pandemic during lockdown scenario, students tried to update themselves as mentioned in *Item No. 3*, with the latest information related to the ongoing pandemic situation on a daily basis. The result indicated that students preferred the Government notification most and it was about to 59.6% out of 470 respondents. It was also quite higher with respect to other sources, i.e., newspaper (12.8%), social media (12.8%), and digital media outlets (14.9%) (refer Table 17.2). Female students curate information from the notification of government news agencies which was quite higher (65%) than male students (53.1%). Whereas for the same purpose, the male students showed higher dependency on non-government electronic media and digital media outlets than female students. But the use of social media for the same purpose was reflected almost similarly in both male and female respondents (see Table 17.2 and Figure 17.3(A)). UG students showed higher affinity to government notification and digital media outlets (61.6% and 16%) in comparison to PG students (55.8% and 12.9); whereas the use of newspaper and social media was higher for Post Graduate respondents than Under Graduate respondents (see Table 17.2 and Figure 17.3(B)). Students belonging to the professional course had greater dependency on Government notification and digital media outlets than students of general course; but the general course students in comparison to the professional students, in the higher percentage had come out in case of using social media (see Table 17.2 and Figure 17.3(C)).

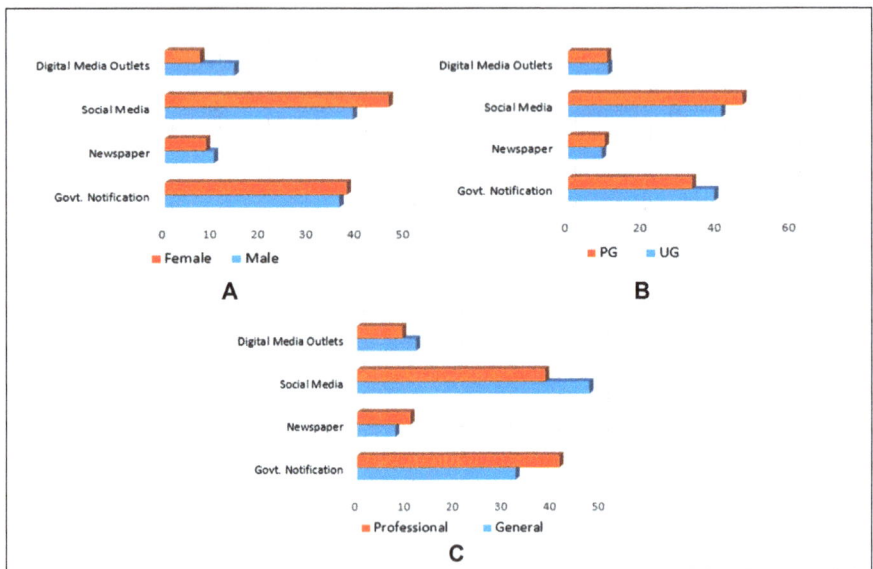

FIGURE 17.2 Chart showing the distribution of percentage of different media use pattern for curating information of first the COVID-19 outbreak in India (A-gender, B-level of education, and C-nature of the course).

The result shows that most of the participants (363 out of 470) frequently searched the website of different government organizations as mentioned in *Item No. 4*, to follow the guidelines for understanding the necessary non-pharmaceutical advocacies related to the COVID-19. The percentage of students those who were searching websites (77.2%) was quite greater than the students those who did not feel the urge to search such websites (22.8%) for the said purpose. As far as the pattern of information curation from specific websites for non-pharmaceutical protective advocacies is concerned, male, and female; UG and PG; and students pursuing general and professional courses had reflected mostly similar to each other (see Table 17.2 and Figures 17.4(A–C)).

During lockdown, the students were worried and very cautious for rapidly changing pandemic situation. Against *Item No. 5*, as per their response, it has been found that they exhibit the tendency to acquire information of latest developments like rate of infection, death rate, rate of recovery, latest protocol of treatment, vaccine formulation, etc. Thus the result reflected here that 46.8% of students at least once in a day, 19.6% of students occasionally, and 33.6% of students searched the media for the specific detail of the current situation and latest developmental about the COVID-19 pandemic. For searching the specific details of the current situation and latest developmental update about the COVID-19 pandemic, the percentage of different responses among group variable in different category: male and female; Under Graduate and Post Graduate; and general and professional had come out very close to each other (see Table 17.2 and Figures 17.5(A–C)).

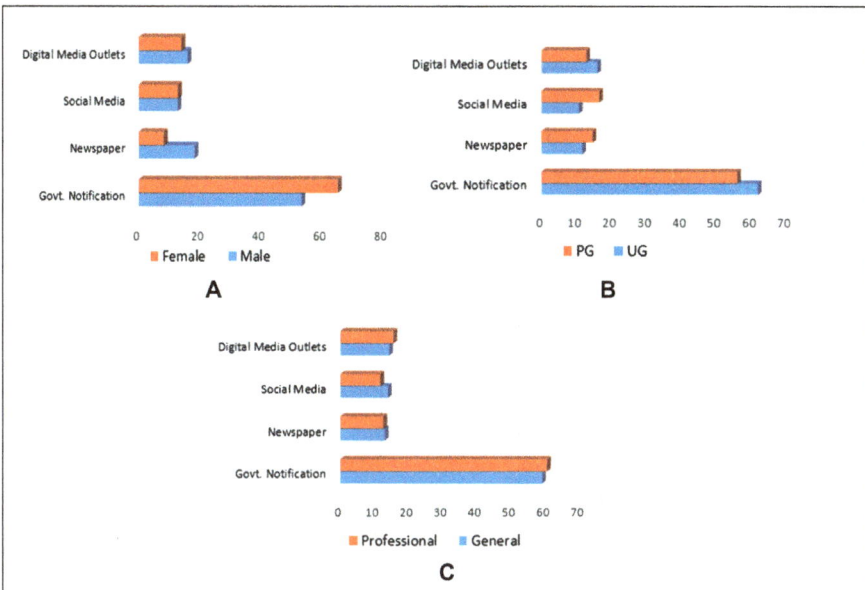

FIGURE 17.3 Chart showing the distribution of percentage of different sources for everyday update of the COVID-19 related information (A-gender, B-level of education, and C-nature of the course).

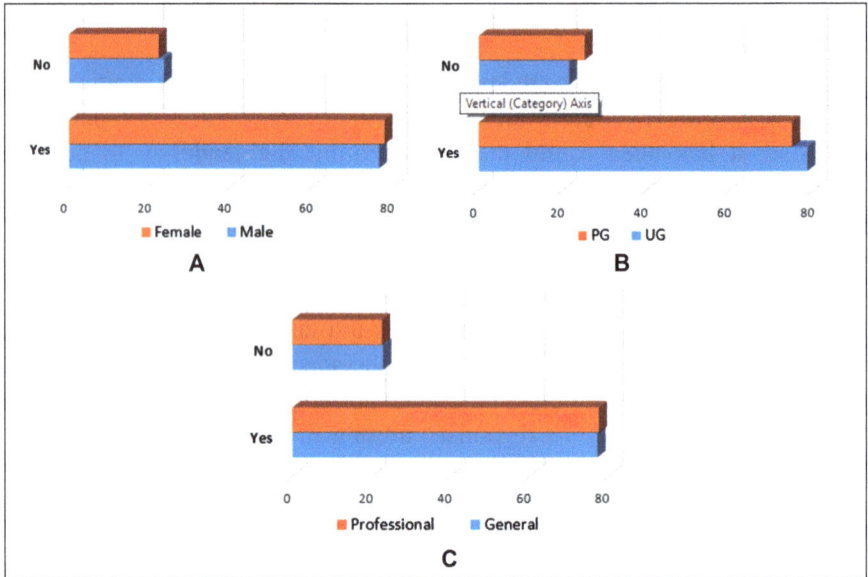

FIGURE 17.4 Chart showing the distribution of percentage of different navigation patterns of organizational websites for non-pharmaceutical advocacy of the COVID-19 (A-gender, B-level of education, and C-nature of the course).

As the situation of immediate social surrounding along with the policy and expertise of local governance usually have a vital role to play in managing and mitigating the COVID-19 related crisis, hence the students were asked to respond to their pattern of frequency of search for local specific information in *Item No. 6*. Thus the result reflected here that 46.6% of students at least once in a day, 17.4% of students occasionally, and 33.6% of students searched the media for the specific information curation of the current situation and latest development. As far as information curation about local specific updates is concerned, the percentage of different responses among group variable in different category viz. male and female; UG and PG; and general and professional had come out almost identical in pattern (see Table 17.2 and Figure 17.6(A–C)).

17.3.3   ASSESSMENT OF PSYCHOSOCIAL REFLECTION

Five items are used to assess the reaction of the University level students on the psychosocial perspectives of the COVID-19 pandemic. Apart from the percentage analysis of the respondent for each of the item, Chi-square test statistics has been employed to observe the influence of the demographic category in respect to each component of psychosocial reflection.

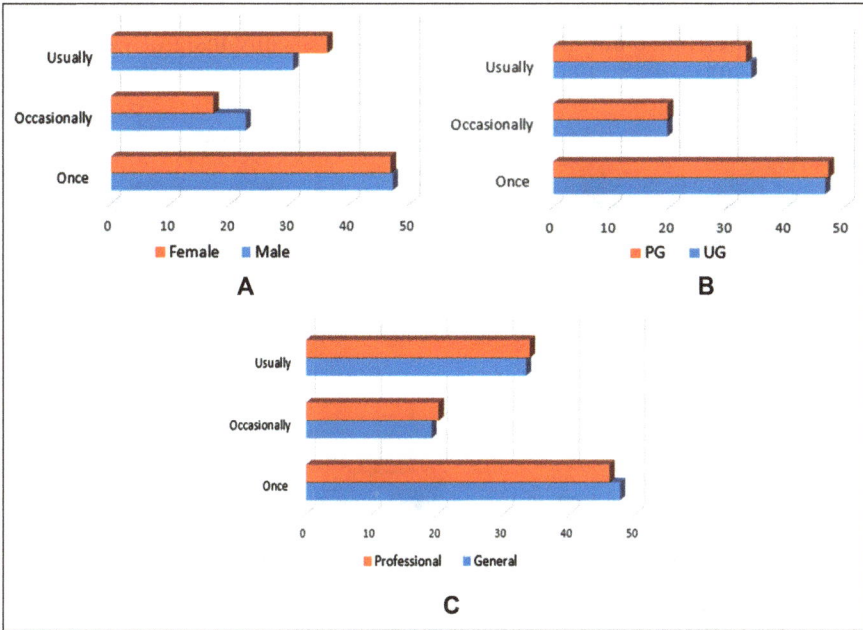

FIGURE 17.5 Chart showing the distribution of the percentage of different searching patterns of everyday for the specific details of the development of global and national level related to the COVID-19 (A-gender, B-level of education, and C-nature of the course).

- **Item 7: *Do you believe the timeliness and transparency of Central and State Government's information regarding public communications of COVID-19?***

  Students' belief on the timeliness and transparency of the information regarding public communications of the COVID-19 provided by the central and state government was reflected in Table 17.3. Most of the participants (66.6%) do not believe the information, provided by the government authority during lockdown period. While only 33.4% of university students believe the government endorsed information.

  The chi-square analysis for item 7 revealed that there was a significant difference ($P<.05$) between male and female students regarding their belief on timeliness and transparency on the information regarding public communications of the COVID-19 provided by the central and state government. The female respondents were more likely to believe (38.9%) towards the transparency of the government's information than male respondents (26.8%). Though there were negligible difference present among different groups of the other two-category variables, i.e., level of education and nature of the course but the differences are statistically insignificant results (P>.05).

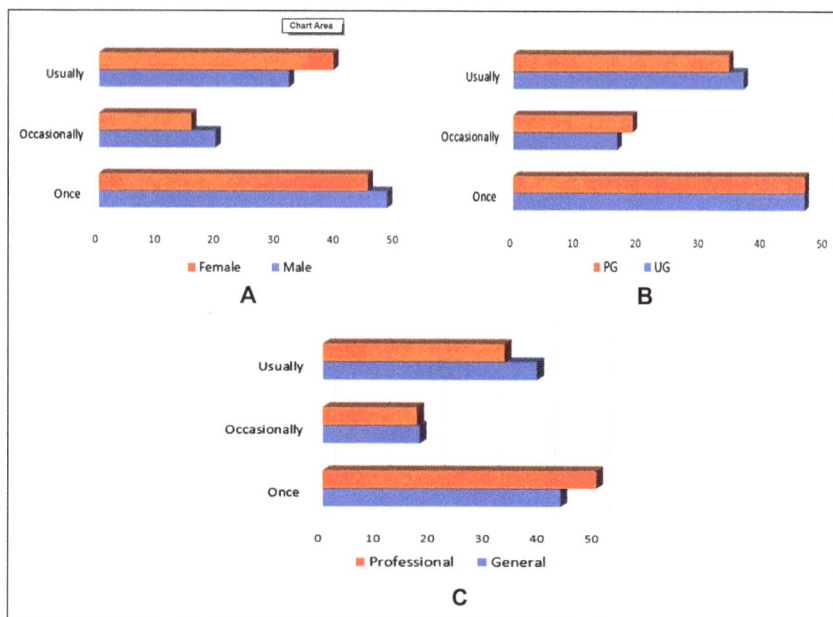

FIGURE 17.6 Chart showing the distribution of percentage of different searching pattern for the updates of the development locally related to the COVID-19 (A-gender, B-level of education, and C-nature of the course).

TABLE 17.3 Percentage and Chi-Square Analysis for Item 7

Category	Overall Responses	Gender			Education			Course		
		M	F	P	UG	PG	P	Gen	Prof	P
Yes	157, 33.4	57, 26.8	100, 38.9	0.01	106, 34.5	51, 31.3	0.48	78, 33.8	79, 33.1	0.87
No	313, 66.6	156, 73.2	157, 61.1		201, 65.5	112, 68.7		153, 66.2	160, 66.9	

– **Item 8: *Do you think that you are never before so fearful about the issues of Personal Hygiene and Public Health?***

Almost like all the other sections of society, young students are also worried and fearful about the chance of infection and hence to some extent, under stress and anxiety. The result, as depicted in Table 17.4, revealed that 78.1% of participants were agreed to admit that they were not so fearful before the COVID-19 outbreak about the issues of personal hygiene and public health. Though only 21.9% were not agreed with the above fact.

TABLE 17.4   Percentage and Chi-Square Analysis for Item 8

Category	Overall Responses	Gender			Education			Course		
		M	F	P	UG	PG	P	Gen	Prof	P
Yes	367,	159,	208,	0.10	239,	128,	0.87	181,	186,	0.89
	78.1	74.6	80.9		77.9	78.5		78.4	77.8	
No	103,	54,	49,		68,	35,		50,	53,	
	21.9	25.4	19.1		22.1	21.5		21.6	22.2	

The Chi-square analysis also suggested that most of the participants from all the group variables agreed with the statement in terms of item 8 that is they are never so fearful and a very few opted the alternate response in all group variables (refer Table 17.4). Thus there were no differences found between the respondents of male and female, UG, and PG, and students pursuing general and professional course in this regard.

– **Item 9: *Do you think that you are paying maximum attention to your personal hygiene than ever before?***

People are always worried about the ongoing COVID-19 pandemic and think individually about how they can protect themselves by certain practices. And this has been reflected as mentioned in Table 17.5 for item 9. Most of the participants (90%) thought that they were paying maximum attention to their personal hygiene during this pandemic scenario than ever before. Though a very limited number of participants (about 10%) were yet to admit the above fact.

TABLE 17.5   Percentage and Chi-Square Analysis for Item 9

Category	Overall Responses	Gender			Education			Course		
		M	F	P	UG	PG	P	Gen	Prof	P
Yes	423,	192,	231,	0.92	279,	144,	0.38	212,	211,	0.21
	90.0	90.1	89.9		90.9	88.3		91.8	88.3	
No	47,	21,	26,	–	28,	19,	–	19,	28,	–
	10	9.9	10.1		9.1	11.7		8.2	11.7	

The result that had come for each group for all the demographic categories (gender, level of education and nature of course) was almost similar (yes = 90±2% and no = 10±2%) to the overall responses in terms of item 8. Thus naturally, the chi-square test statistics revealed that there were no differences between male and female, UG, and PG, and general and professional course pursuing students in terms of paying maximum attention to the personal hygiene prior to the COVID-19. All are mostly paying adequate attention to the personal hygiene.

- **Item 10:** *Are you ready to support your neighbor immediately in all possible ways if he/she is found COVID-19 positive?*
  In the context of supporting the COVID-19 positive patients overcoming the stigma, 65.3% of youth students were ready to support in any of its kind while 34.4% of respondents were not ready to do so. The result shows that female, UG, and general course students were more supportive in attitude than their male counterparts in assisting the neighboring COVID-19 positive patients (see Table 17.6).

TABLE 17.6   Percentage and Chi-Square Analysis for Item 10

Category	Overall Responses	Gender			Education			Course		
		M	F	P	UG	PG	P	Gen	Prof	p
Yes	307,	145,	162,	0.25	206,	101,	0.27	155,	152,	0.43
	65.3	68.1	63.0		67.1	62.0		67.1	63.6	
No	163,	68,	95,	–	101,	62,	–	76,	87,	–
	34.7	31.9	37.0		32.9	38.0		32.9	36.4	

The chi-square analysis for the item 10 was insignificant (p>05) for each category. So, there were no influence of gender, education, and nature of course in this regard.

- **Item 11: *Do you think that you have a scope to contribute in all possible ways like donating, maintaining personal hygiene, staying in home isolation, or even making others aware about the situation and responsibilities to such gravity of crisis of public health?***

  It has been reflected globally that the youth came forward to provide leadership in such social disaster and related psychosocial crisis [5]. Table 17.7 revealed that, during the crisis of public health, 93.4% university students believed that there is ample scope to contribute in all possible ways like donating, maintaining personal hygiene, staying in home isolation, or making awareness among other people and taking responsibility for the society. Still, there were also a negligible percentage of university students (6.6%) who did not believe to have any such scope.

TABLE 17.7   Percentage and Chi-Square Analysis for Item 10

Category	Overall Responses	Gender			Education			Course		
		M	F	P	UG	PG	P	Gen	Prof	p
Yes	439,	194,	245,	0.06	283,	156,	0.14	214,	225,	0.51
	93.4	91.1	95.3		92.2	95.7		92.6	94.1	
No	31,	19,	12,		24,	07,		17,	14,	
	6.6	8.9	4.7		7.8	4.3		7.4	5.9	

The chi-square analysis for item 10 was also insignificant (p>.05) for each category. Therefore, it is evident that there was no significant difference between male and female, UG and PG, and general and professional courses pursuing students in terms of their perception towards the scope of role through which they could contribute for the society during such crisis.

17.3.4   ASSESSMENT OF HYGIENIC PRACTICES

Five items are framed in this section to assess the hygienic practice of the University level students in the COVID-19 pandemic context. Apart from the percentage analysis of the respondent for each of the item, Chi-square test statistics has also been applied to observe the association of the demographic category with respect to each issue of the hygienic practices.

- **Item 12:** *Are you maintaining Hand Washing hygiene as per relevant government advocacy?*

    On the issue of handwashing hygiene, the result showed that more than 89% of students completely followed the government advocacy to maintain proper hygiene, while 9.1% of students partially maintained the same hygienic practice. Though, a very negligible percentage (1.7%) failed to comply with the advocacy in this regard (refer Table 17.8).

TABLE 17.8   Percentage and Chi-Square Analysis for Item 12

Category	Overall Responses	Gender			Education			Course		
		M	F	P	UG	PG	P	Gen	Prof	P
Completely	419,	179,	240,	0.005	278,	141,	0.38	208,	211,	0.74
	89.1	84.0	93.4		90.6	86.5		90.0	88.3	
Partially	43,	29,	14,		24,	19,		20,	23,	
	9.1	13.6	5.4		7.8	11.7		8.7	9.6	
Not at all	8,	05,	03,		05,	03,		03,	05,	
	1.7	2.3	1.2		1.6	1.8		1.3	2.1	

Chi-square analysis revealed that as far as maintaining hand washing hygiene is concerned, there was a prominent distinction existing within different gender groups. In the context of complete maintenance of handwashing advocacy, the percentage of females was greater (93.4%) than males (84%). But the difference was quite less in the respondents' groups depending on education level and nature, of course. So, there was a significant difference ($p<.05$) existing between males and females in maintaining hand washing hygiene. On the contrary, this had been insignificant ($p>.05$) in the other demographic category.

- **Item 13:** *Are you trying to remain confined at home strictly to facilitate lockdown?*

    It is revealed from the response pattern that more than 87% of students tried to maintain completely home confinement while

11.3% of students partially maintained the lockdown. And a very thin percentage (0.9%) was unable to comply with the government order of strict lockdown (Table 17.9).

TABLE 17.9 Percentage and Chi-Square Analysis for Item 13

Category	Overall Res-ponses	Gender			Education			Course		
		M	F	P	UG	PG	P	General	Profes-sional	P
Completely	413, 87.9	172, 80.8	241, 93.8	0.000	277, 90.2	136, 83.4	0.04	201, 87.0	212, 88.7	0.85
Partially	53, 11.3	39, 18.3	14, 5.4	–	29, 9.4	24, 14.7	–	28, 12.1	25, 10.5	–
Not at all	04, 0.9	02, 0.90	02, 0.80	–	01, 0.30	03, 1.8	–	02, 0.90	02, 0.80	–

With respect to their readiness in maintaining the lockdown, female, and UG respondents showed a higher percentage of compliance in comparison to the male and PG students. Therefore, the chi-square analysis revealed that there was a significant difference ($p<.05$) existing within the gender groups according to their level of education. On the other hand, the difference was very less in the groups of students pursuing general and professional courses, and the difference is statistically insignificant ($p>.05$).

- **Item 14:** *Are you following the government advocacy of using mask properly whenever you are compelled to go outside for emergency purposes?*

   To ensure personal protection from the Novel coronavirus infection, the government issued several notifications to ensure the use of masks when people are in compulsion to go outside home for any emergency purpose. In this context, 86.2% of students claimed that they completely followed the advocacy of the government regarding the use of masks in an appropriate manner. Among the others, 11.1% of students tried partially, while 2.8% of students never followed the same when venturing to go outside for emergency purposes (see Table 17.10).

TABLE 17.10   Chi-Square Analysis for Item 14

Category	Overall Responses	Gender			Education			Course		
		M	F	P	UG	PG	P	Gen	Prof	P
Completely	405,	173,	232,	0.02	270,	135,	0.20	197,	208,	0.05
	86.2	81.2	90.3		87.9	82.8		85.3	87.0	
Partially	52,	31,	21,	–	30,	22,	–	27,	25,	–
	11.1	14.6	8.2		9.8	13.5		11.7	10.5	
Not at all	13,	09,	04,	–	07,	06,	–	07,	06,	–
	2.8	4.2	1.6		2.3	3.7		3.0	2.6	

In terms of following the government's advocacy for wearing mask, the result of chi-square revealed that female students showed more willingness than males, and thus, it has been found that gender has a statistically significant association ($p<.05$) with the readiness to follow the mask use protocol. Unlike what has been observed above, the chi-square difference was not significant ($p>.05$) in relation to the respondents of UG and PG and general and professional course students.

- **Item 15: *Do you think it is feasible to maintain physical distancing in spite of the fact that it is very challenging in a country like India?***

   The best way to break the chain of infection is to maintain physical distancing (also termed as social distancing). Though it is very difficult to avoid physical distancing in a country like India, still people are trying to cope up with such neo-normalcy. Almost 57% of student respondents thought that it was possible to maintain physical distancing completely and 40.4% of respondents believed that physical distancing was feasible partially; while only 2.6% of respondents thought that it was not possible to maintain physical distancing even in such pandemic scenario in Indian context (Table 17.11).

   With respect to the feasibility of maintaining physical distancing in India, though the significant difference was absent ($p>.05$) with regards to gender groups, level of education, and nature of the course (general or professional), still the students from female, UG, and general courses showed stronger willingness in terms of affirmative percentage in comparison to the students of male, PG, and professional courses.

TABLE 17.11 Percentage and Chi-Square Analysis for Item 15

Category	Overall Responses	Gender			Education			Course		
		M	F	P	UG	PG	P	Gen	Prof	P
Completely	268,	110,	158,	0.05	180,	88,	0.41	136,	132,	0.53
	57.0	51.6	61.5		58.6	54.0		58.9	55.2	
Partially	190,	95,	95,		118,	72,		88,	102,	
	40.4	44.6	37.0		38.4	44.2		38.1	42.7	
Not at all	12,	08,	04,		09,	03,		07,	05,	
	2.6	3.8	1.6		2.9	1.8		3.0	2.1	

- **Item 16:** *Do you think that you would be able to follow the advocacy regarding the use of mask, for your personal protection, whenever you will go outside, even after the COVID Pandemic crisis would get controlled or over?*

  The result in Table 17.12 shows that, for protection from the infection in future, 88.1% students were ready to completely follow the relevant directives to use mask as hygienic practice even after the post-COVID-19 scenario. On the other only 8.7% of students thought that they would follow the advocacy partially and 3.2% would not be able to follow at all such hygienic practice of wearing mask when the pandemic is over.

TABLE 17.12 Percentage and Chi-Square Analysis for Item 16

Category	Overall Responses	Gender			Education			Course		
		M	F	P	UG	PG	P	Gen	Prof	P
Completely	414,	182,	232,	0.20	265,	149,	0.24	209,	205,	0.29
	88.1	85.4	90.3		86.3	91.4		90.5	85.8	
Partially	41,	24,	17,		30,	11,		16,	25,	
	8.7	11.3	6.6		9.8	6.7		6.9	10.5	
Not at all	15,	07,	08,	–	12,	03,	–	06,	09,	–
	3.2	3.3	3.1		3.9	1.8		2.6	3.8	

The result had shown that such sustenance of hygienic habit of using mask is stronger in case of females, PG, and general course students than male, UG, and professional course pursuing students but the association of gender, education, and nature of the course with the willingness to follow the hygienic practice of using mask in post-COVID-19 scenario is not statistically significant.

17.4   DISCUSSION

The COVID-19 is a crisis, and on the other it is an opportunity to reflect on the so-called normal social design we are practicing till the time. It has given us scope to reflect on our beliefs, values, and priorities of life. We have learnt to re-learn to stand by others and respond to the crisis collectively. This pandemic shows us that the young educated men and women who happen to be the students at College or University have emerged as leaders to support others in need. Despite uncertainty in their academic journey, they engaged themselves in curating information for appropriate decision making and innovations to exercise their social responsibilities. They have proven their abilities to adapt new skills and disseminate such skills in the community. In crisis, people should learn by acting, and the youth students can learn best from failures and mistakes to minimize and mitigate the impact of crisis.

The massive technological development in Web 2.0 not only impacted the peoples' perception of threat further but also influenced the decision-making process. For decision making and action, it is needed to remain informed at its best. Hence it is an important task of social science research to map the pattern of how the educated youth are curating information by selecting media. As there are possibilities of overload of information which may create hindrance ascertaining authentic information [21], therefore, students studying at UG and PG level took engagement with different media for information and instead of accepting media blindly they showed the tendency and ability to filter the information and showed relative choice for media in the COVID-19 context. It is interesting even in the age of social media, this digital youth still preferred the traditional media like Television and Newspaper collectively higher than the other latest formats of media source for information. Females are more inclined to Television than males, and it may be so as they usually spend more time in home and are usually more attached to Television. Male youths are slightly higher exposed to social media for curating the related information. Interestingly, UG level students and students pursuing professional courses preferred traditional media like Television and Newspaper while their counterparts curate infor-mation majorly from social media. It may be so that students of professional courses are more doubtful about the authenticity of facts in social media and UG students are less confident that they could be able to differentiate between fake and real news in social digital platform than PG students. All demographic groups majorly have been navigating relevant websites for self-protection guidelines, and they showed more or less similar pattern of temperament in this regard. As in the United States of America (USA) and UK, it has been found that a good number of people had agreed on the 'myth busters' those who continue to circulate improper and misinformation about the COVID-19 [22]. Here government should have firmer role to prevent such social nuisance.

Irrespective of demographic variation, more than 50% of UG and PG students search for specific updates of the COVID-19 more than once a day and have majorly made it a practice to search the information for global and national level latest development. More or less, a similar media pattern is observed as far as the COVID-related local updates are concerned. Only students of Professional courses have shown slightly less interest than general courses pursuing students for local updates. Maybe students pursuing professional courses have adapted better anxiety management and hence are less frequently searching for local updates. Though gender is usually a major factor but as far as information curation is concerned in the present study, it has not played any remarkable impact.

As far as a psychosocial response is concerned, the Under Graduate and Post Graduate students have shown positive and responsible gestures. Though the majority of respondents irrespective of demographic variable have not shown confidence on the Government authority regarding timeliness and transparency but they had tried to comply with the government advocacy in most of the cases. It may be so that they were worried and frightened about the possibilities of infections, and they admitted that they had not paid so much attention to the self-protective behavior ever before. This finding is in tune with the findings of the study of Cheng [23] in the Malaysian context. Response from administrative authority could have been more prompt, and in responding to the pandemic crisis [24], there is a contradictory finding while most of the UG and PG students (more than 90%) are with the opinion that they have scope to contribute in such period of crisis, but in case of supporting the immediate neighbor in urgency if he/she is found as the COVID positive, more than 34% are still apathetic to extend support. It may be due to social stigma and fear of infection due to lack of proper knowledge [25, 26]. Demographic factors as such have no influence in determining such response. Such pandemic outbreak is an emergency risk communication that is vital to public health and safety [27].

Thus government should explore the alternative ways for educating youth about such outbreaks to overcome social stigmatization.

Predicting hygienic practices of educated youth of India who are pursuing Under Graduate and Post Graduate courses was a major focus of this study. World Health Organization (WHO) in February 2020 asserted "Optimize use of protective equipment and other infection prevention and control measures in health care and community settings-It is critical to protect health care workers and the community from the transmission and create a safe working environment." Such assertion indicates the need of research on self-protective hygienic practices. It has been found that as far as home confinement, hand washing and using mask in desired fashion is concerned, among the respondents, 85 to 90% responded in affirmative and cooperative manner. 'As a susceptible population, a properly fitted face mask plays a crucial importance for the youth' [20]. In terms of using mask, Indian youth has been showing inspiring trends while in Malaysia only 51.2% people are using masks while going out of home which is much less than Indian students but 87% common people are maintaining hand hygiene [21]. Peng [28] also reported majority of university students of China have shown positive and proactive protective practices towards the COVID-19 pandemic. Females have shown better temperament and decision making [29] than males in all above cases, and such difference is statistically significant, thus gender is an influencer as a demographic factor in this regard. This finding is also similar with the earlier research [24, 28, 30]. But as far as home confinement is concerned, as per government directives, UG students have shown higher readiness for complying with the directives than PG level students, and such difference is significant. Other demographic variables are irrelevant here. Interestingly 57% of people completely agreed that maintaining physical distancing is possible, while a substantial portion having opined that it is not possible to comply with the directives of such distancing in the Indian context.

In the context of probability and feasibility to practices in the usage of personal protective hygienic habits even after the COVID-19 pandemic gets over, 88% Under Graduate and Post Graduate expressed their willingness to practice hygienic behavior even in post-pandemic period. It is a very interesting finding and also supported by the study of Mościcka [3]. It has been found in earlier research that less the age is, the easier it is to adapt and retain new habits. Thus such pro-hygienic attitude of the UG and PG Indian students may mark a positive healthy life style and this could be easier to manage such contagious outbreak of communicable diseases in future.

17.5   POLICY IMPLICATIONS

There is speculation in the discourse of evolutionary virology and immunology that the human civilization might have to face much more severe pathogenic outbreaks in the near future, and we should prepare ourselves resilient. Apart from medical intervention, lifestyle, in particular hygienic habits may play a very crucial role in mitigating such contagious diseases at the community level. Therefore, policymakers need to design more effectively targeted campaign materials, especially for the youth.

17.6   CONCLUSION

The present empirical study has attempted to capture some immediate patterns of behavior of Indian UG and PG students in the context of the COVID-19 and tried to generate data to comprehend how the UG and PG students are choosing and screening relevant information, interpreting information in determining their psychosocial response and practicing modes of self-protective behavior. 'Future of the society depends on the health of its youth' [24]. The study suggests that despite their lack of confidence on the government, they responded to the Government advocacies to maintain best practices not only to protect themselves but also to mitigate the COVID-19 pandemic at the community level. But still, a certain portion of the students at the tertiary level are attracted to the probable sources of misinformation like social media and are also showing apathy to the best hygienic practices, which indicate the need of specific elementary health education program at the tertiary level of education across the various disciplines. The findings would further need to be rechecked with a higher sample size accommodating other relevant socio-demographical variables.

KEYWORDS

- **COVID-19 pandemic**
- **hygienic practices**
- **information curation**
- **postgraduate**
- **psychosocial response**
- **undergraduate**

REFERENCES

1. Qiu, J., Shen, B., Zhao, M., Wang, Z., Xie, B., & Xu, Y., (2020). A nationwide survey of psychological distress among Chinese people in the COVID-19 epidemic: Implications and policy recommendations. *General Psychiatry, 33*(2). http://dx.doi.org/10.1136/gpsych-2020-100213.
2. Chew, N. W., Lee, G. K., Tan, B. Y., Jing, M., Goh, Y., Ngiam, N. J., Yeo, L. L., et al., (2020). A multinational, multicentre study on the psychological outcomes and associated physical symptoms amongst healthcare workers during COVID-19 outbreak. *Brain, Behavior, and Immunity*. https://doi.org/10.1016/j.bbi.2020.04.049.
3. Mościcka, P., Chróst, N., Terlikowski, R., Przylipiak, M., Wołosik, K., & Przylipiak, A., (2020). Hygienic and cosmetic care habits in polish women during COVID-19 pandemic. *Journal of Cosmetic Dermatology, 19*(8), 1840–1845. https://doi.org/10.1111/jocd.13539.
4. *Universal Declaration of Human Rights*, (1948). https://www.ohchr.org/EN/UDHR/Documents/UDHR_Translations/eng.pdf (accessed on 28 June 2021).
5. World Bank, (2020). Building a balanced future. *Sustainable Development Series*. https://www.worldbank.org/en/who-we-are/news/campaigns/2020/the-sustainable-development-series-building-a-balanced-future (accessed on 28 June 2021).
6. World Bank Group (Education), (2020). *The COVID-19 Crisis Response: Supporting Tertiary Education for Continuity, Adaptation, and Innovation*. http://pubdocs.worldbank.org/en/621991586463915490/WB-Tertiary-Ed-and-COVID-19-Crisis-for-public-use-April-9.pdf (accessed on 28 June 2021).
7. Rahman, M., Ahmed, S. O., & Mustahsin-ul-Aziz, (2020). *Bangladesh's Unlikely Inventor Creates Face Shields to Tackle Coronavirus*. End poverty in South Asia. https://blogs.worldbank.org/endpovertyinsouthasia/bangladeshs-unlikely-inventor-creates-face-shields-tackle-coronavirus (accessed on 28 June 2021).
8. Chong, M., & Choy, M., (2018). The social amplification of haze-related risks on the internet. *Health Communication, 33*(1), 14–21. https://doi.org/10.1080/10410236.2016.1242031.
9. Ali, P. M., & Sterlin, E., (2020). *Ethics Play Key Role in Universal Health Care Push*. Investing in Health. https://blogs.worldbank.org/health/ethics-play-key-role-universal-health-care-push (accessed on 28 June 2021).
10. Lee, S. A., (2020). Coronavirus anxiety scale: A brief mental health screener for COVID-19 related anxiety. *Death Studies*. https://www.tandfonline.com/loi/udst20 (accessed on 28 June 2021).
11. WeareSocial, (2018). *Digital 2018: Global Overview*. https://wearesocial.com/blog/2018/01/global-digital-report-2018 (accessed on 28 June 2021).
12. Guidry, J. P., Meganck, S. L., Perrin, P. B., Messner, M., Lovari, A., & Carlyle, K. E., (2020). # Ebola: Tweeting and pinning an epidemic. *Atlantic Journal of Communication*, 1–14. https://doi.org/10.1080/15456870.2019.1707202.
13. Merchant, R. M., & Lurie, N., (2020). Social media and emergency preparedness in response to novel coronavirus. *JAMA*. https://jamanetwork.com/journals/jama/fullarticle/2763596 (accessed on 28 June 2021).
14. Gao, J., Zheng, P., Jia, Y., Chen, H., Mao, Y., Chen, S., Wang, Y., et al., (2020). Mental health problems and social media exposure during COVID-19 outbreak. *Plos One, 15*(4). https://doi.org/10.1371/journal.pone.0231924.

15. Wang, C., Liu, L., Hao, X., Guo, H., Wang, Q., Huang, J., He, N., et al., (2020). *Evolving Epidemiology and Impact of Non-Pharmaceutical Interventions on the Outbreak of Coronavirus Disease 2019 in Wuhan, China.* MedRxiv. https://doi.org/10.1101/2020.03.03.20030593.

16. Liu, S., Yang, L., Zhang, C., Xiang, Y. T., Liu, Z., Hu, S., & Zhang, B., (2020). Online mental health services in China during the COVID-19 outbreak. *The Lancet Psychiatry, 7*(4), e17–e18. https://doi.org/10.1016/S2215-0366(20)30077-8.

17. Van, B. T., Basnayake, A., Wurie, F., Jambai, M., Koroma, A. S., Muana, A. T., & Nellums, L. B., (2016). Psychosocial effects of an Ebola outbreak at individual, community, and international levels. *Bulletin of the World Health Organization, 94*(3), 210. https://doi.org/10.2471/BLT.15.158543.

18. Agnew, M., Poole, H., & Khan, A., (2019). Fall break fallout: Exploring student perceptions of the impact of an autumn break on stress. *Student Success, 10*(3), 45. https://doi.org/10.5204/ssj.v10i3.1412.

19. Pan, H., (2020). A glimpse of university students' family life amidst the COVID-19 virus. *Journal of Loss and Trauma*, 1–4. https://doi.org/10.1080/15325024.2020.1750194.

20. Chen, X., Ran, L., Liu, Q., Hu, Q., Du, X., & Tan, X., (2020). Hand Hygiene, Mask-Wearing Behaviors and Its Associated Factors during the COVID-19 Epidemic: A Cross-Sectional Study among Primary School Students in Wuhan, China. *International Journal of Environmental Research and Public Health, 17*(8), 2893. https://doi.org/10.3390/ijerph17082893.

21. Azlan, A. A., Hamzah, M. R., Sern, T. J., Ayub, S. H., & Mohamad, E., (2020). Public knowledge, attitudes and practices towards COVID-19: A cross-sectional study in Malaysia. *Plos One, 15*(5). https://doi.org/10.1371/journal.pone.0233668.

22. Geldsetzer, P., (2020). *Using Rapid Online Surveys to Assess Perceptions During Infectious Disease Outbreaks: A Cross-Sectional Survey on COVID-19 Among the General Public in the United States and the United Kingdom.* medRxiv. https://doi.org/10.1101/2020.03.13.20035568.

23. Cheng, C., (2020). *COVID-19 in Malaysia: Economic Impacts & Fiscal Responses.* https://www.isis.org.my/2020/03/26/covid-19-in-malaysia-economic-impacts-fiscal-responses/ (accessed on 28 June 2021).

24. Odonkor, S. T., Kitcher, J., Okyere, M., & Mahami, T., (2019). Self-assessment of hygiene practices towards predictive and preventive medicine intervention: A case study of university students in Ghana. *BioMed Research International.* https://doi.org/10.1155/2019/3868537.

25. Zhong, B. L., Luo, W., Li, H. M., Zhang, Q. Q., Liu, X. G., Li, W. T., & Li, Y., (2020). Knowledge, attitudes, and practices towards COVID-19 among Chinese residents during the rapid rise period of the COVID-19 outbreak: A quick online cross-sectional survey. *International Journal of Biological Sciences, 16*(10), 1745. https://doi.org/10.7150/ijbs.45221.

26. ISC Research, (2020). *The impact of COVID-19 on education technology in international schools - August 2020.* https://www.iscresearch.com/services/specialist-reports (accessed on 28 June 2021).

27. Toppenberg-Pejcic, D., Noyes, J., Allen, T., Alexander, N., Vanderford, M., & Gamhewage, G., (2019). Emergency risk communication: Lessons learned from a rapid review of recent gray literature on Ebola, zika, and yellow fever. *Health Communication, 34*(4), 437–455. https://doi.org/10.1080/10410236.2017.1405488.

28. Peng, Y., Pei, C., Zheng, Y., Wang, J., Zhang, K., Zheng, Z., & Zhu, P., (2020). *Knowledge, Attitude and Practice Associated with COVID-19 Among University Students: A Cross-Sectional Survey in China* (pp. 1–13). Research square. https://doi.org/10.21203/rs.3.rs-21185/v3.

29. Davies, S. E., Harman, S., True, J., & Wenham, C., (2020). *Why Gender Matters in the Impact and Recovery from COVID-19.* https://www.lowyinstitute.org/the-interpreter/why-gender-matters-impact-and-recovery-covid-19 (accessed on 28 June 2021).

30. Park, J. H., Cheong, H. K., Son, D. Y., Kim, S. U., & Ha, C. M., (2010). Perceptions and behaviors related to hand hygiene for the prevention of H1N1 influenza transmission among Korean university students during the peak pandemic period. *BMC Infectious Diseases, 10*(1), 222. https://doi.org/10.1186/1471-2334-10-222.

31. Al-Hazmi, A., Gosadi, I., Somily, A., Alsubaie, S., & Saeed, A. B., (2018). Knowledge, attitude and practice of secondary schools and university students toward middle east respiratory syndrome epidemic in Saudi Arabia: A cross-sectional study. *Saudi Journal of Biological Sciences, 25*(3), 572–577. https://doi.org/10.1016/j.sjbs.2016.01.032.

32. Ali, K., Zain-ul-abdin, K., Li, C., Johns, L., Ali, A. A., & Carcioppolo, N., (2019). Viruses going viral: Impact of fear-arousing sensationalist social media messages on user engagement. *Science Communication, 41*(3), 314–338. https://doi.org/10.1177/1075547019846124.

33. Anderson, J. L., Warren, C. A., Perez, E., Louis, R. I., Phillips, S., Wheeler, J., Cole, M., & Misra, R., (2008). Gender and ethnic differences in hand hygiene practices among college students. *American Journal of Infection Control, 36*(5), 361–368. https://doi.org/10.1016/j.ajic.2007.09.007.

34. Lau, J. T. F., Yang, X., Tsui, H., & Kim, J. H., (2003). Monitoring community responses to the SARS epidemic in Hong Kong: From day 10 to day 62. *Journal of Epidemiology & Community Health, 57*(11), 864–870. http://dx.doi.org/10.1136/jech.57.11.864.

35. Leung, G. M., Ho, L. M., Chan, S. K., Ho, S. Y., Bacon-Shone, J., Choy, R. Y., & Fielding, R., (2005). Longitudinal assessment of community psych behavioral responses during and after the 2003 outbreak of severe acute respiratory syndrome in Hong Kong. *Clinical Infectious Diseases, 40*(12), 1713–1720. https://doi.org/10.1086/429923.

36. Naser, A. Y., Dahmash, E. Z., Alwafi, H., Alsairafi, Z. K., Al Rajeh, A. M., Alhartani, Y. J., & Alyami, H. S., (2020). *Knowledge and Practices Towards COVID-19 During its Outbreak: A Multinational Cross-Sectional Study.* medRxiv. https://doi.org/10.1101/2020.04.13.20063560.

37. Pabalan, P., (2020). *Youth on COVID19: Young People's Resilience is the Boost We Need Right Now.* Voices. https://blogs.worldbank.org/voices/youthoncovid19-young-peoples-resilience-boost-we-need-right-now (accessed on 28 June 2021).

38. Tang, C. S. K., & Wong, C. Y., (2004). Factors influencing the wearing of facemasks to prevent the severe acute respiratory syndrome among adult Chinese in Hong Kong. *Preventive Medicine, 39*(6), 1187–1193. https://doi.org/10.1016/j.ypmed.2004.04.032.

39. Wenham, C., Smith, J., & Morgan, R., (2020). COVID-19: The gendered impacts of the outbreak. *The Lancet, 395*(10227), 846–848. https://doi.org/10.1016/S0140-6736(20)30526-2.

40. World Health Organization, (2020). *COVID 19 Public Health Emergency of International Concern (PHEIC)* (pp. 1–7). Global research and innovation forum: Towards a research roadmap. Retrieved from: https://www.who.int/blueprint/priority-diseases/key-action/

Global_Research_Forum_FINAL_VERSION_for_web_14_feb_2020.pdf?ua=1 (accessed on 28 June 2021).

41. Zhang, Y., & Ma, Z. F., (2020). Impact of the COVID-19 pandemic on mental health and quality of life among local residents in Liaoning Province, China: A cross-sectional study. *International Journal of Environmental Research and Public Health, 17*(7), 2381. https://doi.org/10.3390/ijerph17072381.

CHAPTER 18

Towards Enhancing Lecturers' Professionalism in a Period of Global Pandemic in Nigerian Universities: Issues and Challenges

DAVID JIMOH KAYODE and SURAIYA RATHANKOOMAR NAICKER

Department of Educational Leadership and Management,
Faculty of Education, University of Johannesburg, South Africa,
E-mail: kayodedj1@gmail.com (D. J. Kayode)

ABSTRACT

Nigeria recognizes education as the instrument of excellence for effecting, promoting, and sustaining national development. However, this laudable goal can only be achieved when quality teaching is taking place in Nigerian universities. The professionalism of teaching in Nigeria higher institutions has been adjudged as a significant determinant of lecturers' professional advancement. Professionalism in higher education in Nigeria focuses on the social and personal improvement of lecturers through understanding challenges that are potent enough to inhibit the realization of individual and institutional goals as well as equipping them with potentials and capabilities which will enhance the attainment of measurable and sustainable results. Quality higher education is therefore critical to Nigeria in getting developed politically, socially, and economically. Professionalism becomes the key for national advancement, especially now that the educational system is confronted with many challenges arising from global uprisings such as pandemics and other political, social, environmental, and economic issues. Allocating resources in teacher professional development is, therefore, the key to the measure of standard of a nation's educational system. The chapter, therefore, examines enhancing lecturers' professionalism towards overcoming challenges arising from global pandemics. This chapter discussed the concept of profession and professionalism, the idea of global pandemics as it affects the educational system. Professionalism was conceptualized into professional competence, commitment to an ethical standard, and professional accountability, and the relationship between professionalism and national development was established. It is therefore recommended that policymakers, university governing boards, and other relevant stakeholders in the administration of higher education in Nigeria should ensure continuous revamping of higher education in Nigeria by ensuring training as and when due and retraining of university teachers towards attaining the threshold of professionalism through exposure to various seminars and conferences building capacities, as well as equipping the university system with adequate instruction enhancing facilities.

18.1 INTRODUCTION

University education is one of the fundamental indicators showing the commitment of a society in its quest for national transformation. University education in developed nations is the center for research, teaching, and learning. It is at this level; an individual inculcates the right type of skills and attitudes in line with societal demands. University education in Nigeria is involved with teaching, administration, research, and development, character, and learning as well as community services for the rapid growth and national transformation [1]. Nigeria depends heavily on university education for economic revamping and technological advancement. The role of university education is playing in the political and social spheres of Nigeria makes it imperative to address issues that could bring the country out of the present pandemic period strong and self-reliant. The COVID 19 pandemic had a significant negative impact on the educational systems of countries across the globe. This has led to closures of universities and other levels of education, not only in Nigeria but also across the world. In April 2020, about 1.723 billion students were said to have experienced disruption in their academics due to pandemics [2]. Closures of schools have far-reaching political, social, and economic consequences, especially in Nigeria, where education has been adopted as an instrument of excellence for effecting rapid national transformation. The closure of schools has defined the need to re-equip our educational system towards mitigating the far-reaching consequences of the COVID 19 pandemic. The growth and technological advancement of Nigeria relies heavily on the quality and quantity of workforce emerging out of Nigeria's university system. University lecturers are central in roles towards producing a high-level workforce for the economy. They are the ones facilitating the transfer of the right type of skills, knowledge, and attitudes towards building a strong and self-reliant nation. This fundamental role being performed by these lecturers make it pertinent for their professional needs to be met at all time, which will further strengthen their level of productivity.

The professionalism of lecturers entails standardization of the teaching profession towards meeting the immediate and future needs of society. It involves adherence to institutional ethical conduct or quality control measures that have been put in place to ensure quality in the system. Professionalism is an ideology that embodies trustworthiness, appealing values of service, integrity, reliable standards, and autonomy [3–5]. After the pandemic era, there would be immediate and urgent needs to carry out reforms in various sectors of the economy. These lecturers are the most significant change agent in educational improvement [6]. Professionalism brings about dynamism in the teaching-learning process. It implements the curriculum at the university level ideal to the contemporary changes in the world. Professionalism extends to changes in classroom practices to new techniques that will further ignite the interest of learners and inculcate in them the right type of attitude towards developing a positive mind.

Unless lecturers provide adequate instructions and create learning environments conducive for the teaching-learning process, students' academic goal attainment will not be at an optimum level. The professionalism of these lecturers is critical to having quality improvement in the university system during and after the pandemic period. Highly equipped staff with economic revamping tools, encouraging incentives from the government, redesigned curriculum to stay relevant to present global challenges, and decentralized decision-making system whereby lectures are involved in decision-making processes would do Nigeria a lot of good in reviving our economy after the pandemic. Professionalism in teaching primarily at the tertiary level of education has helped in building many societies into a modern world through giving priority to skills and knowledge acquisition. Massive investment in university lecturers is paramount to having a community that will emerge strong after the pandemic period. All these should, therefore, be tailored to be in line with societal needs. Professionalism in Nigerian higher institutions of learning are really important for a developing country like Nigeria to rise above all challenges posed by COVID 19. Professionalism in the teaching-learning process will be a useful instrument of change in Nigeria. The shortage of educational facilities and inadequate budget allocation has hindered capacity building in tertiary institutions in Nigeria [7]. It, therefore, calls for more budgetary allocation towards investing in the professional needs of university lecturers in Nigeria Universities, especially during and after the pandemic era.

18.2   CONCEPT OF A PROFESSION

A profession, in its literal sense, is an occupation that requires specialized training or skill. It involves prolonged training and a formal qualification. It is an occupation that requires unique mental ability acquired through the level of official certification. It can further be seen as an activity routinely carried out by a community of persons who comply with ethical standards and are accredited to possess expert knowledge in a recognized field of study. According to Orubite [8], a profession is a paying job in which extensive training of an intellectual character and formal or liberal educational qualifications is required. A profession entails characteristics such as day-to-day decision-making skills, possession of a specialized body of knowledge, clear membership of a particular group, and a set of practices, ethics, and behaviors that members must follow. Sha [9] further declares that the attributes of a specialty include: formal education focused on theoretical understanding, codes of ethics, membership of professional societies, acknowledgment, and acceptance by the public by transparency, qualification, or accreditation. It exemplifies high moral and ethical standards. A profession is a career that depends on advanced intellectual research and training for the offering of eligible services to other members of the community or government for a fixed fee or salary [10]. Yusuf, Afolabi, and Oyetayo [11] further see a profession as a career or vocation that requires technical skills, knowledge of certain areas of learning and qualifications, particularly those with high social status.

18.3   CONCEPT OF LECTURERS' PROFESSIONALISM

Professionalism in teaching, according to Adendorff [12], is better identified and explained, not in terms of salary, rank, or qualifications, but by focusing on the distinguishing types of behavior and decisions that teachers usually take. Professionalism connotes the conduct, behavior, and attitudes of someone at work. It entails a high display of competence and commitment, communication skills, work ethics, flexibility, reputation for integrity, determination, and persistence, accountability, autonomy to practice and confidentiality. Meena [13] sees professionalism as teachers' display of trust in their ability to assess their job, ensure the learning of different learners, teamwork, and collaboration, influence others in enhancing school practice and the autonomy of teachers. It is the strength to provide clarity of job responsibilities in the university system. Campbell [14] argued that the significance of professionalism is characterized by the standards of ethics that regulate not only the desired behavior of professionals but mostly the sense of dedication and duty that they uphold as individual teachers and mutual associates. It is the quality of one's manner of conduct, ethical relations, towards his or her job and display of a high level of mastery over a given task. Tichenor [15] identified five significant professionalism facets for teachers, namely: character, desire for change and continuous development, content knowledge, pedagogical expertise, responsibilities, and working relationships outside of the classroom. Professionalism will no doubt birth workplace success, build good reputations, excellence, and attainment of institutional goals and objectives. Professionalism in academics will help to teach staff to carry out their duties efficiently and effectively, which will assist the learners in the right direction with skills and ideas needed for individual improvement, and improved capacity to contribute towards the survival of individuals and the nation at large.

18.4   CONCEPTUALIZING PROFESSIONALISM IN NIGERIA UNIVERSITIES

18.4.1   PROFESSIONAL COMPETENCE

Academic staff professional competence involves the capacity to plan and direct the job process in a way that motivates lecturers to carry out their teaching adequately, to produce the expected result in terms of lesson presentation, application of suitable teaching methods and proper assessment of students [16].

Professional competence refers to the capability of a professional to perform duties or to perform particular professional tasks, with the expertise of acceptable quality. Nigerian university lecturers are much expected at all times to display a high sense of ingenuity and ability to adapt to changing or dynamic educational environment. The level of professional competency of these varsity lecturers could be measured by looking at content mastery, time management, keeping accurate records, and giving feedback to the students. The outlook must be the one that supports individual competencies and self-improvement. The environment should encourage professional self-development. The competence of a teacher is measured in terms of pedagogical training such a staff is exposed to and how supportive the environment is to put skills into optimal capacity use. There must be a high sense of consciousness towards teaching methods, communication methods, and evaluation of student's academic attainment.

Ekpoh and Ukot [16] raise concerns about the deteriorating level of professional competencies among lecturers in Nigeria federal universities. This, no doubt, is a dangerous trend, especially during the pandemic era. A professionally competent lecturer establishes good interaction with students in classrooms and encourages feedback from students during learning exercises. They are not rigid to a particular method of teaching as they vary their teaching methods to arouse students' interest in the learning process. However, challenges confronting higher education in Nigeria might hinder these university lecturers from displaying a high sense of ingenuity in the courses of discharging their primary assignment at the present pandemic situation.

18.4.2 PROFESSIONAL ACCOUNTABILITY

Academic accountability implies that those who are given responsibility are held answerable for the educational outcomes of the students or are aware of the duty to provide stewardship account in terms of productivity and the quality of the products thereof [17]. Accountability in Nigeria's university system can, therefore, be viewed as a sense of responsibility among university lecturers to be efficient in mobilizing necessary material and human resources in the system for the attainment of educational goals and objectives at both institutional levels and national levels. The measure of accountability in a university system includes accessibility to consulting students, consistency in classroom instruction, guidance, and conducting research, and other academic events such as conferences, seminars, and workshops.

Professional accountability of in Nigeria's university education has a considerable impact on the quality of input and output in the system; the level of professional accountability of a lecture could be measured in his or her ability to put human and material resources to use for greater efficiency and productivity. It measures also include appraisal and assessment of institutional performance concerning the achievement of predetermined objectives. Professional accountability in university education in Nigeria should, therefore, mean accounting for all the resources put in, the process/actions taken, and the output/results to the society that owns it [18].

According to the National Open University of Nigeria [19], accountability in education is seen as an obligation to one's actions in the educational system. A professional is expected to be accountable to relevant stakeholders in the educational system on how scarce resources are put to optimal capacity, how time is maximized to attain optimum results. Hunt [20] sees accountability as the preparedness or willingness, when properly called upon to do so, to provide a justification or clarification to stakeholders involved for one's actions, motives, behaviors, and oversights. It is the submission to an assessment of one's deeds and steps as and when due, accept responsibility of tasks implemented, and recognition of the need to improve where necessary. This is supported by Okoroma [21], who maintained that education accountability has received a great deal of attention because education is usually financed by society through taxation, which would inevitably exert some influence over all aspects of the institutional process. Professional accountability in education is hindered often with goals and objectives that are not measurable, thereby making implementation and goal attainment difficult, a key challenge in the Nigerian university education of today. Another problem is the ever-changing environment which demands readiness to adjust in line with societal demands. The ever-changing climate reflects the current global pandemic ravaging situation, prudence in the allocation of resources demands more of professional expertise during this period.

18.4.3   PROFESSIONAL COMMITMENT TO ETHICAL BEHAVIORS AND STANDARDS

Recently, the quality of Nigerian federal universities' scholarly performance has been evaluated as being of unsatisfactory quality. This low-quality performance is likely to be due to the non-strict adherence of lectures to ethical standards such as professional ethics, professional competence, honesty, or moral obligation. Ekaete [22] asserted that the level of adherence of university lecturers to professional ethics of their job is quite low, which a factor is contributing to a steady decline in the educational system. Such needs immediate attention during the present pandemic ravage.

Ethical standards in Nigeria varieties are quite crucial in such a way that they portray a set of principles established to communicate underlying values behind the creation of such institutions. Katza and Bryne [23] argue that ethical conduct in the workplace represents a detailed collection of acts that demonstrate individual preparedness to abide by codes, rules, and moral principles that primarily create integrity assets through the workforce and the organization. Ethics can, therefore, be seen as acceptable standards of behavior established in an organization to foster discipline and self-control in an organization.

Assessing the level of ethical standards of university lecturers in Nigeria could, therefore, be measured in the willingness to comply with legal frameworks, rules, and adherence to moral standards that primarily generate an asset of integrity among members in the university. It extends to attending to duties as and when due and assigned tasks that are pertinent to the attainment of goals and objectives guiding the establishment of university education in Nigeria. Ethical behavior needs to be sustained in every organization to ensure prompt responses to duties and assigned tasks. Neglect of standards and disregard for institutional ethical standards will create a chaotic atmosphere that will hamper the smooth running of administrative functions. Weak commitment to institutional ethical standards promotes an unethical culture that grooms non-corporative attitudes.

18.5   COVID-19 PANDEMIC IN NIGERIA

The word pandemic is derived from two Greek words: 'pan,' meaning all and, 'demos,' meaning people. Global pandemics do have serious political, environmental, and economic effects on the worldwide economy. It causes instability in the international market which often dip most countries into economic recession. Pandemics have a host of adverse economic, social, and political effects [24]. Nigeria's first confirmed case was announced on 27 February 2020, when the virus was tested positively by an Italian citizen in Lagos [25]. A second case of the outbreak was found in Ewekoro, Ogun State, a Nigerian citizen who interacted with the Italian resident on 9 March 2020. Universities are facing unprecedented challenges as a result of the coronavirus outbreak (COVID 19). The prevalence of the pandemic is represented in Figures 18.1 and 18.2 as well as Table 18.1. Many are struggling to mitigate or cushion the effects of the crisis while trying to deliver efficient and effective course delivery. The biggest challenge being faced by most tertiary institutions, especially in developing countries, was how to move from the traditional model of knowledge transmission to e-learning, as well as sustaining practical courses and training. The challenges extend to keeping students and staff safe, avoiding panic and adherence to compliances, maintaining educational progress with innovative educational solutions such as online classes. It, therefore, suggests that the pandemic must be appropriately managed to lessen the effects on the educational system.

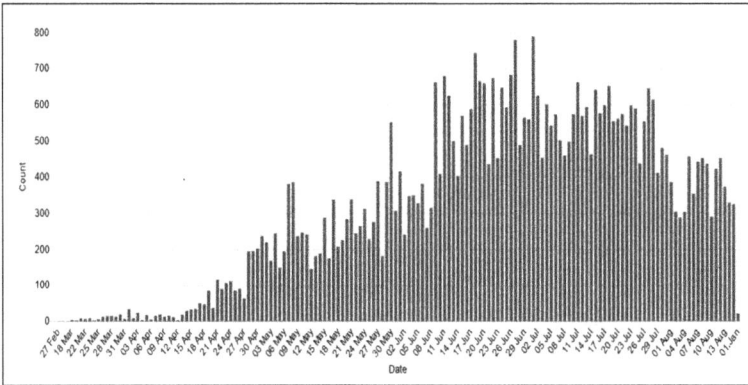

FIGURE 18.1   The occurrence of COVID 19 in Nigeria.
Source: Nigeria Centre for Disease Control [26].

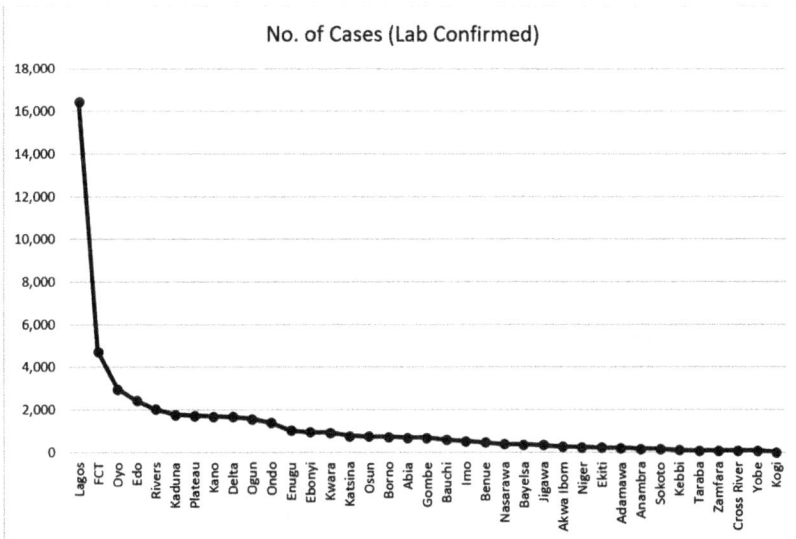

FIGURE 18.2   The cases distribution among the 36 states and the Nigeria federal capital.
Source: Nigeria Centre for Disease Control [26].

TABLE 18.1   COVID 19 Cases Distribution by States and Federal Capital Territory in Nigeria at 15th August 2020

Affected States	Number of Cases (Lab Confirmed)	Number of Cases (on Admission)	Number Discharged	Number of Deaths
Abia	677	126	546	5
Adamawa	185	69	104	12
Akwa Ibom	246	31	207	8
Anambra	156	7	131	18
Bauchi	582	30	538	14
Bayelsa	352	10	321	21
Benue	430	282	139	9
Borno	703	90	577	36
Cross River	73	20	45	8
Delta	1,639	155	1,440	44
Ebonyi	931	52	852	27
Edo	2,423	185	2,138	100
Ekiti	204	108	93	3
Enugu	997	168	810	19
FCT	4,714	3,321	1,347	46
Gombe	676	74	579	23
Imo	506	328	168	10
Jigawa	322	3	308	11
Kaduna	1,766	208	1,546	12
Kano	1,678	258	1,366	54
Katsina	746	265	457	24
Kebbi	90	0	82	8
Kogi	5	0	3	2
Kwara	906	290	593	23
Lagos	16,456	1,788	14,467	201
Nasarawa	374	90	272	12
Niger	229	49	168	12
Nigeria	48,770	11,506	36,290	974
Ogun	1,545	202	1,319	24
Ondo	1,381	579	774	28
Osun	737	304	419	14

TABLE 18.1   *(Continued)*

Affected States	Number of Cases (Lab Confirmed)	Number of Cases (on Admission)	Number Discharged	Number of Deaths
Oyo	2,952	1,389	1,530	33
Plateau	1,708	862	822	24
Rivers	2,005	141	1,808	56
Sokoto	154	0	138	16
Taraba	78	19	55	4
Yobe	67	2	57	8
Zamfara	77	1	71	5

Source: Nigeria Centre for Disease Control [26].

18.6   THE THEORETICAL FRAMEWORK OF THE STUDY

The theory of organizational productivity serves as the theory to back this study. The professionalism of lecturers determines their productive capacity in the system. According to Oluwuo and Nwabueze [27], the theory of organizational productivity theory was propounded by Gilbert in 1947. The theory submits the proposition that the level of productivity in an organization is a function of the level of adequacy of human and material resources available in the production process. Gilbert submits further that when the resources are available in the right quantity and quality, it will facilitate the attainment of organizational goals and objectives. It, therefore, suggests that resources available in an organization must be in the right quality and quantity for organizational goals and objectives to be attained [27]. The theory supports the fact that the professionalism of university lecturers will facilitate the attainment of educational goals and Objectives in Nigeria. As the level of societal challenges increases, so the level of investment in a university academic staff in our various higher educational institutions must also increase. It is expected that during this pandemic period, the quality and quantity of staff must be on the increase side to meet the new expectations and challenges that will be confronting the universities. The professionalism of university lecturers will no doubt yield positive results towards revamping University Education in Nigeria.

18.7 CHALLENGES TO PROFESSIONALISM IN NIGERIA UNIVERSITIES

18.7.1 INADEQUATE FUNDING

Inadequate funding has been a significant problem towards having quality higher education in Nigeria. Funding is considered in every organization as being the drivers of sustainability. A qualitative study by Kayode and Suraiya [28] identified low government allocation, insufficient funding, and infrastructure as a major challenge hindering the efficacy of Nigeria's university education. This financial constraint has made the academic environment not supportive of teaching and learning processes. University lecturers are working under stress and exposing themselves to a lot of physical and environmental hazards. There is no way professionalism could be attained optimally in a difficult situation like this. This issue was raised at the Federal Government of Nigeria/Academic Staff Union of Universities (FGN/ASUU) Re-negotiation Committee in 2009, of which to date, the Federal government has not shown enough commitment towards the funding of education in Nigeria. Federal government allocation to the education sector in the last 10 years has been very poor. The budgetary allocation has always been below 15 to 20% minimum recommended for developing countries by the United Nations Educational, Scientific, and Cultural Organization (UNESCO) (Table 18.2).

18.7.2 THE POOR STATE OF INFRASTRUCTURAL FACILITIES

The deplorable state of infrastructural facilities has been a matter of urgent attention to all stakeholders of the university system. It is one of the items tabled before the federal government by the ASUU. According to ASUU, 163 (23.3%) of the 701 construction projects at universities in Nigeria are abandoned, and 538 (76.7%) are permanently under ongoing projects. Some of Nigerian universities' abandoned ventures are older than 15 years, and some are more than 40 decades old. Around 76% of universities in Nigeria use water well, 45% use pit latrines, and 67% use the bush as toilets. Agabi [31]; Ekankumo and Kemebaradikumo [32] affirm that insufficient support for higher education by current and successive governments in Nigeria has contributed enormously to the collapse in the sector. As stated by Okocha [33], poor internet in Nigeria Universities has brought academic work to a virtual standstill as they have been struggling to shift their activities online as a result of the current global pandemic. As reported by Kayode et al. [34], a large number of universities in Nigeria have little or no internet facilities available to the university communities, and it was emphasized that poor internet connectivity in Nigeria would hinder online lecture delivery. This has made it hard for the lecturers in discharging their duties effectively during this pandemic period.

TABLE 18.2   Budgetary Allocation to Education in Nigeria

Year	Annual Budget	Education Allocation	Percentage of Budget
2009	3.059 trillion	221.19 billion	7.25%
2010	5.160 trillion	249.09 billion	4.83%
2011	4.972 trillion	306.3 billion	6.16%
2012	4.877 trillion	400.15 billion	8.20%
2013	4.987 trillion	426.53 billion	8.55%
2014	4.962 trillion	493 billion	9.94%
2015	5.068 trillion	392.2 billion	7.74%
2016	6.061 trillion	369.6 billion	6.10%
2017	7.444 trillion	550 billion	7.38%
2018	8.612 trillion	605.8 billion	7.03
2019	8.83 trillion	620.5 billion	7.05%

Sources: Refs. [29, 30].

18.7.3   MISAPPROPRIATION OF FUNDS

Budget and Oversight Committee of the Academic Staff Union of the Universities of Obafemi Awolowo University Branch had once accused the university of investing 3.5 billion Naira for the renovation and construction of new lecture halls without due process. The implementation and oversight committee of the federal government set out guidelines for the access of Nigerian public universities to intervention funds. However, the management of Obafemi Awolowo University has not complied with the directives [35]. When resources meant to improve the welfares of lecturers in the university system are mismanaged, the productive capacities of these teaching staff will reduce. Okoroma [36] noted that funding for running institutions often does not get to the institutions. In an ugly situation like this, the psychological state of mind of these lecturers gets disturbed, and this will eventually diminish the attention given to teaching effectiveness. It is saddening that this cankerworm has been seen at all levels of education, with significant squandering and misappropriation of funds worth millions of dollars and billions of Naira [37].

18.7.4   INCESSANT FGN/ASUU DISPUTES AND INTERNAL CRISES

Incessant FGN/ASUU disputes and internal crises are potent barriers to the attainment of educational goals and objectives at both the institutional and national levels. From 1999 till date, there has not been a year ASUU did not go on strike except 2004 and 2012. Frequent disruption in academics dampens the morale of both the teacher and the students. This often leads to so many things in the realm of academics getting compromised. The academic staff of the universities are currently in their 24 weeks of strike action which they have embarked upon shortly before the nation's lockdown. This has negatively affected the lectures, and the university system at large is fulfilling their mandates. The internal crisis is also an issue that affects lecturers' professionalism. These crises can take many dimensions: it can be between the university management and the lecturers, university management and the non-teaching/administrative staffs, it can be between the school management and the students/students union, or between the federal government and the lecturers. An example of such is what is currently happening at the University of Ibadan even before the lockdown where there is a disagreement between the university management and the non-teaching staff on the issue of allow-ances, and the non-teaching staff union has to close the gate of the school in protest to avoid proper functioning of the university. Another case is the case between the governing council and the management of the University of Lagos, where the vice-chancellor was removed. In such a situation, there cannot be effective teaching and learning in the university system.

18.7.5   LACK OF VIBRANT HUMAN CAPACITY DEVELOPMENT PROGRAMS

Lack of or inadequate human capacity development programs is another major issue. No country achieves growth in the economy without the development of the human capital required to drive that growth. Indeed, the development and use of human resources is the key to economic sustainable growth. Training and further training of staff when the need arises still not given priority, thereby limiting the capacities of these lecturers in exploring modern techniques of knowledge transmission. Currently, the ASUU has been on strike even before the global pandemic lockdown due to inappropriate funding of universities by the government, among other demands. Several attempts by the university management to train the academic staff on how they can perform their responsibilities during this lockdown could not be effective because of the current strike actions by the academic staff of the universities.

18.7.6   *LACK OF INFORMATION COMMUNICATION AND TECHNOLOGICAL FACILITIES, AND PRACTICAL EXPERIENCES*

Lack of or inadequate ICT facilities and practical experiences to use the one is available to pose a significant challenge to professionalism in the university system. It is a substantial barrier to transforming our classrooms from traditional methods of learning to modern methods of knowledge transmission. The constant crises between ASUU and the federal government have always been on the issue of funding. On, Wednesday 16 of November 2016, one of the reasons for the ASUU strike was that less than 10% of Nigeria's universities have video conferencing facilities, less than 20% of Nigeria's universities use interactive boards, more than 50% of which do not use the public address system in their overcrowded classrooms and theaters, which are very tricky for lecturers to communicate effectively with students. In most Nigerian universities, Internet networks are non-existent or epileptic and sluggish. ASUU also stated that Nigeria's university library resources are obsolete and still run manually in this era. The Nigerian university library is mostly not automated and quite a disturbing percentage is partially automated. Information communication technology (ICT) integration in the university system will no doubt enhance research. It is alarming to know that in this modern age, many of the universities in Nigeria do not have functional internet facilities and students' results are still processed manually. It is not uncommon to find in these universities inadequate provision of highly efficient computers, multi-media projectors, and electronic whiteboards in classrooms and lecturers' offices. It will be difficult for lecturers to deliver quality research in an environment where there is an acute shortage of water and electricity. Many scholars have been worried about the unfavorable conditions of higher learning institutions in Nigeria [38, 39].

18.7.7   COMPROMISED RECRUITMENT PROCESSES

Politics has introduced nepotism into the university recruitment process, public, and private ones inclusive. Most of the lecturers recruited are not qualified for the positions in which they are assigned roles and responsibilities. This affects their performances when it comes to implementing the contents of the curriculum. Bamiro [40] sees the problem of the de-intellectualization of academia to the low quality of staff in higher institutions in Nigeria. This factor also comes into play in the appointment of principal officers of Universities in Nigeria.

18.8   ENHANCING LECTURERS' PROFESSIONALISM IN GLOBAL PANDEMIC PERIOD

The Federal Republic of Nigeria [41], highlighted the aims of university education in Nigeria as follows: Production of the much-needed high-level workforce essential for the nation's growth and development. They are centers of excellence in teaching, research, and storehouses of knowledge for nurturing the human resources needs of the country, promotion, and encouragement of scholarship and community services, among others. This explains that Nigeria has adopted education as a veritable tool for achieving social, economic, and political development. The attainment of these aims, therefore, warrant inputs of high standards into the Nigeria University system and other levels of education. The lecturers play essential roles in the improvement of the teaching-learning process in the Nigeria University system. They are the ones ensuring active classroom communication takes place by devising learning experiences that help students in becoming useful members of society.

Universities and other educational institutions in the country are currently experiencing devastating epidemics that have disrupted academic and administrative functioning in these higher institutions of learning. However, it should be noted that, despite the ravaging effects of the pandemic, especially in the advanced countries of the world, academic activities continue in places where they are inclined to the scientific digitalized mode of teaching, which has so far, cushioned the effects of COVID 19 on their economies.

The post-pandemic period will unfold new societal demands which all functioning educational institutions must meet. This makes it imperative to have a concerted effort that will incorporate both staff and students in all educational institutions of learning.

Nigeria so far does not have a post-pandemic developmental plan for Nigerian higher institutions. It is crucial to start conceptualizing a way out of this crisis, ensuring the highest degree of professionalism in all facets of our educational system. One of the essential factors that will decide how functioning our higher institutions will be after this pandemic is the lecturers' competencies to operate in virtual learning platforms of high technological complexity. The Post Pandemic era will, therefore, demand a new set of skills and approaches from the lecturers of Universities in Nigeria. There is a need to expose these lecturers to pieces of training that will further enhance their professionalism in the discharge of their duties. There is a need to acquire new knowledge on the latest developments in instructional techniques, which will also prepare the students for future challenges. In light of this, the following are recommended:

1. Re-prioritizing curriculum goals and mechanisms of delivery given the reality on disruptive nature of face-to-face traditional method of learning. It is no thought that with the available resources and facilities on the ground at the university system couple with the student enrollment, a face-to-face lecture may not be visible looking at the guidelines provided by the federal government task force and the Nigeria center for disease control (NCDC). Therefore, online learning will be the only available option when the universities in Nigeria were reopened by the government and ASUU call off their strike actions. The government through the ministry of education (MOE) and the university management must look inwards and make provisions for the takeoff of online course delivery by the lecturers.

2. Lecturers of Universities should be exposed to human capacity building programs using ICT devices on the latest reform on instructional techniques, and ICT facilities should be made available in their right quantity and quality. The government should go into more of partnership with private investors in the areas of organizing workshops, seminars, and conferences which will further equip these lectures with new skills, techniques, knowledge, and experiences that are fundamental to improving on their job performance. The current collaborations of some universities in Nigeria with the

Worcester Polytechnic Institute (WPI) are a welcome development. Although, this could not be effective as those lecturers who called for training have not been paid their salary for the past months. As such, it may be very difficult to achieve the goals of such training if the government and the academic staff union could not settle their differences and the strike actions call-off.

3.   The government should further enhance quality control mechanisms that will improve transparent recruitment processes in the university system. It is no thought that if the recruitment process is faulty, the appropriate candidate may not be taking for the job. As said in the national policy on education that no nation can rise above the quality of its teachers, getting a competent hand into the university system is also paramount. Ethnicity, religiosity, and the federal character commission rules on employment should not be prioritized above the quality of the candidates. This will help the lecturers in discharging the duties effectively if the appropriate and capable persons are employed in the university system.

4.   The government should place a premium on the funding of universities in the country. The budgetary allocation to education yearly is still far below the UNESCO benchmark of 26% of annual budgets. Looking through the government budgetary allocation to the university system, one would ask why Nigeria ably refer as the giant of Africa has been ranked low globally and among its African counterparts. If the yearly allocation to the education sector viz-a-viz the university system is increased, Lecturers will be better equipped and better positioned to transform society in a contemporary world.

5.   Universities should also strive to boost their internal revenue without compromising the quality of instruction. This will augment monthly allocations and grants from the federal government. As much as the government is trying to make education a social service to its citizenry, the government should realize that education is not free anywhere. As such, the government should regulate and introduced affordable tuition fees in all the federal universities in Nigeria. This will help the university management in boosting their internal revenue that can be utilized in providing the infrastructural facilities need for effective teaching and learning in the university system. The university management at an individual level can also form a partnership with industry in the areas of providing facilities for practical training of the students.

18.9   CONCLUSION

This chapter discussed enhancing the professionalism of university lecturers in this pandemic period. The chapter submits that the professionalism of varsity lecturers is vital to meeting the new set of societal demands that will emerge during and after the pandemic. Attainment of quality education in Nigerian universities can only be attained when lecturers are equipped with new skills, techniques, knowledge, and experiences that are fundamental to improving their job performance. This chapter maintains that enhancing the professionalism of university lecturers in Nigeria requires concerted efforts from stakeholders that are internal and external to the university system. The Nigerian university system can be better in quality when there is more budgetary allocation earmarked to exposing lecturers to training that will improve their skills towards making learning become technologically driven. The government should further go into partnership in areas of funding and physical facilities with private investors to assist in equipping our lecturers and university environment with modern facilities to foster innovations and inventions. Innovations and creativity are potent tools that drive an economy towards growth and development, especially during the pandemic period.

KEYWORDS

- **COVID-19**
- **ethical standard**
- **global pandemic**
- **lecturers' professionalism**
- **professional accountability**
- **professional competence**
- **professionalism**

REFERENCES

1. Madumere-Obike, C. U., Ukala, C. C., & Nwabueze, A. I., (2013). *Higher Institution Collaboration with Companies for the Development of Middle-Level Manpower Skills in South-South, Nigeria* (pp. 7007–7015). International Publication of Education, Research and Innovation, Spain.
2. UNESCO, (2020). *COVID-19 Educational Disruption and Response*. UNESCO.

3. Ianinska, G., & Garcia-Zamor, J. C., (2006). Morals, ethics, and integrity: How codes of conduct contribute to ethical adult education practice. *Public Organization Review, 6,* 3–20.

4. Sachs, J., (2003). *The Activist Teaching Profession.* Open University Press, Buckingham.

5. Van, N. S., (2009). *Teacher Codes: Learning from Experience.* International Institute for Educational Planning, Paris.

6. Villegas-Reimers, E., (2003). *Teacher Professional Development; An International Review of the Literature.* Paris: International Institute for Educational Planning. http://www.unesco.org/iiep (accessed on 28 June 2021).

7. Osifila, G. I., Olatokunbo, C. O., & Olaiya, F., (2011). *Human Capital Development Through Universities: The Nigerian Experience (1960–2010).* Lagos, University of Lagos.

8. Orubite, A. K., (2010). Acceptable school norms and unprofessional conduct in Nigerian's schools: Implications for academic standards. *A Paper Presented at the Niger Delta Development Commission (NDDC) Organized Capacity Workshop for Secondary Schools Core Subject Teacher in the Niger Delta Region.*

9. Sha, B. L., (2011). Accredited versus non-accredited: The polarization of practitioners in the public relations profession. *Public Relations Review, 37*(2), 121–128.

10. Dada, S., & Fadokun, J. B., (2010). *Professional Ethics in Teaching: The Training and Developmental Challenges.* Available at http://www.deta.up.ac.za/archive2009/presentations/word/Dada.pdf (accessed on 28 June 2021). (accessed on 28 June 2021).

11. Yusuf, M. A., Afolabi, F. O., & Oyetayo, M. O., (2014). Professionalization of teaching through functional teacher education in Nigeria. *European Scientific Journal, 10*(4), 107–118.

12. Adendorff, M., (2001). *Being a Teacher: Professional Challenges and Choices.* Oxford: CapeTown.

13. Meena, W. E. (2014). The Need for Changing Control of Teacher Colleges in the Quest for Teacher professionalism in Tanzania. *Huria: Journal of the Open University of Tanzania, 17,* 89-95. Available at https://www.ajol.info/index.php/huria/article/view/109478 (accessed on 28 June 2021).

14. Campbell, E., (2003). *The Ethical Teacher.* Open University Press, Philadelphia.

15. Tichenor, M. S., & Tichenor, J. M., (2005). Understanding teacher's perspectives on professionalism. *The Professional Educator, 17*(1, 2), 89–95.

16. Ekpoh, U. I., & Ukot, S. I., (2018). Teaching mentoring and academic staff professional competence in universities. *Educational Extracts, VI*(2), 105–113. ISSN 2320-7612.

17. Uche, C. I., & Clara, O. O., (2011). Academic Accountability, Quality, and Assessment of Higher Education in Nigeria. *East African School of Higher Education Studies & Development, 3*(1), X–XX. Education ISSN: 1816-6822.doi.

18. Uche, C. M., (2010). Assessing the impact of student involvement in community development: The case of the University of Port-Harcourt, Nigeria. *International Journal of Education Research, 5*(1), Winter. 92110.

19. National Open University of Nigeria, (2008). *EDA: 755 Responsibility and Accountability in Education Management.* Lagos: National Open University of Nigeria.

20. Hunt, G., (2002). Public accountability: We are the ones we have been waiting for. *Royal Society of Arts Journal, 3/*6, 10.

21. Okoroma, N. S., (2007). *Perspectives of Educational Management, Planning, and Policy Analysis* (2nd edn.). Port Harcourt: Minson Publishers.

22. Ekaette, E. I., (2019). Teaching staff professional ethics and quality of educational output in federal universities, south-south zone of Nigeria. *American Journal of Educational Research, 7*(8), 548–560.
23. Katza, N., & Bryne, C. E., (2011). Awareness and attitude change: The ethical fallacy. *Journal of Ethics and Corporate Values, 4*(6), 39–51.
24. Davies, S. E., (2013). National security and pandemics. *UN Chronicle, 50*(2), 20–24.
25. *Maclean, R., & Dahir, A. L., (2020). Nigeria Responds to First Coronavirus Case in Sub-Saharan Africa.* The New York Times.
26. Nigeria Centre for Disease Control, (2020). *An Update of COVID-19 Outbreak in Nigeria.* Retrieved from: https://ncdc.gov.ng/themes/common/files/sitreps/915b5907b32 4258ac9899c15b5f466de.pdf (accessed on 28 June 2021).
27. Oluwuo, S. O., & Nwabueze, A. I., (2016). Development of management theories. In: Oluwuo, S. O., & Asodike, J. D., (eds.) *Managing Schools for Productivity: Emerging Perspectives* (pp. 01–40). Port Harcourt: Pearl Publishers International Limited.
28. Kayode, D. J., & Suraiya, R. N., (2019). An investigation into issues impeding higher education effectiveness in public universities. *MOJEM: Malaysian Online Journal of Educational Management, 8*(1), 58–81.
29. National Bureau of Statistics (2017) Annual Abstract of Statistics. Available at https://nigerianstat.gov.ng/elibrary (assessed on 20 June 2021).
30. Sofoluwe, A. O., Oduwaiye, R. O., Ogundele, M. O., & Kayode, D. J., (2018). Accountability: A Watchword for University Administration in Nigeria. *MOJES: Malaysian Online Journal of Educational Sciences, 3*(3), 1–12.
31. Agabi, C. O., (2014). *Teaching and Resources Management in Education.* Port Harcourt: Rodi Printing and Publishing.
32. Ekankumo, B., & Kemebaradikumo, N., (2014). Quality financing of higher education in Nigeria: A nostrum for the provision of quality education. *Journal of Education and Practice, 5*(19), 78–90.
33. Okocha, S., (2020). *Poor Internet Brings Academic Work to a Virtual Stand Still.* Retrieved from: https://www.universityworldnews.com/post.php?story=20200408203452445 (accessed on 28 June 2021).
34. Kayode, D. J., Alabi, A. T., Sofoluwe, A. O., & Oduwaiye, R. O., (2015). Implementation of mobile teaching and learning in university education in Nigeria: Issues and Challenges. In: Zhang, Y., (ed.), *Handbook of Mobile Teaching and Learning.* Springer, Berlin, Heidelberg. https://doi.org/10.1007/978-3-642-41981-2_27-1.
35. The Budget and Monitoring Committee, (2016). *OAU Lecturers Accuse School Management of Misappropriation of Fund Education.* Retrieved from: http://www.nairaland.com/3060164/oau-lecturers-accuse-school-management (accessed on 28 June 2021).
36. Okoroma, N. S., (2004). Principalship and educational accounting in rivers state. *Journal of Research and Development in Education, 2*(1), 134–142.
37. SERAP, (2013). *Education Fund Embezzlement in Nigeria.* Retrieved from: https://www.channelstv.com/tag/education-fund-embezzlement-in-nigeria/ (accessed on 28 June 2021).
38. Asiyai, R. I., (2005). *Trade Union Disputes and Their Perceived Impacts on the University System in Nigeria.* Ph.D. Thesis, Delta State University, Abrak.
39. Odetunde, C., (2004). *The State of Higher Education in Nigeria.* Available at: http://www.nigerdeltacongress.com/sertive/stateofhighereducation (accessed on 28 June 2021).

338

40. Bamiro, O. A., (2012). *The Nigerian University System and the Challenges of Relevance.* Convocation Lecture, University of Lagos, Akoka-Lagos.
41. Federal Republic of Nigeria, (2013). *National Policy on Education* (6th edn., pp. 23–28). Nigerian Educational Research and Development Council (NERDC), Yaba, Lagos.

CHAPTER 19

Remote Learning and COVID-19 Lockdown: Experiences of University Students from the Eastern Cape of South Africa

PIUS TANGA,[1] MAGDALINE TANGA,[2] and ZINTLE NTSHONGWANA[1]

[1]*Department of Social Work, University of Fort Hare, South Africa, E-mail: ptanga@ufh.ac.za (P. Tanga)*

[2]*School of Further and Continuing Education, University of Fort Hare, South Africa*

ABSTRACT

COVID-19 lockdown has disoriented the usual way of life, including the closure of universities, necessitating the ushering in a new way of teaching and learning in South Africa and across the world. The motivation for this chapter stems from the panic that gripped not only educational officials but students in South Africa, especially given the introduction of remote learning, a way many students were not used to. Therefore, the aim of this chapter was to explore the experiences of university students during the COVID-19 lockdown in the Eastern Province of South Africa. The study adopted a qualitative research approach, which is within in the interpretative paradigm and the research design was exploratory case study. A sample of 40 UG students was selected from the four contact universities in the province, University of Fort Hare (UFH), Walter Sisulu University (WSU), Rhodes University (RU), and Nelson Mandela University (NMU). A few students known to the researchers were purposively selected, and the rest were recruited through snowball sampling. Data collection was through in-depth telephone interviews and also through e-mails since face-to-face was not possible during the lockdown. Documentary analysis was also another method of data collection. Data analysis was thematic, and the steps were scrupulously followed. The findings revealed that students were frustrated with the various restrictions. This was emanating from the fact that they were confined in rural and poor infrastructure environment. Consequently, the participants felt hopeless, frightened, and were academically demotivated. The findings further showed that the participants were embarrassed with online or remote learning and could not see a bright future. The participants also adopted some resilience strategies to mitigate the negative challenges posed by COVID-19 lockdown and include reading, exercising, and engaging with others on social media. Finally, the findings revealed that COVID-19 lockdown had its own positive spinoffs and included the fact that participants got support from different stakeholders, learning new digital ways of communication amongst others. The chapter concludes that despite the various challenges, COVID-19 lockdown also brought about some positive outcomes.

19.1   INTRODUCTION

COVID-19 pandemic is a health crisis that has not spared any sector of the South African economy, including education. The pandemic which started in Wuhan, China, in November 2019 and spread to the rest of the world in February/March 2020, has left an indelible mark on all nations' economies. The pandemic has sent shocking waves not only across South Africa and the African continent but throughout the world. At the time of drafting this chapter (August 2020, South Africa had almost 650,000 positive cases of COVID-19 and more than 13,500 deaths. To contain and flatten the COVID-19 curve, the South African government declared a state of emergency and imposed a nationwide lockdown on March 27, 2020, with five stages that were to be followed in easing or opening of the economy. In order not to completely stay without teaching and learning, the department of higher education and training (DHET) together with Universities South Africa and the Council on Higher Education recommended that universities adopt either emergency remote learning (ERL) or the combination of ERL and contact learning (multi-modal). All the universities have either embraced the ERL or the multi-modal learning so as to engage their staff and student. This is what Shakya, Fasano, Marsh, and Rivas [1]; and Pereira et al. [2] call education experiment through new teaching methods. On the other hand, Hodges, Moore, Lockee, Trust, and Bond [3] maintain that colleges and universities have been forced to continue with their programs in these ways so as to keep students and staff safe from the coronavirus pandemic.

South Africa moved from level 3 (Tuesday, August 18, 2020), where universities were expected to bring 33% of their students and staff to campuses to level 2, where this percentage of staff and students to campuses has increased to 66%. Online teaching and learning have brought with it many challenges, as some writers (for example, Ref. [4]) have illustrated from the literature that is reviewed in this chapter. Tanga and Tanga [5] maintain that with 29% of unemployment, livelihood amongst households is threatened. In a similar manner, about 5.5 million South Africans live in informal settlements with four persons per household as well as only 10.4% having access to the internet at home [6]. These factors compound the ERL. The history of the South African educational system is riddled with complexities, which dates back to the apartheid era.

It is well documented that the majority of South African students come from underprivileged backgrounds, and some are studying in rural universities. The Eastern Cape Province is generally referred to as a rural province [7] and has two universities that are classified as rural-based and historically disadvantaged, namely the University of Fort Hare (UFH) and Walter Sisulu University (WSU). While Rhodes University (RU) and Nelson Mandela University (NMU) are regarded as urban-based and previously white universities. This chapter explores the experiences of university students during COVID-19 lockdown in the Eastern Province of South Africa. The chapter has the following objectives:

- To explore challenges regarding students' personal living arrangements and relationships;
- To examine the students' challenges vis-à-vis online learning;
- To investigate the impact of COVID-19 lockdown on students' studies;
- To determine students' coping or resilience strategies.

The first part of this chapter summarizes the research methodology that was used in conducting the study, and this is followed by a detailed and critical literature review. The findings are presented thematically, followed by the discussion and conclusion. The research methodology is the next section, and it detailed the methodological processes and procedures.

19.2   RESEARCH METHODOLOGY

The findings of this chapter are based on empirical and document analysis, hence the adoption of a qualitative research approach that is within the interpretative paradigm, which allows for different methods of data collection. Creswell [8] maintains that a qualitative enquiry examines human actions from the perspective of the social actors themselves (university students). The interpretive paradigm is often used because it provides subjective experiences about the phenomenon being studied [9] and in this case, university students. In this chapter, the interpretive paradigm allowed for the gathering of rich and in-depth data from the participants regarding their experiences during COVID-19 lockdown. In order to gain in-depth and diverse perspectives of the participants, an exploratory case study design was utilized. According to Yin [10], a case study provides a level of detail and understanding of the phenomenon of investigation; in this case, the experiences of students from a South African province, the Eastern Cape. A sample of 40 students was selected from the four contact universities in the province, as shown later in Table 19.1 (UFH, WSU, RU, and NMU. The first few students known to the researchers were purposively selected and the rest were recruited through snowball sampling. All the students were UG students, whose experiences were deemed to be very useful as most PG students are comfortable with online communication with their supervisors, given that the majority of their studies are research-based. Snowball sampling is when research participants recruit other participants for a study, who could have been hard or impossible to find to participate in the study [11] at these difficult times of COVID-19 lockdown. Data was collected through in-depth telephone interviews, and where possible, the interview guide was e-mailed to the students who responded themselves, and documents analysis was another data collection method. In-depth interviews were considered more suitable than other types of interviews as they offer a convenient means of talking with the participants to share their views, ideas, beliefs, attitudes, and perceptions, as Creswell [8] aptly suggested and especially during these challenging times of COVID-19 lockdown. Therefore, there were no face-to-face contacts with the participants.

The primary instrument of data collection was a semi-structured interview guide with a few closed-ended questions on biographic information, and the rest were open-ended questions on topics including living conditions, experiences with self and relationships, challenges regarding online teaching, strategies, or resilience, amongst others. In addition, document analysis was another method of data collection. It involved the exploration of various relevant COVID-19 documents relating to students' COVID-19 lockdown experiences. According to Bowen [12], document analysis is a form of qualitative research that enables the researcher to interpret documents and gives them voice and meaning on an investigated topic. Data that was collected from primary sources of data (telephone interviews and e-mails) and document analysis was analyzed thematically and using the six-step framework proposed by Braun and Clarke [13]. Thematic analysis has been defined as the process of identifying patterns or themes within qualitative data that has been collected through qualitative data methods [14]. The following steps were followed in the process of thematic analysis; becoming familiar with the data, generate initial codes, search for themes, review themes, define themes, and write-up. Data and methodological triangulations were used to cross-check, validate, and verify information collected from interviews and documents. This ensures the credibility of the findings and trustworthiness. All the different participants from four universities in the province brought multiple perspectives (multiple sources according to Kumar [15]) in the exanimation and interpretation of the information, which helped to curb bias and enhanced the provision of reliable information. Dependability of the data was ensured through peer review of the information and chapter draft. The following ethical principles, as suggested by Babbie [9], were strictly observed: confidentiality and anonymity, informed consent, voluntary participation, and avoidance of harm. As part of the research methodology, the biographic information is presented in Table 19.1.

19.2.1 BIOGRAPHICAL INFORMATION OF THE PARTICIPANTS

Table 19.1 illustrates that most participants who took part in the study were females while males were few. Table 19.1 further shows that the majority of the participants reported that they were originally from the Eastern Cape Province. Some of the students were either residing in Limpopo, Kwazulu Natal, Gauteng, Mpumalanga, Western Cape, or Free State. The reason why the Eastern Cape Province has many participants is that the focus of the study was on university students from the Eastern Cape. Many of them were in their 3rd year of study, whilst others were either in 1st, 2nd, or 4th year of study. Lastly, most students were under the faculty of Social Sciences and Humanities, and some of them were either in Education, Health Sciences or

Science and Agriculture faculties. The literature review which comes next is presented in subsections so as the cover the research objectives and from where some of the themes are generated.

TABLE 19.1 Characteristics of the Participants

Gender	Province of Origin	Year of Study	Program of Study/ Department	Faculty	University
F	UKZN	3rd yr.	Social sciences	FSSH	UFH
M	Eastern Cape	2nd yr.	Computer science	SAA	UFH
M	Gauteng	3rd yr.	Journalism	FH	NMU
F	Eastern Cape	3rd yr.	Social sciences	SSH	UFH
M	Eastern Cape	4th yr.	Bachelor of Arts	SSH	UFH
F	Eastern Cape	3rd yr.	Social work	SSH	WSU
M	Eastern Cape	4th yr.	Psychology	SSH	UFH
M	Eastern Cape	2nd yr.	Sociology	SSH	UFH
M	Mpumalanga	3rd yr.	Education	Education	UFH
M	Mpumalanga	4th yr.	Education	Education	UFH
F	Eastern Cape	2nd yr.	Social work	SSH	UFH
M	Eastern Cape	3rd yr.	Geology	SAA	UFH
F	Western Cape	4th yr.	Psychology	SSH	UFH
F	Eastern Cape	2nd yr.	Philosophy	SSH	UFH
F	Eastern Cape	2nd yr.	Psychology	SSH	WSU
F	Eastern Cape	3rd yr.	Agriculture	SAA	UFH
M	Limpopo	3rd yr.	Education	Education	UFH
F	Eastern Cape	2nd yr.	of Nursing	Health science	UFH
F	Eastern Cape	3rd yr.	Criminology	SSH	WSU
F	Eastern Cape	3rd yr.	Computer science	SAA	UFH
M	Free State	1st yr.	Biological sciences	FS	Rhodes
M	Gauteng	4th yr.	Social work	FH	NMU

TABLE 19.1 *(Continued)*

Gender	Province of Origin	Year of Study	Program of Study/ Department	Faculty	University
F	Eastern Cape	3rd yr.	Further and continuing educ.	Education	UFH
M	Eastern Cape	3rd yr.	Further and continuing educ.	Education	UFH
F	Eastern Cape	2nd yr.	Geography	FH	WSU
F	Eastern Cape	2nd yr.	Biochemistry	FH	Rhodes
F	Gauteng	4th yr.	Nursing	Medical science	WSU
M	Free State	3rd yr.	Further and continuing educ.	Education	UFH
F	UKZN	4th yr.	Social work	FSSH	UFH
M	Limpopo	2nd yr.	Further and continuing educ.	Education	UFH
M	UKZN	3rd yr.	Agri. economics	SAA	UFH
M	Free State	2nd yr.	Computer science	Sciences	NMU
F	Limpopo	4th yr.	Pharmacy	Health science	NMU
F	Mpumalanga	4th yr.	Further and continuing educ.	Education	UFH
M	Gauteng	1st yr.	Social work	FH	WSU
F	Eastern Cape	3rd yr.	Social work	FSSH	UFH
M	Eastern Cape	4th yr.	Further and continuing educ.	Education	UFH
F	Mpumalanga	1st yr.	Social sciences	FH	NMU
F	Limpopo	3rd yr.	Social sciences	FH	WSU
F	Eastern Cape	2nd yr.	Chemistry	SAA	UFH

19.3 LITERATURE REVIEW

This section addresses students' challenges regarding their personal arrangements and relationships during lockdown. It also provides a discussion of challenges vis-à-vis online learning. The impact of COVID-19 lockdown on studies as well as the students' coping strategies is also discussed in this section. Although existing studies focused on various socio-economic groups, there has been a dearth of literature that focuses on the well-being of university students, who are perceived as a significant group in many communities. This gap is important in research because university students in their young adulthood stage encounter serious transitions characterized by changes, adjustments, confusion, and exploration, and during this period, the choices they make may have long-lasting consequences. Furthermore, Bask and Salmela-Aro [16] argue that the social experiences of university students are relatively limited when compared to those who are employed, their self-consciousness and psychological endurance are generally low, and this makes them more vulnerable to psychological problems.

19.3.1 CHALLENGES REGARDING PERSONAL LIVING ARRANGEMENTS AND RELATIONSHIPS

Due to COVID-19 and the closure of institutions of higher learning, students were forced to leave their residences, return back to their home, and engage in remote learning. Online learning from home has brought a number of challenges which affect students' academic work. A discussion of the challenges that students encounter from remote learning in their homes are given in subsections.

19.3.1.1 POOR HOUSING AND OVERCROWDED FAMILIES

Solari and Mare [17] explored the effects that overcrowded houses have on the well-being of children; they indicate that the home environment has received less attention in terms of how it affects individuals' lives in significant ways. Home environment enables and allows children to learn roles and interact with others, therefore, the general household physical characteristics and the degree of housing specifically may be an important mechanism in explaining their well-being. Studies indicate that living in a home that is overcrowded may have an impact on individuals' well-being in many ways. Firstly, the absence of a comfortable and quiet environment affects children's academic performance as they encounter challenges in both reading and studying. Secondly, when there is limited space, various schedules held by household members may distract others' sleep. Poor sleep quality can lead to difficulties in focus during the day and can affect the mood and behaviors. Moreover, children in overcrowded households have higher chances of catching illnesses/it is easy for them to catch illnesses which can impede with their everyday activities and studies [18]. Evidence on the role of housing on the well-being of individuals has been found in studies indicating how important housing is in terms of accessing other essential services such as public transport and health care [19]. Learning is a crucial element in the lives of children, but it becomes a challenge when they are exposed to low socio-economic conditions.

19.3.1.2 LOSS OF INCOME, HUNGER, AND FOOD INSECURITY

According to Statistics South Africa [20], South Africa is amongst countries with the highest rate of income inequality and extremely high levels of absolute poverty globally. South Africa's Gini index/ratio is estimated to be 0.68 [21]. About 56% of the population in South Africa lives in poverty and nearly 28% of them are in extreme poverty, below the food poverty line. In addition, at the national level, South Africa is perceived to be food secured but many households are food insecure. Approximately 20% of households in South Africa are estimated to have poor or extremely poor access to food [20]. In South Africa, food insecurity is associated with the socio-economic status of the household as indicated by income, employment status and food expenses [22]. For that reason, total income in the household is essential in reaching food security, however, with high levels of unemployment and poverty, it is challenging for many households in the country (South Africa) to purchase enough food for the entire family [23, 24]. It is a struggle for the majority of the population to sustain a decent income, as the estimated average income of poor was below R524 per month in 2012 [25]. All these have a negative impact on the students' academic progress as most of them cannot really learn on an 'empty stomach.'

According to Smit [26], due to national lockdown to control the spread of COVID-19, approximately 3 million South Africans have lost their jobs. During lockdown, an additional 1.5 million employees have lost their income. Furthermore, the National Income Dynamics Coronavirus Rapid Mobile

Survey [27] reported that 47% of the households lack basic needs such as food. According to the Wave 2 survey, which was conducted by Statistics South Africa [28] between 29 April and 6 May 2020, findings indicated that 8.1% of the respondents have lost their jobs or had to shut down their businesses due to COVID-19 lockdown. On Presidential virtual Imbizo, President Cyril Ramaphosa assessed the damage that COVID-19 has on the economics of the country and the subsequent national lockdown as it resulted in losses of jobs as companies embarked on substantial retrenchments [29].

19.3.1.3   LACK OF ACADEMIC AND SOCIAL SUPPORT

According to Agnew et al. [30], as many universities have transitioned to remote learning, some students suffered from poor psychological health because of the interruption of academic routine. When universities closed due to lockdown, many students had to terminate their internships on campus and their research projects. In addition, disturbances caused by lockdown jeopardized their study programs and internships, they also delayed their graduations and their competency on the job market, and as a result, they suffer from anxiety. According to Konishi et al. [31], academic development is associated with social development. However, the academic journey has repeatedly been regarded as the main cause of stress. The search and actual use of support as well as the belief of its possible accessibility are regarded as the factors that can ease the pressure and strain involved in the pursuit of education. They operate as protective elements that prevent low academic achievement and school disengagement [32, 33]. Numerous studies indicate that a high perception of support favors academic achievement [34, 35]. Previous studies revealed that the withdrawal or dropout depends on their well-being as university students and has a major impact on their mental and physical well-being. According to Li et al. [36], social support improves the self-confidence of students which in turn promotes their academic progress and relieves emotional exhaustion. According to Rueger et al. [37], people with a high level of academic and social support are likely to have high self-confidence. On the contrary, individuals may feel rejected and devalued due to lack of support from their families and friends, and that leads to negative self-assessments, which in turn cause low self-confidence. Fang [38] argues that self-confidence can act as a stimulus/motivation to students so that they can accomplish their academic goals. It is eminent that all the students who find themselves in this situation, may have very little or no motivation to pursue their studies, especially during this COVID-19 era where students need all possible support to learn.

19.3.2   CHALLENGES VIS-À-VIS ONLINE LEARNING

According to Beqiri, Chase, and Bishka [39], although students may struggle with the traditional approach to solve difficult problems but they have access with immediate assistance from either a lecturer or their classmates. In addition, Beqiri et al. [39] also maintain that remote learning could be a lonely experience as students usually help each other in class. It is obvious that the students in the selected universities are exposed to very little or no access to their peers or lecturers as maintained by these writers. Consequently, during remote learning, it is assumed that students feel lonely and abandoned without instant access to help or knowledge, which may lead to dropout. Therefore, it is important to examine the challenges students faced regarding e-learning, and their coping strategies. Other challenges highlighted by Tanga, Ndhlovu, and Tanga [40] include time management and time consuming and overwhelming, which seems to be the main concern as some students were juggling commitments in terms of classes, work, and family. These authors also reported students' inability to access e-learning materials, long processes in the delivery of e-learning devices and inadequate software applications for remote learning by the institutions.

According to Morrison, Ross, and Kemp [41], if the accessible two-way communication's quality is poor, students may lose interest in the instruction due to poor quality and destructions, which may lead to frustration. The absence of a lecturer is perceived as another disadvantage to remote learning, particularly for students with certain learning modalities. For instance, students who learn through tactile modality, they are best when touching, moving, and doing in facilitating their experience in learning. For such students, virtual/online learning is not a perfect environment, as they identify their learning experience through abstract symbols, decontextualized, and cast on a screen that is two dimensional [42]. Remote learning is out of the physical realm of campus, therefore allows students to work on their pace. However, weekly lectures which may serve as a pacing mechanism may fail in an online classroom and students may fall behind [41]. Morrison et al. further state that online learning leads to a high rate of student's dropout compared to normal campus routine. On average, fully online courses have lower success rates compared to face-to-face learning.

For example, with online learning, there is a minimal support and guidance provided to students, and for assignments and exam completion, they have to seek for their own learning material. To some students, this is a discouraging and stressful experience, and therefore, it is the objective of this study to find out the support students received during remote learning.

19.3.2.1 POOR BASIC INFRASTRUCTURE IN TOWNSHIPS

According to World Bank [43], South Africa's geographical division includes that of townships and informal settlements, which involve large communities that are under developed. A township can be defined as an area, usually in an urban environment that is underdeveloped, it is the residential areas that were reserved for non-whites (Africans, Coloureds, and Indians) who used to work in the areas that were restricted for whites only during apartheid period [44–46]. Today, South African townships are remnants of the apartheid system. According to Thulo [46], the effects of past abandonment, overpopulation, and isolation from urban areas are still evident, mostly represented by poor infrastructure and essential resources and a high level of unemployment. Statistics South Africa [47] reported that approximately 1.25 million households live in informal settlements. South African government is investing a lot of money into making its townships more livable; however, the struggle continues, and the majority of blacks are poverty-stricken [48, 49]. Nearly 50% of the South African urban population lives in townships and informal settlements, and about 38% of them are working age citizens. South African townships and villages lack basic infrastructure that students need to function, and many communities and households are not conducive spaces for a fulfilling learning experience [50]. There are large numbers of households that cannot access services such as electricity in informal settlements in cities and peri-urban areas, and that in turn affect students' engagement in online learning.

19.3.2.2 ELECTRIFICATION AND NETWORK CHALLENGES IN RURAL AREAS

In South Africa, nearly 31% of the population lives in rural areas. More than 60% of households in these areas have no access to electricity. This means that there are more than 50% of non-electrified households in those rural communities [51–54]. Approximately 48% (6.7 million) South African households belong to an underprivileged group [55]. In most rural areas, the network is poor or non-existence [56, 57]. Moreover, in such communities, poor telecommunication infrastructure creates challenges, and residents cannot access the benefits of services that information communication technology (ICT) provides [58]. This may likely be a negative influence on remote learning with most students who find themselves in these areas.

19.3.3   STUDENTS' COPING STRATEGIES

Anxiety is extremely prevalent among university students. The main three concerns among students are academic performance, pressure to succeed and plans post-graduation [59]. Heavy course loads, pressure to obtain a high-grade point average, complex interpersonal relationships also put students under pressure [60]. During an epidemic/pandemic state, students are experience additional stressors such as fear of being infected. However, each person has their way of coping and reducing the intermingling stress plaguing their minds [61].

19.3.3.1   CREATING A POSITIVE MIND-SET IN BUILDING OWN RESILIENCE

In times of crisis, positive emotions can induce novel and creative thoughts, which will then lead to exploration and experimentation. Eventually, students develop effective coping strategies and increase their resilience against negative life experiences [62]. Short-term effects of a positive mindset keep depression at bay, and long-term benefits can lead to positive crisis growth. Therefore, to cope with the crisis and emotional strain, the majority of students are trying to look at a bright a side. Tanga, Ndhlovu, and Tanga [40] reported that some students think the lack of commuting gives them more time to explore writing a higher quality research report. Therefore, the students perceived isolation as an opportunity to read more and write their research reports. It was also stated that some students also saved money by staying at home (Tanga, Ndhlovu, and Tanga). For some students, spending the quarantine with their families, bonding with them can take the stress away.

19.3.3.2   SMALL ACTIVITIES OR DISTRACTIONS TO BREAK MONOTONY

Remote learning can actually bring monotony to some students. Therefore, it is beneficial for one to take a break or distraction as a motivation [63]. Students have a lot of time; therefore, some have started finding new hobbies and developing new skills such as cooking skills while others have been reading literature, watch documentaries and movies just to keep their minds busy and relieve stress [40]. Some students have started mediating to ease the anxiety. Isolation can lead to a very dormant lifestyle, so, students make sure that they exercise on a regular basis. According to Esch and Stefano [64], the specific physiological ways to explain the impact that exercise has on reducing stress has not been outlined. Human and animal studies show that physical activeness improves the way the body responds to stresses because of the response in hormonal changes and the exercise affects neurotransmitters in the brain that affect mood and behaviors [65]. In addition to the potential physiological mechanisms, it is possible that exercise functions as a time-out or break from stressors.

Constant communication with family, friends, and peers has also been identified as a way of distraction and breaking monotony [66]. According to Mushtag and Khan [67], regular communication with advisors, colleagues, friends, and family has a positive impact on the academic performance of students. It is obvious that during this period of pandemic, families have been perceived as the best support system as it strengthened bonds between students and their family members [40]. Communication with loved ones is important for the student's mental health, especially during times of crisis where they can support each other throughout and share positive moments. According to Griffiths et al. [66], people often perceive sources of informal help as useful and helpful for dealing with depression. Another important tool of communication is social media, which attracts different perceptions. Social media has kept many students abreast with happenings across the country and around the world, as well as chatting with family and friends [40].

According to Ahmad and Murad [68], social media allows people to share their positivity with friends and family and is also a source of funny and interesting material which can brighten one's mood. It allows people to connect irrespective of their locations. The positive impact that social media platforms such as Facebook have on people can never be denied because they allow people to interact, communicate, and socialize with one another around the world [69, 70]. The use of social media is associated with even higher levels of awareness of events that stressful that unfold on the people's lives [71]. Social media provides an ambient understanding of immediate connection with the public and for the interactive sharing of important information. Even though social media platforms help to strengthen guest loyalty and satisfaction, they can also lead to negativity, incorrect information, and unnecessary censure [72]. Nonetheless, social media has proved by the literature as supporting students during COVID-19 pandemic to chat and communicate in ways that anxiety and stress are reduced. The literature review has painted a dark picture of students' academic circumstances and the positive spinoffs during COVID-19 pandemic. The literature has also shown that the length and breadth of COVID-19 is just beginning and needs more literature on the topic. This chapter contributes in its own small way towards the understanding of students' experiences during this pandemic, especially in a province of South Africa which is rural in nature and given the complexities of remote learning. The findings of the study are presented in the next section and subsections of this chapter.

19.4 FINDINGS

The findings of this chapter are generated from the participants as well as document analysis. A summary of the findings is presented in Table 19.2 according to themes, subthemes, and categories.

Four major themes emerged from the responses of participants regarding their experiences on remote learning of university students in the Eastern Cape during COVID-19. They include personal frustration, academic frustration, resilience measures, and Positive spinoff of COVID-19 lockdown. These themes are presented in the section below:

- **Theme 1: Personal Frustrations with Various Restrictions:** In the process of interpreting and analyzing data from the different levels of students, two sub-themes emerged relating to personal frustrations with various restrictions.
- Subtheme 1: 'We Were Confined in Rural and Poor Infrastructure Environment' (Resource Constraint): The discussion with the students from different levels of studies at different universities, it emerged that half of the students who participated in the study were residing in rural areas and townships where infrastructure is poor, inadequate, and under-maintained. This is what the literature refers to as 'resource constrain environment.' Some mentioned that they were living with extended family members such as aunts, uncles, grandparents, and

cousins. The majority of female students reported that they ended up shouldering a greater burden, typically given unequal division of household chores, so they never had time to focus on their studies as they had to clean the house, fetch water from the river and cook for the family. The findings also showed that students were experiencing poor network connectivity as a result; some had poor or lost communication with their friends, families, and supervisors. Most notably, the high-pressure environment of confinement, combined with financial stress as some students had not received their school allowances that include meals, book allowance, and living allowance, and the data that institutions promised them delayed students' proper engagement with remote learning. They could not afford to buy the prescribed books and data. The following are excerpts from some of the participants:

COVID-19 lockdown forced us to stay at home, and couldn't travel. At first, it was hard to even go to town, so for a month I didn't go anywhere. I haven't seen my family, friends, and my boyfriend. It has caused a lot of strain in my relationships because of the distance. It's really hard to do e-learning because at home there are kids, and they keep on interrupting. Besides them, I'm from deep rural areas, so I'm struggling with network problems, and there's no other way I can solve that [Student 15, 2nd year, Female, EC].

Ever since lockdown began, my life became so difficult. I have adapted to the fact that home is going to be my new learning environment. However, it is not a good place where I can do my research peacefully because there so many disturbances such as having to complete house chores, having to educate family members about the virus. On the other hand, data is expensive, and I cannot afford to buy large GBs to continue with my school work as the university has not yet provided data bundle to us [Student 16, 3rd year, EC].

- Subtheme 2: Hopelessness, Frustration, and Fear Characterized Stay at Home: Life during lockdown has reshaped students' personal relationships in unprecedented ways, forced them to be away from their loved ones. For many students, COVID-19 lockdown has been a unique social experience that has had a major impact on their relationships with their families and friends. Some believed that their relationships with others have been strengthened while others have come under severe strain. Many students found themselves confined for prolonged periods of time with other people (family members) and have come into conflict with each other, as they are not used to stay together for longer periods. Domestic violence has been reported to have increased during these times. Others have experienced lockdown alone, resulting in profound social isolation, as some of the daily interactions have intensified and others had not been possible at all. Most students have reported that lockdown has necessitated close, constant contact with their families and partners, but social distancing measures have isolated them from their friends and wider communities as they could not even attend the funerals of their loved ones. Consequently, staying at home is frustrating and the future seems hopeless and therefore, a characterization of fear in many students. Examples of words verbatim from some of the participants are presented below:

I have lost my uncle who was living in another town and due to the limited number of people to attend gatherings, I couldn't attend his funeral. I'm very sad because we were very close, so missing his funeral is a very disturbing thing that will take time to heal. I am really fearful of this pandemic, and we don't know what the future holds for us as students [Student 1, 3rd year, female, year, KZN].

In all honesty, I experienced the "lockdown" in the literal sense of the word. We were basically stranded (lack of a better word), if I may put it that way, and we had to abide by the given restrictions of how to conduct our everyday lifestyle, routines changed, habits changed, our whole living lifestyle as a person in fact changed. I felt imprisoned at some point until I had to succumb to the fact, I had no choice but to abide so it was a torture, really. It is a frightful experience and it seems as if life is hopeless [Student 11, 2nd year, Female, EC].

- Subtheme 3: Academically Demotivated: Most students stated that they were academically demotivated due to challenges they have encountered in remote learning and lockdown. They have lost the drive, energy, and perseverance in accomplishing their 2020 academic goals. It was difficult for them to continue with their studies as they did not receive emotional encouragement and advice from knowledgeable individuals, physical, and financial support. They lost hope in completing studies for the 2020 academic year as they are academically behind. The findings also revealed that students have not completed first semester courses although it is already the second semester, and this creates anxiety. They perceived 2020 as a very challenging year, especially final year students who are overwhelmed by assignments, practical, experiments, and research. Some students were looking forward to attend academic conferences and present their papers, engage in high level debates with other scholars and peers. Health Science students, final years in Education and Social Work could not complete fieldwork practicum and they were unable to go to the field and collect data for their research projects due to lockdown regulations. Science students were also unable to do their lab work/experiments due to the closure of universities.

Some of us learn by hearing and interacting with lecturers, other students, and oneself, but now all that had to change and we were forced to have online groups which are not so effective nor efficient because sometimes you find that you need to combine an assessment but someone within the group is experiencing network problems or doesn't have data for that [Student 13, 4th year, Female, WC].

I'm so demotivated; I have lost hope in everything. I mean now I'd be on the second semester studying and preparing for tests towards my continuous assessment. I would have written mid-year exams and have passed. I mean now I don't see any hope of getting fee waivers in this online learning. Next year I'm doing my final year and I haven't studied anything that can contribute to that. I mean, my major will require this year's information and I just don't know how things will be [Student 1, Female, EC].

- – **Theme 2: Academic Frustrations:** A second theme emerged from the findings, academic frustrations. Three subthemes emanated from this theme.
- • Subtheme 1: Online or Remote Learning an Embarrassment: The findings showed that the transition to online learning left students embarrassed as many of them had poor network connection since they were living in rural areas. Some have indicated that they do not have access to the internet, which makes it difficult/impossible for them to access academic material such as e-books, e-mails, and Blackboard, which is the university teaching and learning platform. However, many stated that accessing Blackboard is a challenge/struggle on its own as they were not used to study through it. Others indicated that they were never taught/ trained on how to use Blackboard to access

study material and assessments. Furthermore, some students reported not having or owning laptops, especially 1st-year students, as they were hoping to purchase them with their book allowance, but the universities delayed to load their allowances. Some reported that they never received data from their institutions, therefore could not do any academic work online. On the other hand, lecturers are putting more pressure on them as they want to finalize the first semester. The following two:

I'm struggling to use Blackboard; as a result, I haven't managed to send my assignments or anything through it, it's frustrating. Teaching and Learning Centre taught us on how to use Blackboard when I was doing 1st year and there was only one course that required us to use Blackboard to send assignments and most of the time, it was group assignments, so I didn't really learn to use it independently [Student 4, 3rd year, Female, EC].

I stay in deep rural areas where the network is very poor, so it's not easy for me to participate in group discussions or online lectures. Sometimes we spend days without electricity. As a 3rd year student in social work, we were supposed to be doing community work, but the universities closed and we had to go home [Student 6, 3rd year, Female, Eastern Cape].

- Subtheme 2: 'No Light in the Tunnel' Regarding Completing the Academic Year: Many students complained that they have lost hope in completing the 2020 academic year; they feel that the universities have no plan in place to start face-to-face lectures and assessment is on moratorium. These students indicated that they are used to contact learning as it allows them to interact and engage with other students. It is also easy for them to access study materials, labs, and libraries. The students also mentioned the fact that they usually have study groups in preparing for tests and examinations in order to share knowledge and help each other. They described contact learning as the best learning method that accommodates students with different learning abilities and challenges. In contrast, they described online learning as having many challenges that hinder students from engaging in academic activities. Some revealed that they have lost hope of returning to campus as they have not yet received permits. They reported being behind academically and with no hopes that things will be back to normal this year. They believed that completing the academic year is important as some of them were in their final years and were hoping to seek for employment by 2021; however, 2020 for them was a lonely and frustrating academic year. Hence, they 'see no light in the tunnel.' A student reported as follows:

Personally, I feel like the government has failed our educational system, especially for students within the black communities or lower class. Our needs have been neglected, we have been waiting for data and laptops since the beginning of this pandemic, and nothing has changed. Data has only recently been uploaded, but other schools have been going on with the calendar year of 2020, and some are commencing with semester 2 whilst some are still fighting for PPE and data and gadgets. Therefore, for me, I see no light in the tunnel for us students at this university [Student 17, 3rd year, Male, Limpopo].

Another participant said that:

COVID-19 lockdown and closure of the universities left us academically stranded because many of us have lost contact with each other and our lecturers who were our strong support system. Ever since lockdown began, things are running very slowly academically as we have embarked on e-learning and it seems as if we won't engage in contact learning anytime soon and it's a challenge to many of us [Student 18, 2nd year, EC].

- Subtheme 3: Qualifications Might be Perceived in Poor Light by Employers; Hence Blink Future: Many students believed that universities do not have a proper plan to save the academic year; but rather rushing to complete the year. They were of the view that most universities were not ready for online learning, but due to pressure, they opted for it. In addition, students stated a number of challenges with online learning, yet they are expected to perform well academically. Some revealed that they could not go to the field for their data collection and problem of sending ethical clearance applications via e-mail. Consequently, the students stated that it will be difficult for them to get employment as many companies will question and perceive their qualifications as of poor quality. They further described their future as unclear and uncertain. This is captured in the words of this student who stated that:

If we manage to finish the 2020 academic year and graduate, I believe that employers won't take our qualifications serious. In fact, they will question them because we were just rushing to finish the academic year without acquiring knowledge and skills needed in the labor market [Student 19, 3rd year, EC].

- **Theme 3: Resilience Not to be Defeated by COVID-19 Pandemic:** A third theme emerged from the findings, resilience not to be defeated by COVID-19 pandemic. A presentation of various coping mechanisms that students used during lockdown is provided, and three subthemes emerged.
- Subtheme 1: Distraction with Reading of Academic and Non-Academic Materials: During interviews, some of the students reported that staying at home was stressful and was a challenging experience for them. Therefore, in distracting negative thoughts and energy, they were reading both academic and non-academic materials, and these include books, magazines, newspapers, and journal articles. They read articles related to their research projects and course work to gain new ideas, broaden their convictions, and increased their knowledge. This improved their understanding of their courses; it also enforced independence in terms of thinking and finding scientific solutions to problems. They were confident that reading these materials has improved their vocabulary, thinking skills, and writing skills. Through reading, they reported being inspired and motivated to continue with their studies whilst at home. The following are excerpts from some of the participants:

Academically, I read articles related to my course so that I will be able to engage during online discussions; this also broadens my knowledge about the course. It also introduced me to self-reliance as I sometimes add a lot of information on the notes that our lecturers send to us [Student 5, 4th year, Male, EC].

Since I did not have data to connect and do academic work, I read magazines, newspapers, and books just to learn and motivate myself [Student 7, 4th year, Male, EC].

- Subtheme 2: Exercising and Adhering to COVID-19 Regulations: The majority of students reported that life during lockdown was difficult because everyone was expected to stay at home, healthy, and safe, while at the same time adhering to new norms, which are COVID-19 regulations. Some of them stated that they resorted to exercising during lockdown, as a way of keeping their psychological and physical well-being healthy. They engaged themselves in long walks and were jogging to reduce stress and risk of chronic diseases. With their exercises, they were adhering to COVID-19 regulations as they were exercising in isolation and maintaining good personal hygiene, including washing hands thoroughly after the exercise. Many believed that their academic stress levels were normal as they would do the exercises twice a day (morning and afternoon). A student who is a soccer lover reported that:

I formed a soccer team of young boys that keeps us busy because we exercise every afternoon, and this team also aims at keeping them off the streets since schools are closed. It also helps them not to commit criminal activities; it is also a way of relieving and overcoming stress brought by COVID-19 [Student 12, Male, 3rd year, EC].

Another participant stated that:

I've managed to make this far by adhering to the COVID-19 given guidelines, social distancing, wearing of masks, self-medication for precaution and staying home, etc. I've kept up with regular workout routines to keep me going and that has helped stimulate my mental health too [Student 18, 2nd year, Female, EC].

- Subtheme 3: Engaging in Social Media and Listening to News: Lockdown with its movement restrictions has made it difficult/impossible for families to visit each other. Many students stated that staying at home prompts feelings of isolation and loneliness. Therefore, in keeping socially connected and promoting deeper forms of human connection, they would do phone calls and video-chatting with their families and friends. Some reported that they use the internet to access information about what is happening and be updated. They also mentioned that they were using a variety of media such as Facebook and Twitter for entertainment and engagement on different topics/issues that affect the country. Some were using YouTube channels to improve and learn new skills. Others used media for entertainment and to watch news, TV shows and sport, and listen to music. Below are excerpts from some participants on the above subtheme.

I keep contact with the family and friends via social media and video call, and that helps as we provide support to each other. We also do video calls as friends and talk about school work, where we engage on a certain topic that has been done in class [Student 9, 3rd year, Male, Mpumalanga].

I'm more active on social media platforms, especially WhatsApp and Facebook. It's easy to communicate with different people, on different topics, and they keep me posted and updated about what is happening around the world [Student 11, 2nd year, Female, EC].

Another student said that:

Since I came back from varsity, I've been keeping myself busy by listening to and watching news just to get updated about coronavirus and other things. Social networks also help me to relieve stress because in them I find entertainment and I also watch sport and listen to music [Student 10, 4th year, Mpumalanga].

- **Theme 4: Positive Spinoff of COVID-19 Lockdown:** COVID-19 had some unintended positive impact on the academic journeys of students during lockdown. Several subthemes on how students perceived lockdown positively are presented.
- Subtheme 1: Feeling Supported: Some students reported that as they were at home, away from campus life and environment, it was not easy to adapt to the online learning but the support and motivation they received from their parents and supervisors kept them going. Those who never received data from their institutions mentioned the understanding, financial assistance, and emotional support they have received from their parents. They further reported the financial assistance from the government, R350 COVID grant, which made a huge difference in their lives as they were struggling to buy data. So, with the R350, they managed to buy data and some few essentials during lockdown as this was a monthly allowance. Students, specifically from WSU and NMU, mentioned the support that their universities have provided to them during lockdown. These universities have issued out laptops with data for students to be able to start online classes, engage with other students and learn on their own as they had the needed tools of learning. Examples of direct quotations from some participants are as follows:

When we vacated residences, the university negotiated with different mobile networks to provide data bundles to students, then I am one of the students who is receiving data from MTN through support from the school.

I am now doing my school work well, communicating, and interacting with others well virtually through the use of gadgets [Student 3, 3rd year, Male, Gauteng].

My supervisor is helping me with everything that is school related. She is always calling me to check my life during this difficult time. I'm doing my work well, and my supervisor is also supervising my work well. I'm also receiving a lot of support from my parents and siblings as they keep motivating me to do my school work under these difficult conditions [Student 13, 4th year, Female, WC].

- • Subtheme 2: Learning New Digital Ways of Communication That Enhances Learning: The participants revealed that the transition from face-to-face teaching and learning to online has introduced students to new digital ways of communication. Students mentioned that they were having group discussions via Zoom or Microsoft teams, which made it easier for them to interact with other students and lecturers. They were able to take notes of the discussions or record the discussions and later listen to them. Furthermore, assignments were accessed and submitted through Blackboard, a thing that is foreign to many a few months ago. Final year students who took part in the study reported that supervision and consultations with supervisors were running smoothly, as they were consulting via Zoom. These students further revealed that, at first, they were uncertain about online learning as they were not used to it, but as time goes by, they have learned and realized that it is the better way to learn and communicate with supervisors and classmates. A student report that:

Online learning introduced us to other better ways of communication as we are submitting our assessments via Blackboard, and I find it very easy and convenient, especially if one has good internet and network connection [Student 17, 3rd year, Male, Limpopo].

Another participant said that:

I thought online learning wouldn't work since we were new to it, but it makes things easier to interact with other students whilst we are home; Microsoft teams and e-mails help us to interact with other students and to communicate with our supervisors. Whenever I want to consult, I do that, and I sometimes record the meeting and later listen to it [Student 18, 2nd year, Female, EC].

- Subtheme 3: Becoming More Independent/Self-Reliance: Some students stated that lockdown and online learning allowed them to be more independent as they could not physically interact with their classmates and lecturers. They reported that they were used to the traditional method of learning, but lockdown has introduced them to academic independence and self-reliance. They had time to focus more on their studies, did thorough research on what they wanted to research on. Others had time to read through online resources, understand their courses and made notes for themselves. For others, lockdown, and remote learning has motivated them as they have enough time to write more academic papers for publication. Two students expressed their views regarding this subtheme as follows:

I have been doing a lot of reading just to keep my mind busy. I have also managed to focus more on my studies, as a final year student, I have a research project, so I had more time to do at least three chapters during lockdown. I got time to get deep on the chapters of the module because there's no lecturer to summarize them and I have to make notes on my own which made me to get more information [Student 3, 3ʳᵈ year, Gauteng].

I've used lockdown period to learn new things, for example, I've learned how to write an article and managed to write a paper with my supervisor. It is a milestone that I think I wouldn't have achieved if I was at school because I wouldn't think of it since I'm still an undergraduate student [Student 3, 3ʳᵈ year, Male, Mpumalanga].

- Subtheme 4: Engagement in Community Development: Few students used lockdown as an opportunity to engage in community development. They participated in community projects, where they delivered key prevention messages to communities and ensured that people have information about the virus. These projects allowed them to promote awareness of social distancing and preparedness to handle issues relating to the pandemic. They were scaling up all community awareness activities by sharing messages and advice to reduce the spread of COVID-19 through distributing flyers. The students expressed satisfaction as they believed that they made a difference in the lives of their community members. They have also noted and learned that, in order to improve the well-being of others, one does not need education or a degree, but they must be passionate and patient. Lastly, they perceived this as an eye-opener as it provided them the opportunity and ideas on how they can work together as a community and fight other societal problems. Excerpts of two students are presented below:

This is my final year so I was supposed to do teaching practical but schools were closed so I have decided to join a project in my community where we distribute flyers on COVID-19 around different communities [Student 10, 4th year, Mpumalanga].

Engaging in community projects was an eye-opener for me because it gave me a purpose in life. We even shared ideas on how we can start other projects that will help our communities [Student 15, 2nd year, Female, EC].

19.5 DISCUSSION

The findings of this study show that students were confronted with a number of challenges with online learning. Most of them reside in remote areas where there is no electricity and network, and that had a negative impact on their academic progress as they could not participate in digital group discussions. UNDESA [73] found that electricity provides multiple services. It helps students to access multiple ICT services; it also allows students to study for longer hours, which in turn affect their academic performance. The study also found that most students were from financially disadvantaged families, they could not focus on their academic work as they were living in overcrowded family households, where they were expected to perform household duties/chores. These findings echo Lacour and Tissington [74]; and Tanga and Maphosa [75], who found that poor socio-economic conditions have a negative impact on student's educational achievement. Pillay [76] also found that learners who are living in overcrowded households tend to perform poorly in school. The findings further show that lockdown did not only delay students' academic progress, it also affected their psychological and emotional well-being, as many of them reported hopelessness, frustration, and fear as they have lost contact with their friends and families due to COVID-19 regulations. According to Basner et al. [77], confinement has negative behavioral and psychological impact on the lives of people. The transition to online learning left students academically demotivated as they were away from the campus environment, where it is easy to access information, share information with classmates, and consult with their lecturers and supervisors. Literature reveals that if students are not motivated, it is difficult or impossible for them to improve their academic performance. Moreover, students who are academically demotivated are likely to disengage other students from academics [78]. Furthermore, motivation is perceived as a significant factor for enhanced learning outcomes of all students, therefore if students lack motivation, it leads to poor academic performance [79].

Due to challenges that many students have encountered, they felt that remote/online learning is an embarrassment as most of them did not have internet and were not familiar with Blackboard. These findings are consistent with Andersson and Grönlund [80] who found that low internet connectivity or speed is one of the factors that impede the practice of e-learning. Furthermore, literature shows that unreliable electricity power supply makes the e-learning method very difficult for students to access the internet [81]. However, studies revealed that e-learning benefits students as it provides support to learning processes and the distribution of education and training, as well as the evaluation of content and skills [40]. It allows them to collaborate with and engage other students, it also allows for a consistent delivery of content [82, 83]. Again, the findings show that many students have lost hope in completing their studies as they believed that universities are not prepared for online learning. According to Mitchell [84], universities globally were mainly not prepared for a sudden switch to online learning. Many universities appeared not to have a risk management strategy in place that would allow them to respond to a pandemic, specifically the capacity to offer e-learning and provide support to students. Many students believed that their qualifications might be questioned or may be perceived as poor quality by the employers, and that might expose them to the already high rate of graduate unemployment in South Africa. Mohamedbhai [85] reported that almost all African countries have lately been experiencing the challenge of graduate unemployment, and in some countries, the rate is alarming. In South Africa, the unemployment rate is reported to be above 29% [40].

As the COVID-19 continues to threaten the lives of many across the globe, students have adopted coping mechanisms that help them to cope with the pandemic's lockdown. They distract themselves by reading academic and non-academic materials. Studies revealed that reading is an essential life skill, and there is a correlation between reading and academic success of students [86, 87]. Similarly, Duff, Tomblin, and Catts [88] suggest that reading can offer key opportunities for the advancement in vocabulary development. Also, the findings indicate that in keeping their psychological, mental, and physical well-being healthy, students were exercising and adhering to COVID-19 regulations. Literature revealed that physical activity has significant health benefits. Studies also indicate a positive association between exercising and general well-being. Exercising has been confirmed to have positive effects on physical activity participation on cognition, including the treatment and prevention of depression [89–91]. Equally, being physically inactive is associated with a high risk of chronic diseases. Furthermore, studies found that in either case of disease prevention or treatment, physical activity and regular exercise provide a higher quality of life and maybe increase longevity [92]. Students also spend most of the time in social media platforms. According to News 18 [93], in April 2020, 4.57 billion people made use of the internet, almost 60% of humanity. Among them, 3.81 billion were active on social networks. Studies revealed that all social networking platforms could cause or at least promote narcissistic behavior among users [94]. However, Greetham et al. [95] found that social media helps people to socialize, be connected with their friends, and be updated. Gibney and McGovern [96] conducted a study on the relationship between social interaction and mental health. They studied the impact of social support network type on mental health, and the findings showed no evidence that being in such a network exacerbates the distress with traumatic life events.

The findings of this study indicate that universities and government played a significant role in supporting students during lockdown. Universities provided gadgets for students to be able to start online learning. It has been found that lecturers and supervisors continued to provide support to students as they embarked on remote learning. Studies have emphasized the important role of supervisor support and psychological capital on students' behavior and academic progress [97, 98]. In parallel, past studies have also highlighted the considerable impact of supervisor support for harnessing students' academic behaviors. Furthermore, Caesens and Stinglhamber [97] found that the impact of supervisor's support significantly improved students' engagement. The government on the other hand, has financially supported people with R350 grant for essentials. The government has provided R500 billion in economic supports for the package to mitigate the impact of the novel coronavirus pandemic; this grant is a social relief of distress for six months for unemployed individuals [99]. Universities also ensured that all registered students for the 2020 academic year receive computer devices and data. Universities have made arrangements with mobile network operators to load the data to students so that they will be able to catch up on the academic work. However, some universities have been slow in the provision of these essential tools and infrastructure. This can be explained from the universities' historical backgrounds, which date back to the apartheid era. Consequently, these universities are still plagued with infrastructure and other financial constraints.

Also, the findings reveal that remote learning has introduced students to new digital ways of communication that enhance learning. Students were able to communicate and engage with other students and their supervisors through Zoom or Microsoft teams. Literature indicates that communication between students, their classmates, and lecturers is enhanced through incorporating technology to keep students up to date [100, 101]. It has also been found that digital technology can increase the ease and frequency of student-lecturer communication and can provide meaningful information. Moreover, incorporating digital tools as a communication method enables lecturers and students to quickly engage [102–104]. Lockdown and online learning have been found to have a positive impact on students, as they became more independent academically. Studies revealed that through online learning, students become academically matured [105]. Finally, the findings show that some students used lockdown as an opportunity to engage in community development. According to Sibanda [106], participation in community development is an important science for individuals' definitions of self-esteem and self-identity in development that concerned them. Participating in community development serves as a link between individuals and larger societal structures. In addition, community participation helps communities to build capacity and empower the communities through engagement.

19.6 CONCLUSION

The enormous challenges that were brought by the pandemic show that few students have perceived COVID-19 lockdown positively. This is because they had time to partake in community projects and made great contributions to their communities. It enabled students to broaden their knowledge, as they had time to study and focused more on their research projects. During the pandemic period, the government also played a vital role in supporting people financially to cope with the effects of the lockdown, as many have lost sources of income. However, many students perceived lockdown as a lonely and frustrating experience as many of them were stuck in remote areas where there is poor infrastructure. Universities, on the other hand, found the transition to online learning as the only solution to save the academic year. It introduced many universities and students to digital communication, allowed learning to continue whilst students are home. In contrast, it brought numerous challenges to students, especially those who were living in rural areas where there are huge problems with network and internet connections.

It brought frustration and despair to many as they have lost contact with their academic and social support systems (friends, lecturers, and services within the institution). However, many of them have adopted habits that help them to cope with the COVID-19 lockdown and remote learning.

It is suggested that further studies could examine the perceptions of student and academic staff on the use of the different digital platforms used in remote learning. Also, the experiences of lecturers regarding COVID-19 lockdown and remote learning or what is now commonly ERL will also be worth pursuing in future research.

KEYWORDS

- **COVID-19 lockdown**
- **digital platforms**
- **emergency remote learning**
- **internet connectivity**
- **remote learning**
- **university students**

REFERENCES

1. Shakya, T., Fasano, S., Marsh, M., & Rivas, S., (2020). *For Teachers and Students, Remote Learning During COVID-19 Poses Challenges, Stokes Creativity.* Accessed from: https://www.goodmorningamerica.com/news/story/teachers-students-remote-learning-covid-19-poses-challenges-70770744 (accessed on 28 June 2021).
2. Pereira, J. A., Pleguezuelos, E., Merí, A., Molina-Ros, A., & Masdeu, C., (2007). Effectiveness of using blended learning strategies for teaching and learning human anatomy. *Medical Education, 41*(2), 189–195.
3. Hodges, C., Moore, S., Lockee, B., Trust, T., & Bond, A., (2020). *The Difference Between Emergency Remote Teaching and Online Learning.* Educause Review. Accessed from: https://er.educause.edu/articles/2020/3/the-difference-between-emergency-remote-teaching-and-online-learning (accessed on 28 June 2021).
4. Mthethwa, A., (2020). *Remote Learning Challenges Delay Resumption of Universities.* Accessed from: https://www.dailymaverick.co.za/article/2020-04-22-remote-learning-challenges-delay-resumption-of-universities/ (accessed on 28 June 2021).
5. Tanga, M., & Tanga, P. T., (2019). The impact of teachers' strikes on students' quality of education and further education in the Eastern Cape Province of South Africa. *Dirasat: Educational Sciences, 46* (2), 467–484.

6. Abrams, E. M., & Szefler, S. J., (2020). COVID-19 and the impact of social determinants of health. *The Lancet Respiratory Medicine, 8*(7). https://doi.org/10.1016/S2213-2600(20)30234-4.

7. Tanga, P. T., & Tangwe, M. N., (2014). The interplay between economic empowerment and HIV and AIDS amongst migrant workers in the textile industry in Lesotho. *SAHARA-J: Journal of Social Aspects of HIV/AIDS: An Open Access Journal, 11*(1), 187–201. doi: 10.1080/17290376.2014.976250.

8. Creswell, J., (2013). *Research Design: Qualitative, Quantitative and Mixed Methods Approach* (2nd edn.). Thousand Oaks, CA: Sage.

9. Babbie, E., (2015). *The Practice of Social Research* (14th edn.). Cape Town: Cengage Learning.

10. Yin, R. K., (2018). *Case Study Research and Applications: Design and Methods* (6th edn.). Los Angeles: Sage Publications.

11. Everitt, B. S., & Skrondal, A., (2010). *The Cambridge Dictionary of Statistics*. Cambridge: Cambridge University Press.

12. Bowen, G. A., (2009). Document analysis as a qualitative research method. *Qualitative Research Journal, 9*(2), 27–40. doi: 10.3316/QRJ0902027.

13. Braun, V., & Clarke, V., (2006). Using thematic analysis in psychology. *Qualitative Research in Psychology, 3*, 77–101.

14. Clarke, V., & Braun, V., (2013). Teaching thematic analysis: Overcoming challenges and developing strategies for effective learning. *The Psychologist, 26*(2), 120–123.

15. Kumar, R., (2014). *Research Methodology: A Step-by-Step Guide for Beginners* (4th edn.). London: Sage Publications.

16. Bask, M., & Salmela-Aro, K., (2013). Burned out to drop out: Exploring the relationship between school burnout and school dropout. *European Journal of Psychology of Education, 28*(2), 511–528.

17. Solari, C., & Mare, R. D., (2012). Housing crowding effects on children's wellbeing. *Social Science Research, 41*(2), 464–476. doi: 10.1016/j.ssresearch.2011.09.012.

18. Leventhal, T., & Newman, S., (2010). Housing and child development. *Children and Youth Services Review, 32*, 1165–1174.

19. Gingrich, J., & Ansell, B., (2014). Sorting for schools: Housing, education and inequality. *Socio-Economic Review, 12*(2), 329–351.

20. Statistics South Africa (Stats SA), (2014). *Poverty trends in South Africa. An examination of absolute poverty between 2006 and 2011.* Report No. 03-10-06. Pretoria: Statistics South Africa. Accessed from: http://www.statssa.gov.za/publications/Report-03-10-06/Report-03-10-062015.pdf (accessed on 28 June 2021).

21. Statistics South Africa (Stats SA), (2017). *Poverty Trends in South Africa: An Examination of Absolute Poverty Between 2006 and 2015.* Report No. 03-10-062015. Pretoria: Statistics South Africa. Accessed from: http://www.statssa.gov.za/?p=10341 (accessed on 28 June 2021).

22. Chopra, M., Davlaud, E., Pattinson, R., Fonn, S., & Lawn, J. E., (2009). Saving the lives of South Africa's mothers, babies and children: Can the health system deliver? *The Lancet, 374*(9692), 835–846.

23. Shisanya, S., & Hendricks, S., (2011). The contribution of community gardens to food security in the Maphephetheni uplands. *Development Southern Africa, 28*(4), 509–526.

24. Hendricks, S., (2014). Food security in South Africa: Status quo and policy imperatives. *Agreka, 53*(2), 1–24.

25. National Planning Commission (NPC), (2012). *National Planning Commission Office of the Presidency*. Pretoria: National Development Plan.
26. Smit, S., (2020). *Three Million Jobs Lost and Hunger Surging Amid COVID-19 Crisis-Survey*. Mail & Guardian. Accessed from: https://mg.co.za/news/2020-07-15-three-million-jobs-lost-and-hunger-surging-amid-covid-19-crisis-survey/ (accessed on 28 June 2021).
27. National Income Dynamics Coronavirus Rapid Mobile Survey (Nids-Cram, (2020). *2020 Coronavirus Rapid Mobile Survey: An Overview of Results and Findings*. Accessed from: https://www.dailymaverick.co.za/article/2020-07-15-overview-chapter-of-the-2020-coronavirus-rapid-mobile-survey-results-and-findings/ (accessed on 28 June 2021).
28. Statistics South Africa, (2020). *Statistics South Africa on Respondents Losing Jobs or Businesses Due to Coronavirus COVID-19 Lockdown*. Accessed from: https://www.gov.za/speeches/respondents-lost-jobs-20-may-2020-0000 (accessed on 28 June 2021).
29. Feketha, S., (2020). *Ramaphosa Concerned Over Gender-Based Violence Continuing 'with Little Restraint.'* Accessed from: https://www.iol.co.za/news/politics/ramaphosa-concerned-over-gender-based-violence-continuing-with-little-restraint-51019774 (accessed on 28 June 2021).
30. Agnew, M., Poole, H., & Khan, A., (2019). *Fall Break Fallout: Exploring Student Perceptions of the Impact of an Autumn Break on Stress*. Student success. Retrieved from: https://doi.org/10.5204/ssj.v10i3.1412.
31. Konishi, C., Hymel, S., Zumbo, B. D., & Li, Z., (2010). Do school bullying and student-teacher relationships matter for academic achievement? A multilevel analysis. *Canadian Journal of School Psychology, 25*(1), 19–39.
32. Mackinnon, S. P., (2012). Perceived social support and academic achievement: Cross-lagged panel and bivariate growth curve analyses. *Journal of Youth and Adolescence, 41*(4), 474–485. doi: 10.1007/s10964-011-9691-1.
33. Perry, J. C., Liu, X., & Pabian, Y., (2010). School engagement as a mediator of academic performance among urban youth: The role of career preparation, parental career support, and teacher support. *The Counselling Psychologist, 38*(2), 269–295. doi: 10.1177/0011000009349272.
34. Murray, C., & Zvoch, K., (2011). The inventory of teacher-student relationships: Factor structure, reliability, and validity among African American youth in low-income urban schools. *The Journal of Early Adolescence, 31*(4), 493–525. doi: 10.1177/0272431610366250.
35. Bordes-Edgar, V., Arredondo, P., Robinson, K. S., & Rund, J., (2011). A longitudinal analysis of Latina/o students' academic persistence. *Journal of Hispanic Higher Education, 10*(4), 358–368. doi: 10.1177/1538192711423318.
36. Li, J., Wang, W., Sun, G., & Cheng, Z., (2018). How social support influences university students' academic achievement and emotional exhaustion: The mediating role of self-esteem. *Learning and Individual Differences, 61*, 120–126. doi.org/10.1016/j.lindif.2017.11.016.
37. Rueger, S. Y., Malecki, C. K., & Demaray, M. K., (2010). Relationship between multiple sources of perceived social support and psychological and academic adjustment in early adolescence: Comparisons across gender. *Journal of Youth and Adolescence, 39*(1), 47–61.
38. Fang, L., (2016). Educational aspirations of Chinese migrant children: The role of self-esteem contextual and individual influences. *Learning and Individual Differences, 50*, 195–202.

39. Beqiri, M. S., Chase, N. M., & Bishka, A., (2010). Online Course Delivery: An empirical investigation of factors affecting student satisfaction. *Journal of Education for Business, 85*(2), 95–100. doi: 10.1080/08832320903258527.

40. Tanga, P. T., Ndhlovu, G. N., & Tanga, M., (2020). Emergency remote teaching and learning during COVID-19: A recipe for disaster for social work education in the eastern cape of South Africa? (Forthcoming in *African Journal of Social Work*).

41. Morrison, G. R., Ross, S. M., & Kemp, J. E., (2007). *Designing Effective Instruction* (5th edn.). New York: John Wiley & Sons.

42. Monk, L., (2010). The human touch. In: Noll, J. W., (ed.), *Taking Sides: Clashing Views on Educational Issues*. Boston: McGraw Hill.

43. World Bank Study, (2014). *Economics of South Africa Townships, Special Focus on Diepsloot*. Washington, DC: World Bank Group.

44. Pernegger, L., & Godehart, S., (2007). *Townships in the South African Geographic Landscape-Physical and Social Legacies and Challenges*. Accessed from: http://www.treasury.gov.za/divisions/bo/ndp/TTRI/TTRI%20Oct%202007/Day%201%20-%20 29%20Oct%202007/1a%20Keynote%20Address%20Li%20Pernegger%20Paper.Pdf (accessed on 28 June 2021).

45. Marnewick, C., (2014). *Information and Communications Technology Adoption Amongst Township Micro and Small Business: The Case of Soweto*. Accessed from: http://www.sajim.co.za/index.php/SAJIM/article/view/618/769 (accessed on 28 June 2021).

46. Thulo, L., (2015). *Gauteng SOPA 2015: What it means for SMEs*. Accessed from: http://www.smesouthafrica.co.za/Gauteng-SOPA2015-What-it-means-for-SMEs (accessed on 28 June 2021).

47. Statistics South Africa, (2012). *The South Africa I know, the Home I Understand / Statistics South Africa*. Accessed from: http://www.statssa.gov.za/Census2011/Products/Census_2011_Pictorial.pdf (accessed on 28 June 2021).

48. Aiken, N. T., (2013). *Identity, Reconciliation and Transitional Justice: Overcoming Intractability in Divided Societies*. Abingdon: Routledge.

49. Powell, C., (2014). *Rethinking Marginality in South Africa: Mobile Phones and the Concept of Belonging in Langa Township*. Cameroon: Langaa.

50. Mzileni, P., (2020). How COVID-19 will affect students. Mail & Guardian [23 African University. *African Journal of Health Professions Education, 4*, 123–127. Accessed from: https://mg.co.za/education/2020-04-23-how-covid-19-will-affect-students/ (accessed on 28 June 2021).

51. White, S., & Koopman, S., (2011). *Off-Grid Electrification in Rural Areas of South Africa, Energize*. Accessed from: http://www.ee.co.za/wpcontent/uploads/legacy/Energize_2011_/09_SeT_01_Eskom_off-grid.pdf (accessed on 28 June 2021).

52. Municipal Institute of Learning, (2013). *Toward an Integrated Urban Development Framework: A Discussion Document*. Municipal Institute of Learning, Republic of South Africa. Accessed from: http://sacitiesnetwork.co.za/wpcontent/uploads/2014/08/urban-policy.pdf (accessed on 28 June 2021).

53. Madzhie, L., (2013). *Integrated National Electrification Program [Presentation]*. Department of Energy, Republic of South Africa. Accessed from: http://mfma.treasury.gov.za/Media_Releases/ReviewO (accessed on 28 June 2021).

54. Noah, A., (2012). *Eskom's Electrification Program* [Presentation to National Electrification Indaba], Distribution Division, Eskom. Accessed from: https://pmg.org.za/files/131008eskom.ppt (accessed on 28 June 2021).

55. University of South Africa (2012). *Income and Expenditure of Households in South Africa, Bureau of Market Research*. Information Blurb, University of South Africa. Accessed from: http://www.unisa.ac.za/contents/faculties/ems/docs/Press429.pdf (accessed on 28 June 2021).

56. Sørensen, C., (2013). Digital platform and infrastructure innovation. In: Higashikuni, H., (ed.), *Mobile Strategy Challenges (In Japanese)*. Tokyo: Nikkan Kogyo Shimbun Ltd.

57. Rey-Moreno, C., Blignaut, R., Tucker, W. D., & May, J., (2016). An in-depth study of the ICT ecosystem in a South African rural community: Unveiling expenditure and communication patterns. *Information Technology for Development, 22*(1), 101–120.

58. Sekyere, E., Tshitiza, O., & Hart, T., (2016). *Levering m-governance innovations for active citizenship engagement*. Accessed from: http://www.hsrc.ac.za/uploads/pageContent/7504/HSRC%20Policy%20Brief%2018%20-%20Levering%20m-governance_PRESS.pdf (accessed on 28 June 2021).

59. Beiter, R., Nash, R., McCrady, M., Rhoades, D., Linscomb, M., Clarahan, M., & Sammut, S., (2015). The prevalence and correlates of depression, anxiety, and stress in a sample of college students. *Journal of Affective Disorders, 173*, 90–96. https://doi.org/10.1016/j.jad.2014.10.054.

60. Chernomas, W. M., & Shapiro, C., (2013). Stress, depression, and anxiety among undergraduate nursing students. *International Journal of Nursing Education, 10*(1). https://doi.org/10.1515/ijnes-2012–0032.

61. Elphinstone, B., & Conway, S., (2020). *Time Well Spent, Not Wasted: Video Games are Boosting Well-Being During the Coronavirus Lockdown*. The Conversation. Accessed from https://theconversation.com/time-well-spent-not-wasted-video-games-are-boosting-well-being-during-the-coronavirus-lockdown-135642 (accessed on 28 June 2021).

62. Tugade, M. M., & Fredrickson, B. L., (2011). Resilient individuals use positive emotions to bounce back from negative emotional experiences. *Journal of Personality and Social Psychology, 86*(2), 320–333. https://doi.org/10.1037/0022-3514.86.2.320.

63. Grey, P. H., (2017). *Five Sneaky Motivation Killers to Avoid in Graduate School*. Science Magazine. Accessed from: https://www.sciencemag.org/careers/2017/09/five-sneaky-motivation-killers-avoid-graduate-school (accessed on 28 June 2021).

64. Esch, T., & Stefano, G. B., (2010). Endogenous reward mechanisms and their importance in stress reduction, exercise and the brain. *Archives of Medical Science, 6*(3), 447–455.

65. Greenwood, B. N., & Fleshner, M., (2011). Exercise, stress resistance, and central serotonergic systems. *Exercise Sport Science Review, 39*(3), 140–149.

66. Griffiths, K. M., Crisp, D. A., Barney, L., & Reid, R., (2011). Seeking help for depression from family and friends: A qualitative analysis of perceived advantages and disadvantages. *BMC Psychiatry, 11*(196), 1–12.

67. Mushtaq, I., & Khan, S. N., (2012). Factors affecting students' academic performance. *Global Journal of Management and Business Research, 12*(9), 2249–4588.

68. Ahmad, A. R., & Murad, H. R., (2020). The Impact of social media on panic during the COVID-19 pandemic in Iraqi Kurdistan: Online questionnaire study. *Journal of Medical Internet Research, 22*(5), 1–20.

69. Kietzmann, J. H., Hermkens, K., McCarthy, I. P., & Silvestre, B. S., (2011). Social media? get serious! Understanding the functional building blocks of social media. *Business Horizons, 54*(3), 241–251. doi: 10.1016/j.bushor.2011.01.005.

70. Xiang, Z., & Gretzel, U., (2010). Role of social media in online travel information search. *Tourism Management, 31*(2), 179–188. doi: 10.1016/j.tourman.2009.02.016.
71. Hampton, K., Rainie, L., Lu, W., Shin, I., & Purcell, K., (2015). *Social Media and the Cost of Caring*. Pew Research Center Internet and Technology. Accessed from http://www.pewinternet.org/2015/01/15/social-mediaand-stress (accessed on 28 June 2021).
72. Revathy, V. R., Aram, I. A., & Sharmila, V. S., (2018). Social media as a means to overcome stress and depression among women. *Journal of Media and Communication Studies, 10*(6), 46–64. doi: 10.5897/JMCS2018.0605.
73. United Nations Department of Economic and Social Affairs (UNDESA), (2014). *Electricity and Education: The Benefits, Barriers, and Recommendations for Achieving the Electrification of Primary and Secondary Schools*. Accessed from: sustainabledevelopment.un.org/content/documents/1608Electricity%20and%20Education.pdf (accessed on 28 June 2021).
74. Lacour, M., & Tissington, L. D., (2011). The effects of poverty on academic achievement. *Educational Research and Reviews, 6*(7), 522–527.
75. Tanga, M., & Maphosa, C., (2018). Socio-economic background and students' poor academic performance in South African Universities. *International Journal of Educational Science, 33*(1–3), 27–37.
76. Pillay, J., (2017). The relationship between housing and children's literacy achievement: Implications for supporting vulnerable children. *South African Journal of Education, 37*(2), 1–10. doi: 10.15700/saje.v37n2a1268.
77. Basner, M., Dinges, D. F., Mollicone, D. J., Savelev, I., Ecker, A. A., Jones, C. W., Hyder, E. C., et al., (2014). Psychological and behavioral changes during confinement in a 520-day simulated interplanetary mission to Mars. *PLOS One Journal, 9*(3), 1–10.
78. Center on Education Policy, (2012). *Student Motivation: An Overlooked Piece of School Reform*. Washington DC: Graduate School of education and human development.
79. Saeed, S., & Zyngier, D., (2012). How motivation influences student engagement: A qualitative case study. *Journal of Education and Learning, 1*(2), 252–267. doi: 10.5539/jel.v1n2p252.
80. Andersson, A., & Grönlund, Å., (2009). A conceptual framework for e-learning in developing countries: A critical review of research challenges. *The Electronic Journal on Information Systems in Developing Countries (EJISDC), 38*(8), 1–16.
81. Mtebe, J. S., & Raisamo, R., (2014). Investigating perceived barriers to the use of open educational resources in higher education in Tanzania. *The International Review of Research in Open and Distributed Learning (IRRODL), 15*(2), 1–24. doi: https://doi.org/10.19173/irrodl.v15i2.1803.
82. Bell, S., Douce, C., Caeiro, S., Teixeira, A., Martín-Aranda, R., & Otto, D., (2017). Sustainability and distance learning: A diverse European experience? Open learning: *The Journal of Open, Distance and E-Learning, 32*(2), 95–102. doi: 10.1080/02680513.2017.13196382017.
83. Vasquez-Colina, M. D., Russo, M. R., Lieberman, M., & Morris, J. D., (2017). A case study of using peer feedback in face-to-face and distance learning classes among pre-service teachers. *Journal of Further and Higher Education, 41*(4), 504–515.
84. Mitchell, N., (2020). *Universities Not Ready for Online Learning - U-Multirank*. Accessed from: https://www.universityworldnews.com/post.php?story=20200609183303614 (accessed on 28 June 2021).

85. Mohamedbhai, G., (2020). *COVID-19: What Consequences for Higher Education?* Accessed from: https://www.universityworldnews.com/post. php?story=20200407064850279 (accessed on 28 June 2021).

86. Dogan, E., Ogut, B., & Kim, Y. Y., (2015). Early childhood reading skills and proficiency in NAEP eighth-grade reading assessment. *Applied Measurement in Education, 28*(3), 187–201. doi: 10.1080/08957347.2015.1042157.

87. Schwabe, F., McElvany, N., & Trendtel, M., (2015). The school-age gender gap in reading achievement: Examining the influences of item format and intrinsic reading motivation. *Reading Research Quarterly, 50*(2), 219–232.

88. Duff, D. J., Tomblin, B., & Catts, H., (2015). The influence of reading on vocabulary growth: A case for a Matthew effect. *Journal of Speech, Language, and Hearing Research, 58*, 853–886.

89. Coombes, J. S., Law, J., Lancashire, B., & Fassett, R. G., (2015). Exercise is medicine: Curbing the burden of chronic disease and physical inactivity. *Asia Pacific Journal of Public Health, 27*(2), 601–605.

90. Garber, C. E., Blissmer, B., Deschenes, M., Franklin, B. A., Lamonte, M. J., Lee, I. M., Nieman, D. C., & Swain, D. P., (2011). American College of Sports Medicine position stand. Quantity and quality of exercise for developing and maintaining cardiorespiratory, musculoskeletal, and neuromotor fitness in apparently healthy adults: Guidance for prescribing exercise. *Medical Science Sports Exercise, 43*(7), 1334–1359.

91. World Health Organization, (2010). *Global Recommendations on Physical Activity for Health*. Geneva: World Health Organization. Accessed from: https://www.who.int/ dietphysicalactivity/publications/9789241599979/en/ (accessed on 28 June 2021).

92. Pedersen, B. K., & Saltin, B., (2015). Exercise as medicine: Evidence for prescribing exercise as therapy in 26 different chronic diseases. *Journal of Medicine & Science in Sports, 25*(3), 1–72. www://doi.org/10.1111/sms.12581.

93. News 18, (2020). *More People are Turning to Social Media, Music and E-Sports During COVID-19 Lockdown*. Accessed from: news18.com/news/tech/more-people-are-turning-to-social-media-music-and-e-sports-during-covid-19-lockdown-2606813.html (accessed on 28 June 2021).

94. Pantic, I., (2014). Online social networking and mental health. *Cyberpsychology, Behavior, And Social Networking, 17*(10), 652–657.

95. Greetham, D. V., Hurling, R., Osborne, G., & Linley, A., (2011). Social networks and positive and negative affect. *Procedia Social and Behavioral Sciences, 22*, 4–13.

96. Gibney, S., & McGovern, M., (2011). Social networks and mental health: Evidence from SHARE. *Journal of Epidemiology Community Health, 65*(1), 9–17.

97. Caesens, G., & Stinglhamber, F., (2014). The relationship between perceived organizational support and work engagement: The role of self-efficacy and its outcomes. *European Review of Applied Psychology / Revue Européenne de Psychologie Appliquée, 64*(5), 259–267. https://doi.org/10.1016/j.erap.2014.08.002.

98. Wilks, S. E., & Spivey, C. A., (2010). Resilience in undergraduate social work students: Social support and adjustment to academic stress. *Social Work Education, 29*(3), 276–288.

99. Felix, J., (2020). *Five Million People Have Received R350 COVID-19 Grant*. News 24. Accessed from: https://www.news24.com/news24/southafrica/news/five-million-people-have-received-r350-covid-19-grant-so-far-lindiwe-zulu-20200730 (accessed on 28 June 2021).

100. Olmstead, C., (2013). Using technology to increase parent involvement in schools. *Tech Trends, 57*(6), 28–37. doi: http://dx.doi.org.pearl.stkate.edu/10.1007/s11528-013-0699-0.

101. Patrikakou, E. N., (2016). Parent involvement, technology, and media: Now what? *School Community Journal, 26*(2), 9–24.

102. Palts, K., & Kalmus, V., (2015). Digital channels in teacher-parent communication: The case of Estonia. *International Journal of Education and Development using Information and Communication Technology, 11*(3), 65–81.

103. Kraft, M. A., & Rogers, T., & Society for Research on Educational Effectiveness, (2014). Teacher-to-parent communication: Experimental evidence from a low-cost communication policy. *Society for Research on Educational Effectiveness*, 1–9.

104. Flowers, T. M., (2015). *Examining the Relationship Between Parental Involvement and Mobile Technology Use (Order No. 3670518).* Available from Education Database; ProQuest Dissertations & Theses Global (1650707837). Accessed from: http://pearl.stkate.edu/login?url=http://search.proquest.com.pearl.stkate.edu/docview/1650707837?accountid=26879 (accessed on 28 June 2021).

105. Roddy, C., Amiet, D. L., Chung, J., Holt, C., Shaw, L., McKnzie, S., Garivaldis, F., et al., (2017). Applying best practice online learning, teaching, and support to intensive online environments: An integrative review. *Frontiers in Education, 2*(59), 1–10. doi: 10.3389/feduc.2017.00059.

106. Sibanda, D., (2011). *The Role of Community Participation in Development Initiatives: The Case of the Danga Ecological Sanitation Project in the Zvishavane District, Zimbabwe* (Master's Thesis), University of the Western Cape. Accessed from: https://etd.uwc.ac.za/bitstream/handle/11394/2634/Sibanda_MA%28DVS%29_2011.pdf?sequence=1&isAllowed=y (accessed on 28 June 2021).

107. Eurostat, (2017). '*Overcrowding Rate by Household Type'*. Accessed from: http://bit.ly/2yWEFNo (accessed on 28 June 2021).

108. Rey-Moreno, C., Tucker, W. D., Cull, D., & Blom, R., (2015). Making a community network legal within the South African regulatory framework. In: *Proceedings of the Seventh International Conference on Information and Communication Technologies and Development ACM*.

CHAPTER 20

The Sociology of a COVID-19 Virtual University

MARIAM SEEDAT-KHAN[1] and ARADHANA RAMNUND-MANSINGH[2]

[1]*Department of Sociology, University of KwaZulu Natal, Durban, South Africa*

[2]*Human Resource Cluster, MANCOSA Honoris United Universities, Durban, South Africa, E-mail: raakheemansingh17@gmail.com*

ABSTRACT

The precipitous closing of schools, universities, and colleges across the globe has impacted significantly on the teaching ecosystem. The COVID-19 pandemic has metamorphosed the academy radically. Notwithstanding this histrionic shift, the augmented teaching concomitant loads of online assessments, reconfiguration of teaching templates, research, and student consultations, and academic advising has extended the workday beyond any universally accepted standards. This unrecognizable teaching milieu has impacted deleteriously on women in the academy. Socially constructed virtual COVID-19 classrooms expeditiously superseded the substitution of traditional face-to-face lectures. The demands for a remodeled university environment, novel teaching systems, and inventive conjectural method-ologies propelled teaching and learning specialists to work assiduously. The response to COVID-19 necessitated proficiencies in a cutting-edge technical experience together with complementing pecuniary and clerical capitals to support academics in virtual classroom deliveries. COVID-19 has demanded dexterities to compress academic content for virtual platforms. The failure to safeguard academics individual private space has expedited irretrievable impairment on their physical and mental health. The destruction of work-life balance, unprecedented role overload imposed on women, has heightened gender exploitation in the academy. This chapter embraces two meaningful teaching and learning approaches. The first is centered on first-hand COVID-19 classrooms. It assumes a qualitative desktop methodological approach, which examines the impact of virtual teaching and learning on academics at universities in COVID-19 virtual classrooms. The second is a clinical approach that measures seven universal performance areas that are noteworthy to aspects of teaching and learning approaches for academics. The outcomes of this study indicate the challenges experienced by women who undertake the responsibility to maintain exemplary academic standards. Within the analysis of scholarship and the formulation of a clinical model, this chapter examines the impact of role overload and learning to teach virtually in a gendered virtual space. We seek to provide sociological understandings and offer clinical interventions, deliberating the impact, complexities, challenges, and the position of women in the academy in these unprecedented times.

20.1 INTRODUCTION

On 1 March, 2020, patient zero arrived in South Africa after an Italian vacation with a group of friends. The COVID-19 zoonotic pandemic that began in Wuhan-China was proliferating worldwide at an unprecedented pace, claiming human lives indiscriminately. Universities around the world are guided by existing enterprise risk management policies that outline carefully constructed responses and measures for student discontent, natural disasters, fire, security threats, and a multitude of associated risks. The absence of a pandemic enterprise risk management response at universities around the world has imposed unparalleled weight on academics. The pandemic has unrelentingly disordered every segment of the academy, with women experiencing the greatest burden. This chapter cognizes seven critical areas of significance in an attempt to understand gendered work in academia pre-COVID-19 and a response to COVID-19, considering significant guidelines and clinical interventions. These include:

- Personal academic progression;
- Teaching responsibilities;
- Administrative duties;
- Research efficiency and promotions;
- Academic advising of PG students;

- Accessing research funding; and
- Community engagement.

These seven areas exemplify a pervasive portion of the sociological scholarship, which deliberate intensifying intersections of a COVID-19 state of crisis.

20.2   SCHOLARSHIP AND MODEL

20.2.1   PERSONAL ACADEMIC PROGRESSION

The idiosyncratic strains have distorted the function of women academics, who have of late altogether imported their already excessive pre-COVID-19 workload into the familial personal space. The most significant lockdown challenge that women are experiencing is the act of balancing work and home, which has plagued academics for decades. It is not uncommon for women to work 20-hour days, to meet intensified academic demands. COVID-19 is recognized as an intersecting thread that binds women in embedded struggles.

While a limited portion of disengaged academics uses idem theoretical content repetitively, enthusiastic academics engage with critical, current, and decolonized sociological content, newly constructed for each academic semester. These academics initiated the semester with a set of lecture plans, aligned to the module templates of the course, making effective use of online platforms (Moodle, Blackboard, Learn) prepared for the delivery and execution of a successful academic year.

The augmented responsibilities imposed excessive expectancies on academics forced into teaching on virtual systems with makeshift approaches for which they have not been adequately prepared. The responsibility foisted primarily on women has been rigorous. As a consequence, the procedure of best practice optimal 'online learning' strategies has yet to be identified, leaving academics scrambling for 'emergency online resources' [1].

The obligation to convert teaching and assessment models, reconfigure academic supervision models and amend critical research interventions have encumbered women in the academy. Within a space of two months, academics had to review and revise their curriculum delivery based on the precipitous changes on the cusp of lockdown. Ramnund-Mansingh and Seedat Khan [2] have identified the gravity of gender inequity in the academy and its devastating impact on women in South Africa. The intellectual inventiveness has created extraordinary work-life challenges, with women experiencing disproportionate workloads. The gratuitous teaching workload and associated assessment template formulations have stretched the workday for women punitively.

The relocation into virtual COVID-19 blended approach classrooms has obliterated the fundamental separation between academic workspace and the solitude of academics' individual homes. The encroachment of the academy into personal physical spaces intersects at personal and professional levels. The impact of this virtual university underpins epistemological shifts as academics are duty-bound to assume planning, assessment, coordination, development, teaching philosophies, and design of capricious COVID-19 classrooms. The COVID-19 pandemic and university responses around the world have failed to provide solutions that prioritize the historical marginalization of career trajectories of women in the academy. The failure to consider the systemic, entrenched patriarchal tradition in higher education is not surprising. Women's rights and equality have continuously been placed on the back burner in favor of prioritizing contemporary political, social, health, and economic emergencies. The onset of the COVID-19 pandemic has immersed women into one of the most unprecedented exploitative labor configurations since the 1950's.

The work and time invested in content preparation at the start of the 2020 academic year have been voided. The transformation of the teaching facilitation platforms has contributed to days spent on having to recreate written academic assessments and re-organize presentations and classroom activities initially primed for face-to-face lectures. "There are unparalleled opportunities for cooperation, creative solutions, and willingness to learn from others and try new tools" [3]. Assessments and traditional exams required realignment to blended methodologies to safeguard accurateness and authenticity of accurate online assessments and health safety COVID-19 protocols. Furthermore, academics are required to ensure students have cognized the module outcomes. Female academics have been hit particularly hard during the COVID-19 lockdown as all indications point to career stagnation for years to come, high levels of stress and possibly burnout, while 20-hour days persist (Table 20.1).

TABLE 20.1 Clinical Sociology Model on a COVID-19 Response of Considerations for Promoting Gender Equity in the Academy—Personal Academic Progression

Clinical Considerations for Promoting Gender Equity in the Academy: A COVID-19 Response

Personal Academic Progression

Pre-COVID-19	COVID-19 Response	Gender-Specific Challenges	Guidelines	Clinical Intervention
Completion of PhD	No modifications; No concessions; Academics are required to meet prescribed deadlines.	Women experience role overload, making PhD completion challenging.	Establish a COVID-19 gender response support network to ensure equity among all staff at all levels. *Professor; Associate Professor; Senior Lecturer; Lecturer.*	Systematic processes prescribed by human resources, to facilitate completion.
Researcher rating	No modifications; No concessions; Academics are required to meet prescribed deadlines.	Women experience role overload, making rating challenging.	Establish a COVID-19 gender response support network to ensure equity among all staff at all levels. *Professor; Associate Professor; Senior Lecturer; Lecturer.*	Systematic processes prescribed by human resources, to facilitate rating with guidance and mentorship.
Promotion	No modifications; No concessions; Academics are required to meet prescribed deadlines.	Women experience role overload, making travel promotion requirements challenging. Familial responsibility, young children.	Establish a COVID-19 gender response support network to ensure equity among all staff at all levels. *Professor; Associate Professor; Senior Lecturer; Lecturer.*	Systematic processes prescribed by human resources, to facilitate promotion with guidance and mentorship.
Fellowships	No modifications; No concessions; Academics are required to meet prescribed deadlines.	Women experience role overload, making travel for protracted periods challenging familial responsibility, young children.	Identify and deliver shorter fellowship experiences to ensure equity among all staff at all levels. *Professor; Associate Professor; Senior Lecturer; Lecturer.*	Equitable access among all staff at all levels. *Professor; Associate Professor; Senior Lecturer; Lecturer.*

TABLE 20.1 *(Continued)*

Clinical Considerations for Promoting Gender Equity in the Academy: A COVID-19 Response

Pre-COVID-19	COVID-19 Response	Gender-Specific Challenges	Guidelines	Clinical Intervention
Personal Academic Progression				
Sabbatical	No modifications; No concessions; Academics are required to meet prescribed objectives outlined in the sabbatical agreement.	Women experience role overlap making travel for protracted periods challenging familial responsibility, young children.	Identify equitable among all staff at all levels. *Professor; Associate Professor; Senior Lecturer; Lecturer.*	Equitable access among all staff at all levels. *Professor; Associate Professor; Senior Lecturer; Lecturer.*
Increase proficiencies	No modifications; No concessions; Academics are required to meet prescribed deadlines for proficiencies.	Requests for administrative tech support are overlooked.	Equitable response to requests and access to available funds for specialist skills and training.	Equitable access among all staff at all levels. *Professor; Associate Professor; Senior Lecturer; Lecturer.*

20.2.2   *TEACHING RESPONSIBILITIES*

With just over 60 days of lockdown before universities resumed their curriculum, how well prepared were they? While private institutions seamlessly transitioned as their infrastructure was already in place for distance learning; having a sound technological foundation, students lost minimal time in the semester. Even months after re-opening, public universities contend with failed blended approaches. Data connectivity remained a challenge for students in both public and private institutions. Aside from a technical infrastructure that is not complete and many rural areas are to contend without connectivity from the lack of cellular towers in these geographic regions; many South Africans simply cannot afford the exorbitant data costs. In assessing the successful continuation of the curriculum, researchers have failed to fully cognize the extensive challenges experienced by academics.

What thenceforth are the experiences of South African women in Social and Human Science faculties, where first-year level modules commonly include 1600 students. Women in the academy are overwhelmed by considerable teaching loads, particularly those of the substantial first-year modules [4]. The physical and now virtual teaching has evolved, demanding additional preparation time, advanced technological proficiencies, and intensified administration responsibilities. Academics skillfully executed first-year modules with 1600 students allocating them into four separate lecture areas contingent on the capacity at university. Online virtual teaching models allow academics to attend to all 1600 students in one virtual classroom.

The challenge lies in the delivery and response to overwhelming student support. South African university students frequently require support specifically in the context of English language proficiencies and understanding of academic content. These challenges intersect with student pandemic anxieties and place female academics under immeasurable difficulty to help students emotionally and academically.

Female academics are perceived as nurturing, maternal figures, and approachable as a source of academic support and guidance [5]. The effect of workloads both at home and paid work keeps women struggling to focus. Studies by Ramnund-Mansingh and Seedat [6] on female academics confirm that they experience high levels of stress manifested as physical and emotional illnesses, as opposed to their male counterparts. These include mental health problems such as depression and anxiety as well as physical burnout. This is impacted by their disproportionate day, where they are constrained by a full academic day, homework of attending to domestic duty and children while returning to the overflow of academic work late at night. Stieg [7] contends that *"in the survey of 3,117 people conducted from 13 April to 17, women were two times more likely to report symptoms like a racing heartbeat, problems sleeping, and feeling overwhelmed than men. Women are disproportionately feeling overwhelmed."*

A study [8] conducted on female university professors who work at online universities reviews the exposure to stress factors which contribute to excessively high levels of stress and burnout. This is a significant study for academics faced with online teaching using a blended approach, during COVID-19. Mental fatigue and role ambiguity play a substantial role in their physical and emotional wellbeing. García-González et al. [8] declares that "excessively rigid scheduling in online teaching and the bureaucratization of the evaluation systems that cause the pace of work to be imposed by the educational system." The student-centric approach translates into the absence of autonomy for the female academic who is attempting to juggle and organize her entire household around her online teaching schedule during COVID-19. This resulted in burnout, the physical manifestation of further illnesses such as back pain and visual fatigue (Table 20.2).

20.2.3 ADMINISTRATIVE RESPONSIBILITIES

Sustained efforts to maintain and establish gender equity in the academy have been threatened by the onset of a pandemic via the formation of the COVID-19 virtual classroom. The unequal division of academic teaching and administrative workloads and associated undertakings remain the responsibility and added burden of women in the academy. This teaching workload has been exacerbated by the pandemic resulting in the creation of COVID-19 virtual classrooms all over the world. Women are burdened and exploited virtually. Deep racial and 'invisible' gendered, patriarchal structural impairments function to denounce the distinctiveness of women academics. Academics work, whether virtual or physically at university includes a measure of institutional housekeeping. Women are burdened with the structure and organization of committee and departmental meetings, virtual departmental social events, and administrative duties associated with these [9]. There are no resources or recognition for institutional housekeeping but is viewed as 'women's work' which is "much like unpaid domestic housekeeping typically performed by women in family units" (Table 20.3) [10].

TABLE 20.2 Clinical Sociology Model on a COVID-19 Response of Considerations for Promoting Gender Equity in the Academy—Teaching Responsibilities

Clinical Considerations for Promoting Gender Equity in the Academy: A COVID-19 Response				
Teaching Responsibilities				
Pre-COVID-19	**COVID-19 Response**	**Gender-Specific Challenges**	**Guidelines**	**Clinical Intervention**
Fulfill assigned teaching workload aligned to academic level (*Professor; Associate Professor; Senior Lecturer; Lecturer*)	Increased workload on women at *Senior Lecturer; and Lecturer.*	Role overload, with associated administrative responsibilities. Time demands. Student support.	Establish a COVID-19 teaching response support network to ensure equity among all staff at all levels. *Professor; Associate Professor; Senior Lecturer; Lecturer.*	Weekly virtual support meeting with constructive support on teaching challenges *Professor; Associate Professor; Senior Lecturer; Lecturer.*
Measure student academic performance for each assigned module.	Online assessments and evaluations	Inundated with special requests from students. Time demands.	Establish a COVID-19 administrative response team, with additional human resources.	Subsidize funds for the employment of additional administrative, human resources.
Ensure quality proficiency independent student evaluations for each module. Time demands.	Online assessments and evaluations	Difficult to co-ordinate determined by virtual attendance. Time demands.	Establish a COVID-19 administrative response team, with additional human resources.	Subsidize funds for the employment of additional administrative, human resources.
Ensure quality proficiency independent peer evaluations for each module.	Online assessments and evaluations	Difficult to co-ordinate determined by the availability of senior academics. Time demands.	Establish a COVID-19 academic response team, with *Professor; Senior Associate Professor; Senior Lecturer; Lecturer.*	Minimum mandatory peer evaluations per semester.
Develop and design new academic content and programs.	Rationalization of academic programs.	Compromise's innovation. Time demands.	Establish and support new areas of scholarship and expertise.	Identify teams of specialists to include: *Professor; Associate Professor; Senior Lecturer; Lecturer.*

TABLE 20.2 *(Continued)*

Clinical Considerations for Promoting Gender Equity in the Academy: A COVID-19 Response

Teaching Responsibilities				
Pre-COVID-19	COVID-19 Response	Gender-Specific Challenges	Guidelines	Clinical Intervention
Include efficient and relevant teaching methods.	Virtual Platforms	Role overload, increased demands for intricate proficiencies and dexterities. No physical contact.	Establish a COVID-19 academic information communication system support team, for *Professor; Associate Professor; Senior Lecturer; Lecturer.*	Accessible information communication system support team, during teaching hours.
Include efficient and relevant use of technology.	Training for all academic staff; online assessments; online lectures, compression of data; online delivery and engagement.	Role overload, increased demands for intricate proficiencies and dexterities. No physical contact. Time demands.	Establish a COVID-19 academic information communication system support team, for *Professor; Associate Professor; Senior Lecturer; Lecturer.*	Accessible information communication system support team, during teaching hours
Prescribed teaching templates	Modified assessment templates.	Administration imposed on women. Time demands.	Establish a COVID-19 administrative response team, with additional human resources.	Develop proficiencies among staff at *Professor; Associate Professor; Senior Lecturer; Lecturer.*
Student consultations	Increased student demands.	Inundated with special requests from students. Time demands.	Establish a COVID-19 academic response team, with Professor; *Associate Professor; Senior Lecturer; Lecturer.*	Minimum mandatory consultations per semester.

TABLE 20.3 Clinical Sociology Model on a COVID-19 Response of Considerations for Promoting Gender Equity in the Academy—Teaching Responsibilities

Clinical Considerations for Promoting Gender Equity in the Academy: A COVID-19 Response				
Administrative Responsibilities				
Pre-COVID-19	**COVID-19 Response**	**Gender-Specific Challenges**	**Guidelines**	**Clinical Intervention**
Fulfill administration aligned to academic level (*Professor; Associate Professor; Senior Lecturer; Lecturer*).	No modifications; No concessions; Academics are required to meet prescribed administration practice.	Increased administrative responsibility. Virtual operations; Absence of physical assistance and support.	Adhere to existing protocol for data protection.	Provide resources and training to deliver requests virtually. Provide additional administrative support.
Fulfill teaching administration responsibilities, academic counseling	No modifications; No concessions; Academics are required to meet prescribed administration practice.	Increased administrative responsibility. Virtual operations; Absence of physical assistance and support.	Adhere to existing protocol for data protection.	Provide resources and training to deliver requests virtually. Provide additional professional support.
Maintaining student records	No modifications; No concessions; Academics are required to meet prescribed administration practice.	Increased administrative responsibility. Virtual operations; Absence of physical assistance and support.	Adhere to existing protocol for data protection.	Provide resources and training to deliver requests virtually. Provide additional administrative support.
Administering teaching assistants	No modifications; No concessions; Academics are required to meet prescribed administration practice.	Increased administrative responsibility. Virtual operations; Absence of physical assistance and support.	Adhere to the terms and conditions of employment contracts	Provide resources and training to deliver requests virtually.

TABLE 20.3 *(Continued)*

Clinical Considerations for Promoting Gender Equity in the Academy: A COVID-19 Response

Administrative Responsibilities

Pre-COVID-19	COVID-19 Response	Gender-Specific Challenges	Guidelines	Clinical Intervention
Chair and or membership and or representation on research, teaching, learning, national, international departmental role.	No modifications; No concessions; Academics are required to meet prescribed committee obligations	Women underrepresented in management roles. Women overlooked for senior positions.	Establish a COVID-19 gender response support network to ensure equity among all staff at all levels. *Professor; Associate Professor; Senior Lecturer; Lecturer.*	Initiate co-chairing with *Professor; Associate Professor; to mentor Senior Lecturer; Lecturer.*
Participation in examination and assessment processes and associated administration	No modifications; No concessions; Academics are required to meet prescribed augmented administrative obligations	Increased administrative responsibility. Virtual operations; Absence of physical assistance and support.	Establish a COVID-19 gender response support network to ensure equity among all staff at all levels. *Professor; Associate Professor; Senior Lecturer; Lecturer.*	Provide resources and training to deliver requests virtually. Provide additional administrative support.
Serve on approved University Committees	No modifications; No concessions; Academics are required to meet prescribed committee obligations	Women underrepresented in management roles. Women overlooked for senior positions.	Establish a COVID-19 gender response support network to ensure equity among all staff at all levels. *Professor; Associate Professor; Senior Lecturer; Lecturer.*	Initiate co-chairing with *Professor; Associate Professor; to mentor Senior Lecturer; Lecturer.*

20.2.4   RESEARCH EFFICIENCY AND PROMOTIONS

Promotions in the academic space are reliant on a sum of key performance areas, and the most significant is research and publication productivities. The actuality of COVID-19 has augmented the drudgery for female academics, and the consequences are predicted to outlast the pandemic by decades. It can be conjectured that the numbers of female academics reaching higher academic ranks, such as professorship, will be considerably decreased. The domino effect of the privation of publications will be excessively experienced. The unpublished analysis by Sugimoto [11] corroborates that a meager 31% of coauthors on scientific research papers are women between the years 2008 to 2017, which reinforces the underrepresentation of women in the contribution to research. Zimmer's [11] study conducted in the United States established a significant decrease in the number of women listed as first authors for publications dated March to May 2020. With role overload from prodigious childcare and housework burdens, universities, and funding bodies must take into consideration the gendered effect the pandemic has on research when making assessments on promotions and tenure [12].

The negative resonant impact of the decreased publications will further entrench women within the lowest academic ranks. Zimmer [11]; and Matthews [12] studies corroborate the equivalent professional suicide that female academics are undergoing. The study by Zimmer [11] specifically interpreted statistics on 2000 COVID-19 related medical studies and the proportion of female first authors were 20% lower than medical studies published during 2019. Matthews [12] analysis concluded that globally 60,000 scientific journals confirmed a disturbing reduction in putative publications where female academics are identified as the first author.

The analysis cognizes trends from January to February between 2015 to 2020. There has been a steady increase of women publishing as first authors from 2015 with 31% to 2019 with 34%. Conversely, the onset of COVID-19 in March 2020 led to the reconfiguration of universities. There has since been waning in the already low publications statistics authored by women. From 34% in February 2020, the numbers indicated a decline in the historical trends of previous years, which plummeted significantly to 26% in May 2020 [12].

The negligible advancements secured over in science, technology, engineering, and math (STEM) are expected to be impacted unfavorably. Women have long been underrepresented in areas of STEM research, due to the gender bias social construction of these research areas. The already truncated statistics continue to diminish at a faster rate during the pandemic, thereby impacting on women's careers and research outputs [11]. In addition, research societies, and journal editors have established that scientific research submissions by male academics have remained unaffected, and submissions by male academics have increased since COVID-19 safety protocol lockdowns and regulations have been implemented. The publications or acceptance of papers from male academics in the health science faculties were reported as significantly high during the lockdown period. This is problematic for a number of reasons. The gendered lens at which we are viewing research on the COVID-19 virus is skewed. The virus affects men and women differently, and the female narrative needs to be heard (Table 20.4) [11].

20.2.5   ACADEMIC ADVISING OF POSTGRADUATE (PG) STUDENTS

The multiplicity of gender, race, and identity has been acknowledged within the COVID-19 classroom. It must be recognized that the experience of academics is not homogenous. Literature unfailingly indicates gender differentiation in the way that academics experience their lives, as well as strategies they adopt to deal with issues of race, gender, and identity [13–17].

South African universities must urgently address gender inequities as they persist as traditionally male directed institutions [17–19]. Walker [17] maintains *"gender is a critical analytical lens for viewing South African universities"* and *"it cannot be taken as a given that gendered relations outweigh racialized identities…but this is not to discount gender as a shaping practice in academic relations, for both Black and White women."* Significant to this unaffected précis are structural and cultural influences which allocate women to large classes while men escape these challenging responsibilities.

Internationally statistics exhibit an increase in the representation of women in academia, but Black women in particular, remain in lower levels of the overall hierarchy [18, 19] and are often associated with the heaviest workloads [28]. The allocation of honors research projects to women is common practice; senior academics shy away from this level of academic advising. The likelihood or possibilities of publications is negligible, with students requiring excessive attention, support, and guidance. Male academics are unquestionably favored as preferred recipients of masters and doctoral candidates; which present opportunities for scientific research publications associated with academic advising at advanced levels of study (Table 20.5) [2].

TABLE 20.4 Clinical Sociology Model on a COVID-19 Response of Considerations for Promoting Gender Equity in the Academy—Research Efficiencies and Promotions

Clinical Considerations for Promoting Gender Equity in the Academy: A COVID-19 Response				
Research Efficiency and Promotions				
Pre-COVID-19	**COVID-19 Response**	**Gendered Specific Challenges**	**Guidelines**	**Clinical Intervention**
Research productivity aligned to academic level (*Professor; Associate Professor; Senior Lecturer; Lecturer*)	No modifications; No concessions; Academics are required to meet prescribed research productivity units.	COVID-19 restrictions on social distancing. Access to research participants and associated risk to familial household. Mobility determines financial responsibilities. Risk in relation to familial household.	Establish a COVID-19 research response support network. *Professor; Associate Professor;* Co-author with *Senior Lecturer; Lecturer.*	Weekly virtual support meeting with constructive support on publications in progress *Senior Lecturer; Lecturer.*
Professional profile in the academic fraternity.	No modifications; No concessions; Academics are required to intensify their research profile.	Cancellation of local, national, and international conferences. Loss of research funds.	Establish a COVID-19 research response support fund.	Subsidize lost research funds for *Senior Lecturer; Lecturer*
Guest/editor of a scientific journal/ book	No modifications; No concessions; Academics are required to meet prescribed research productivity units.	Existing academic networks determine opportunity and accessibility to scientific journals and books. Social distancing and virtual engagements further reduce opportunities. Limited networks of experts in the field.	*Professor; Associate Professor,* required to invite *Senior Lecturer; Lecturer* as observers.	*Senior Lecturer; Lecturer* teamed with *Professor;* *Associate Professor* to submit a proposal for a *special edition journal or a book* based on a doctoral study.

TABLE 20.4 *(Continued)*

Clinical Considerations for Promoting Gender Equity in the Academy: A COVID-19 Response

Research Efficiency and Promotions

Pre-COVID-19	COVID-19 Response	Gendered Specific Challenges	Guidelines	Clinical Intervention
Publication of journal articles/ book chapters	No modifications; No concessions; Academics are required to meet prescribed research productivity units.	Absence of mentorship and support. Social distancing and virtual engagements further reduce opportunities. Financial limitations and costs of publication and editing fees. Existing academic networks determine opportunity and invitations associated opportunities and requests.	Establish a COVID-19 research response support network. *Professor; Associate Professor;* Co-author with *Senior Lecturer; Lecturer.*	Weekly virtual support meeting with constructive support on publications in progress *Senior Lecturer; Lecturer.*
Academic honors	No modifications; No concessions; Academics are required to exceed research productivity units.	Limited exposure to executive members of sociological associations; poor mentorship; lack of research funds compromises the ability of women to compete.	All *Senior Lecturer; Lecturer* faculty must have subsidized membership to sociological associations.	*Senior Lecturer; Lecturer* teamed with *Professor; Associate Professor* to become active members of working groups and research committees.
Membership and executive roles in local, national, continental, and international sociological associations	No modifications; No concessions; Academics are required to maintain membership and pursue leadership roles.	Cost of annual membership; funded by research publications in scientific journals and books.	All *Senior Lecturer; Lecturer* faculty must have subsidized membership to sociological associations.	*Senior Lecturer; Lecturer* teamed with *Professor; Associate Professor* become active members of working groups and research committees. Secure membership to a local organizing conference committee. Accept one executive role at a national level, graduating to an international executive role.

TABLE 20.4 (Continued)

Clinical Considerations for Promoting Gender Equity in the Academy: A COVID-19 Response

Research Efficiency and Promotions

Pre-COVID-19	COVID-19 Response	Gendered Specific Challenges	Guidelines	Clinical Intervention
Academic local, national, and international scientific partnerships.	No modifications; No concessions; Academics are required to establish and formalize scientific partnerships.	Cost of attending meetings, conferences; funded by research publications in scientific journals and books. Impacts adversely on networking opportunities to establish partnerships.	Subsidize one national/ international conference per annum for *Senior Lecturer; Lecturer.*	Membership to a research committee and attend all sessions to establish significant networks. Volunteer as a regional representative.
Academic mentorship	No modifications; No concessions; Academics are required to establish and formalize mentorship initiatives.	The absence of a formal mentorship process; debilitates career trajectory, academic growth, and advancement.	Assign a mentor to every *Senior Lecturer and Lecturer.*	Contract between mentor and mentee with weekly meetings and communications.
Conference participation; session chair; organizer; presenter; keynote speaker; conference committee.	No modifications; No concessions; Academics are required to continue participating in conference at multiple levels.	Cost of attending meetings, conferences; funded by research publications in scientific journals and books. Impacts adversely on networking opportunities to attend and participate in academic meetings.	Subsidize one national/ international conference per annum for *Senior Lecturer; Lecturer.*	Membership to a research committee and attend all sessions to establish significant networks. Volunteer as a regional representative. Participate in doctoral workshops.

TABLE 20.5 Clinical Sociology Model on a COVID-19 Response of Considerations for Promoting Gender Equity in the Academy—Academic Advising of Post Graduate Students

Clinical Considerations for Promoting Gender Equity in the Academy: A COVID-19 Response				
Academic Advising of Postgraduate Students				
Pre-COVID-19	**COVID-19 Response**	**Gender-Specific Challenges**	**Guidelines**	**Clinical Intervention**
Fulfill assigned supervision workload aligned to academic level *(Professor; Associate Professor; Senior Lecturer; Lecturer)*	No modifications; No concessions; Academics are required to meet prescribed supervision workload.	COVID-19 restrictions on social distancing. Access to research participants and associated risk to familial household of students. Mobility determined by the financial resources of students.	Establish a COVID-19 supervision response support network. *Professor; Associate Professor; Senior Lecturer; Lecturer.*	Weekly virtual support meetings with constructive support on supervision challenges in progress *Professor; Associate Professor Senior Lecturer; Lecturer.*
Graduate assigned masters and PhD students associated to academic level *(Professor; Associate Professor; Senior Lecturer; Lecturer)*	No modifications; No concessions; Academics are required to meet prescribed supervision workload.	COVID-19 restrictions on social distancing. Access to students that require face to face advising, learning disabilities and or physical disabilities and access to technology.	Flexible guidelines to accommodate unprecedented COVID-19 circumstances.	Suspended registrations, limit the allocation of additional students.
Publish with PhD students to academic level *(Professor; Associate Professor; Senior Lecturer; Lecturer)*	No modifications; No concessions; Academics are required to meet prescribed supervision publication workload.	Advisors with limited publications and experience.	Establish a COVID-19 research response support network. *Professor; Associate Professor; Co-supervise with Senior Lecturer; Lecturer.*	Monthly virtual support meeting with constructive support on publication related supervision in progress *Senior Lecturer; Lecturer.*

20.2.6 ACCESSING RESEARCH FUNDING

On a 'regular' day in pre-COVID-19 times, female academics faced insufferable discrimination in the uneven distribution of research funding [20]. The role overload experienced has been exacerbated by the pandemic. Every negligible form of help that women require include schools, daycare, caregivers and or domestic staff, were deemed non-essential services and inaccessible throughout lockdown. Subsequently lockdown levels were reduced, high at-risk individuals with comorbidities were restricted from procuring support in the home. The routine academic workload as onerous and previously produced complex challenges on work life balance for women [5].

The pandemic imposed significantly complex weights. A survey conducted in the United States and Europe in April 2020, consisting of 4500 researchers confirmed that having a young child under the age of five was the most prevalent factor for the decrease in research hours and output. This relates directly to women as more women had young children, and this impacted on their research [12]. Women contend with domestic roles, partners, elder care, child care and facilitate homeschooling in her 20-hour day. TUAC [21]; and Matthews [12] substantiate women often begin engaging with academic writing, proposal formulation at 8 pm. At this stage, exhaustion ceases any possibilities of meeting a funding deadline, and investing several hours preparing a suitable research proposal for consideration. Teaching preparation, online activities and marking results in inadequate sleep and irregular sleep patterns night, repeating their tedious routine daily. Working from home fast becomes a seven-day workweek as to catch up with research funding backlogs.

In Austria, UK, and Poland, parents can apply for leave without fear of any deleterious impact on their career trajectories in the academy, even if the leave is time constrained or unpaid. Conversely, associated imbalanced *"gender pay-gaps, women might be much more affected if decisions on unpaid leave have to be taken by families"* [21]. In Japan, this was managed differently as financial support was introduced *"to employers who let their employees take additional paid leave during COVID-19-measures"* [21]. Additionally to the domestic chores, there was a significant increase in the academic workload, as all work and preparation for teaching had to be amended and adjusted for online consumption.

The female academic needs to be a pillar of strength to her family, her partner, children, and students who are also facing high levels of anxiety and uncertainty. With all of the responsibilities, how do female academics conduct research or publish? (Table 20.6).

TABLE 20.6 Clinical Sociology Model on a COVID-19 Response of Considerations for Promoting Gender Equity in the Academy—Assessing Research Funding

Clinical Considerations for Promoting Gender Equity in the Academy: A COVID-19 Response

Accessing Research Funding

Pre-COVID-19	COVID-19 Response	Gender-Specific Challenges	Guidelines	Clinical Intervention
Secure research funding from local, national and international donors. aligned to academic level *(Professor; Associate Professor; Senior Lecturer; Lecturer).*	No modifications; No concessions; Academics are required to meet prescribed areas of performance.	Funding limitations due to COVID-19 safety protocol, impacting on fieldwork and associated ethical requirements; compromised existing grant agreements.	Flexible guidelines to accommodate unprecedented COVID-19 circumstances. Establish a COVID-19 academic information communication system research training Professor; *Associate Professor; Senior Lecturer; Lecturer.*	Defer funding initiatives. Migrate to desktop, secondary research and or quantitative methods.
Proficiencies in grant applications aligned to academic level *(Professor; Associate Professor; Senior Lecturer; Lecturer).*	No modifications; No concessions; Academics are required to meet prescribed areas of performance.	Funding limitations due to COVID-19 safety protocol, impacting on fieldwork and associated ethical requirements; compromised existing grant agreements.	Flexible guidelines to accommodate unprecedented COVID-19 circumstances. Establish a COVID-19 academic information communication system research training Professor; *Associate Professor; Senior Lecturer; Lecturer.*	Defer funding initiatives. Migrate to desktop, secondary research and or quantitative methods.

TABLE 20.7 Clinical Sociology Model on a COVID-19 Response of Considerations for Promoting Gender Equity in the Academy—Community Engagement

Clinical Considerations for Promoting Gender Equity in the Academy: A COVID-19 Response				
Community Engagement				
Pre-COVID-19	**COVID-19 Response**	**Gender-Specific Challenges**	**Guidelines**	**Clinical Intervention**
Provide Academic Professional service to a community of practice aligned to academic level (*Professor; Associate Professor; Senior Lecturer; Lecturer*).	No modifications; No concessions; Academics are required to meet prescribed practice.	COVID-19 restrictions on social distancing. Access to community and associated risk to familial household. Mobility determined by resources and co-morbidities of academic.	Promote the intellectual project. Adhere to ethical standards.	*Professor; Associate Professor* to collaborate with; *Senior Lecturer; Lecturer* to provide mentorship and access to networks.
Delivery of consultation assistances to communities, business, and industry that aligned to academic level (*Professor; Associate Professor; Senior Lecturer; Lecturer*).	No modifications; No concessions; Academics are required to meet prescribed practice.	COVID-19 restrictions on social distancing. Access to community and associated risk to familial household. Mobility determined by resources and co-morbidities of academic.	Promote the intellectual project. Adhere to ethical standards.	*Professor; Associate Professor* to collaborate with; *Senior Lecturer; Lecturer* to provide mentorship and access to networks.
Occupy leadership positions in national or international sociology through consultation, policy development, reviews, and clinical interventions.	No modifications; No concessions; Academics are required to meet prescribed practice.	Limited exposure to executive members of sociological associations; poor mentorship; lack of research funds compromises the ability of women to compete.	Promote the intellectual project. Adhere to ethical standards.	*Professor; Associate Professor* to collaborate with; *Senior Lecturer; Lecturer* to provide mentorship and access to networks.

TABLE 20.7 (Continued)

Clinical Considerations for Promoting Gender Equity in the Academy: A COVID-19 Response

Community Engagement

Pre-COVID-19	COVID-19 Response	Gender-Specific Challenges	Guidelines	Clinical Intervention
Publish public intellectual opinion-editorial pieces aligned to areas of specialization.	No modifications; No concessions; Academics are required to meet prescribed practice.	Absence of mentorship and support. Social distancing and virtual engagements further reduce opportunities. Existing academic networks determine opportunity and invitations associated opportunities and requests.	Establish a COVID-19 research response support network. *Professor; Associate Professor;* Co-author with *Senior Lecturer; Lecturer.*	Featured profiles of individual academic proficiencies and expertise accessible to the corporate affairs division of the university
Facilitate and establish relationships and research that advance the academic project for students, academics, and university.	No modifications; No concessions; Academics are required to meet prescribed practice.	COVID-19 restrictions on social distancing. Access to global networks, require funds to participate in sociological forums, conferences, and congress.	Promote the intellectual project. Adhere to ethical standards.	Provide mentorship and dexterities on developing a global presence in the sociological community.
Deliver keynote address within a sociological space.	No modifications; No concessions; Academics are required to meet prescribed practice.	COVID-19 restrictions on social distancing. Membership to local and global networks, require funds to participate in sociological forums, conferences, and congress.	Promote the intellectual project. Adhere to ethical standards.	Featured profiles of individual academic proficiencies and expertise accessible to the corporate affairs division of the university

20.2.7   COMMUNITY ENGAGEMENT

Higher education institutions globally have identified community engagement as a key performance indicator for academics and strategic value for the institution is partnering with communities and industry. Community engagement is an integral collaboration between higher education institutions and communities. This results in a partnership of mutual reciprocity for the exchange of knowledge and resources [22].

Although it is mutually beneficial to all parties, the obstacles enlisted by COVID-19 has detrimentally impacted this engagement and interaction. Limited interaction and support transpired on online platforms and universities took to outreach programs during this difficult time for many. Community engagement includes research projects for improvement or advancement. The global pandemic foiled plans of international travels, conferences, and scientific projects are at risk of non-completion. Trends by Marinoni and de Wit [23] on the response to community engagement during COVID-19 have been that one-third of the prospective engagement had decreased, but over half of the community engagements continued irrespective of the crisis. Academics have several roles to play expressly during COVID-19. However, it is encouraging to note that amidst these difficult times, specific academics continue to embark on these endeavors (Table 20.7).

20.3   CONCLUSION

According to Kelsky [24], despite significant academic privileges, benefits, job security, and research and development opportunities, now is the time to explore innovative and diverse academic options. Women must, however, continue to navigate prejudiced conventions consistent with institutions embedded in patriarchy, reverberated by the intellectual dominance over women.

The fundamental institutionalized nature of gender, race, socio-economics, and geographic location in the academy, has collectively impacted on women as a gendered sector. This is consistent for minority groups that are similarly underrepresented in human, social, and health sciences at senior academic ranks. These include but are not limited to first nation people in Canada, Native Americans, Hispanics, and black populations around the world who are excessively affected by socio-economic factors associated with the pandemic. Sugimoto in Ref. [11] articulates those academics from minority populations are likely to experience a decline in research productivity, based on increased risk exposure resulting in them becoming sick or increased familial sick care responsibilities.

However, that validity requires a protracted period of time to determine specific empirically grounded reasons for the decline in publication outputs among minority women in the academy. Frederickson in Zimmer [11] adds that it is critical to have diverse convergence of researchers during the vaccine design and trials, to allow for greater reliability and holistic results, while Taylor in Zimmer [11] declares that different people would have varying approaches in the recruitment of individuals for drug trials. Women fought unremittingly to gain access into universities as intellectual equals; substantial advances are endangered by the expeditious COVID-19 teaching responses and transformations, in socially constructed virtual universities.

Prevailing gender, race, and identity paradigms traverse at a professional level in the academy. This chapter underlines significant variables of gender, race, and identity intersections for academics, with a focus on women. Universities must authorize rationalizations to support and recognize marginalized women that continue to experience incongruences vis-à-vis recognition, permanent appointments, and challenges in their career trajectory to a professorship. Varied consequences of exertions to survive gender. Specific challenges: inconsistent career advancement for different sociological areas of investigation have been noted in the literature, as well as frustration, stress, and long-term reductions in feelings of commitment to work. Female academics are often met with contract appointments and workloads consistent with higher teaching volumes. This immediately disadvantages her from higher progression in academia, as research is one of the key indicators for this. The expectation is that research can be conducted at home. However, for women, this is a mammoth task due to her multitude of responsibilities [25].

Women have traditionally endured unremitting inequitable circumstances in the academic space [2]. The traditional dominance of the preponderant old boys' network efficaciously sustains a gendered bias environment. The virtual COVID-19 classroom has expedited the assimilation of gender, race, and academic identity intersections into the personal spaces of women in the academy resulting in unprecedented workloads. The impact on the mental health of women has been long recognized [26]. The amplified workload, increased teaching-related administration, strains to procure extensive virtual teaching proficiencies; and intricate virtual assessment dexterities, coupled with amplified demands from large numbers of students; have exposed the ubiquitous and unremitting suppression of women in the academy.

KEYWORDS

- academics
- idiosyncratic strains
- natural disasters
- online
- resources
- virtual systems
- work overload

REFERENCES

1. Petrie, C., Aladin, K., Ranjan, P., Javangwe, R., Gilliland, D., Tuominen, S., & Lasse, L., (2020). *Spotlight: Quality Education for all During COVID-19 Crisis*. Research initiative between Hundred and OECD.
2. Ramnund-Mansingh, A., & Seedat-Khan, M., (2020a). Move over Ms. Professor! *Journal of Higher Education Service Science and Management (JoHESSM), 3*(1).
3. Doucet, A., Netolicky, D., Timmers, K., & Tuscano, F. J., (2020). *Thinking About Pedagogy in an Unfolding Pandemic*. Independent report to UNESCO.
4. Seedat, K. M., Ramnund-Mansingh, A., & Johnson, B., (2020). Welcome to university: Have a seat please! *Journal of Higher Education Service Science and Management (JoHESSM), 3*(2).
5. Ramnund, A., (2019). Exploring the link between institutional culture and the career advancement of female academics in higher education: A case study of the University of Kwazulu-Natal, South Africa. *PhD Thesis Submission*.
6. Ramnund-Mansingh, A., & Seedat-Khan, M., (2020b). Understanding the career trajectories of Black female academics in South Africa: A case study of the University of Kwazulu-Natal. *Perspectives in Education, 38*(2), 56–69.
7. Stieg, C., (2020). *Facebook's Sheryl Sandberg: Preventing Burnout 'Needs to be a Priority'* Retrieved from: https://www.cnbc.com/2020/05/08/sheryl-sandberg-preventing-burnout-must-be-priority-amid-covid-19.html (accessed on 9 July 2021).
8. García-González, M. A., Torrano, F., & García-González, G., (2020). Analysis of stress factors for female professors at online universities. *International Journal of Environmental Research and Public Health, 17*(8), 2958.
9. Swanson, D. H., & Johnston, D. D., (2003). Mothering in the ivy tower: Interviews with academic mothers. *Journal of the Motherhood Initiative for Research and Community Involvement, 5*(2).
10. Bird, S., Litt, J., & Wang, Y., (2004). Creating status of women reports: Institutional housekeeping as women's work. NWSA Journal, 16, 194–206.
11. Zimmer, K., (2020). *Gender Gap in Research Output Widens During Pandemic*. The Scientist. Retrieved from: https://www.the-scientist.com/news-opinion/gender-gap-in-research-output-widens-during-pandemic-67665 (accessed on 28 June 2021).

12. Matthews, D., (2020). *Pandemic Lockdown Holding Back Female Academics, Data Show*. Retrieved from: https://www.timeshighereducation.com/news/pandemic-lockdown-holding-back-female-academics-data-show (accessed on 28 June 2021).

13. Gupta, N., & Sharma, A. K., (2002). Women academic scientists in India. *Social Studies of Science, 32*(5, 6), 901–915.

14. Johnsrud, L. K., (1995). Korean academic women: Multiple roles, multiple challenges. *Higher Education, 30*(1), 17–35.

15. Prozesky, H., (2006). Gender differences in the journal publication productivity of South African academic authors. *South African Review of Sociology, 37*(2), 87–112.

16. Thorstad, R. R., Tamara, L., Anderson, M., Hall, E. L., Willingham, M., & Carruthers, L., (2006). Breaking the mold: A qualitative exploration of mothers in Christian academia and their experiences of spousal support. *Journal of Family Issues, 27*(2), 229–251.

17. Walker, M., (1998). Academic identities: Women on a South African landscape. *British Journal of Sociology of Education, 19*(3), 335–354.

18. Boshoff, N., (2005). The representation of women academics in higher education in South Africa: Progress in the pipeline? *South African Journal of Higher Education, 19*(2), 359–377.

19. Petersen, N., & Gravett, S., (2000). The experiences of women academics at a South African university. *South African Journal of Higher Education, 14*(3), 169–176.

20. Bailey, T., & Mouton, J., (2004). *Synthesis Report - Women's Participation in Science, Engineering, and Technology*. Supported by the Department of Science and Technology and National Advisory Council on Innovation. Pretoria.

21. Trade Union Advisory Committee to OECD, (2020). *Impact and Implications of the COVID 19-Crisis on Educational Systems and Households*. TUAC Secretariat Briefing. Retrieved from: https://tuac.org/news/the-impact-and-implications-of-the-COVID-19-crisis-on-educational-systems-and-households/ (accessed on 28 June 2021).

22. Eckel, Peter, Barbara Hill, & Madeleine Green, (1998). "En Route to Transformation." On Change: Occasional Paper Series No. 1 of the ACE Project on Leadership and Institutional Transformation. American Council on Education. Washington, 1–10.

23. Marinoni, G., & De Wit, H., (2020). *A Severe Risk of Growing Inequality Between Universities*. University World News. Retrieved from: https://www.universityworldnews.com/post.php?story=2020060815405140 (accessed on 28 June 2021).

24. Kelsky, K., (2020). *The Professor is in: Fear, Anxiety, and the Faculty Career*. Retrieved from: https://www.chronicle.com/article/The-Professor-Is-In-Fear/249197 (accessed on 28 June 2021).

25. Barrett, L., & Barrett, P., (2011). Women and academic workloads: Career slow lane or cul-de-sac? Higher Education, 6, 141–155.

26. Asakura, T., & Chen, L., (1993). Study on life stress and health of Asian international students. *Bulletin of Tokyo Gakugei University the 5th Department, Art Health Sports Science, 45*, 97–103.

27. *Education in South Africa: Achievements Since 1994*, (2001). Department of Education. Retrieved from: https://www.dhet.gov.za/Reports%20Doc%20Library/Education%20in%20South%20Africa%20Achievements%20since%201994.pdf (accessed on 28 June 2021).

28. South African Government Gazette No. 18207. 15 August. "Education White Paper 3: A Programme for Higher Education Transformation," (National Commission on Higher Education). 1997. [Online]. Available at: https://www.justice.gov.za/commissions/FeesHET/docs/1997-WhitePaper-HE-Tranformation.pdf (accessed on 24 July 2021).

CHAPTER 21

School and University Closures in COVID-19: Impacts on Educational Processes and Systems

CHANDRA LAL PANDEY,[1] BAL CHANDRA LUITEL,[2] and LINA GURUNG[2]

[1]*Community Development Program, School of Arts, Kathmandu University, Dhulikhel, Nepal, E-mail: chandra.pandey@ku.edu.np*

[2]*School of Education, Kathmandu University, Dhulikhel, Nepal*

ABSTRACT

Schools and universities have been closed for over 6 months, almost, all over the world. Millions of school children and university students are not able to attend their educational institutions and forced to stay home either in isolation or in quarantine. Many of the educational institutions, particularly in developed countries, have been running their classes online; however, a large number of students in South Asia, including Nepal, are not able to attend either face to face classes because of lockdown or virtual classes because of hardware and software technologies inaccessibility. Social and physical distancing and lockdown have been considered effective intermediate measures until humanity will have developed vaccines to control/fight against the novel coronavirus. These measures have been able to control the disease spread to some extent; however, they have also deprived millions of students from their fundamental rights of acquiring education. To continue classes during COVID-19, there is a buzzword—online classes—in the market now, and many of the schools and universities have started to offer courses through online platforms. However, no study has been conducted thus far to understand the challenges and prospects of pandemic such as COVID-19 and the shift of teaching-learning from face-to-face to online modes. In this chapter, we document existing online teaching and learning practices in Nepal and beyond, identify the research and practice-informed best practices, expecting them they can play catalyst roles during COVID-19 and similar pandemic in the future.

21.1 INTRODUCTION

The medical and scientific community demonstrated marvelous efforts in the understanding and control of novel coronavirus however, there are still gaps in terms of the molecular basis of the physical stability and transmissibility of the virus, foolproof infection control, and an effective vaccine with no immune enhancement. The novel coronavirus pandemic requires strong national and international solidarity to ensure that the world becomes able to face the pandemic and address its impacts in all sectors, including education. Schools and universities have been closed for over 6 months, almost, all over the world due to the pandemic of COVID-19. Over 1.6 billion of school children and university students are not able to attend their educational institutions and forced to stay home either in isolation or in quarantine. Many of the educational institutions, particularly in developed countries, have been running their classes online (although they also have a number of issues pertaining to access, quality, and inclusion) however a large number of students in South Asia including Nepal are not able to attend either face to face class because of lockdown or virtual classes because of the inaccessibility of hardware and software technologies. Social and physical distancing and lockdown have been considered effective intermediate measures until humanity will have developed vaccines to control/fight against it. These measures have been able to control the disease spread to some extent; however, they have also deprived billion-plus of students from their fundamental rights of acquiring education. To combat this, in this context, most of the schools and universities have started or are mulling to offer courses through online platforms. However, no study has been conducted thus far to understand the challenges and prospects of pandemic such as COVID-19 and the shift of teaching-learning from face-to-face to online distant modes. In this chapter, we identify key gaps of the shifts from face-to-face classes to online learning and lack of infrastructure maintaining physical and social distances, disconnect between students' and teachers' access to hardware and software information technologies and proficiency in using them, and the digital divide, leading to inequity in neo-education system assumed to be effective during the pandemic situations. We document existing teaching and learning practices in Nepal and beyond, identify the research and practice informed best practices to be used during pandemic, expecting that they can play catalyst roles during COVID-19 and similar pandemic in the future.

21.2   BACKGROUND OF THE STUDY

World Health Organization (WHO) declared the novel coronavirus disease (COVID-19) outbreak in 2019, reporting that it is caused by severe acute respiratory syndrome (SARS) and terming it to be a global pandemic on March 12, 2020 [1]. Regular hand wash using soaps, use of hand sanitizer and respiratory masks, avoiding crowds, maintaining physical and social distancing were key measures advised by WHO [1] for the public to be used against the novel coronavirus. Most of the governments around the world have closed educational institutions to maintain social and physical distancing to prevent the spread of the COVID-19 pandemic. Governments of the world imposed two types of closures of educational institutions, which are 'nationwide closure' and 'localized closure.' For example, most of the countries in South Asia, Latin America, Europe, and Africa are closing educational institutions nationwide while China, Russia, the United States of America (USA), among a few others, have localized closures only. Due to these nationwide and localized closures, according to a UNESCO (United Nations Educational, Scientific, and Cultural Organization) report, more than 1.6 billion school and university students across 191 countries have been severely affected [2]. Initial estimations were that COVID-19 would disappear in a few months time and the world would move in normalcy, however, the trends of the spread of the novel coronavirus and its recurrence in the form of multiple new waves has led the world towards a new direction—adaptive new normal. However, a recent study done in the United Kingdom (UK) questions whether the closures of schools and universities actually help prevent the novel coronavirus because when children are at home, they are likely to get out often and mix up with other children with the more likelihood of helping the virus spread [3].

The educational institutions closure measures, either nationwide or localized are unprecedented globally in recent history, but it is still not very clear about how long countries can maintain such preventive measures. Current realities demonstrate that physical and social distancing measures will need to be in place for many months or even years, thereby hinting at an urgent need to identify how countries can safely return students to education for learning. Education is one of the strongest predictors of the health, wealth, and development of a country and impacts of long-term closure of educational institutions may bring a number of challenges of overall national goals and development [4]. Thus, the extended lockdown due to COVID-19 has brought a number of significant challenges, in all areas of human and natural environment nexus, to address including the transformative potentials of education for all (EFA). As far as educational processes are concerned, the COVID-19 has forced and directed the world to innovate alternative pathways to move things ahead in a new normal situation. This thinking is equally applicable to educational systems and a number of schools and universities all over the world are engaged in innovating new measures of teaching and learning continuity although the key feature of school's physical space as and for equalizing privileges for students from different ethnic and socioeconomic strata remains as challenge. For examples, many of them are mulling to utilize or are already utilizing the benefits of modern information and technology as alternative teaching tools, methods, and techniques. However, there is a lack of proper ICT (Information and Communication Technology) facilities in most of educational institutions and at homes of the students and teachers in low-income and middle-income countries, which has caused major educational discontinuity in these countries. In addition to it, girls, children with disabilities and marginalized communities have further been restricted to access to education because of the inaccessibility of ICT and distant education facilities. Given the ongoing debates around education through ICT as a means for transformative initiatives versus potential for status quo, inequity, and exclusion, there is a need for a study that looks into the questions pertaining to the status, process, and experiences of students, teachers, parents, and concerned officials, thereby offering solutions that are grounded in the contexts, needs, and sustainability.

The review of literature exhibits that, at least, there are two diverging views on the use of ICT tools for teaching and learning. One group of scholars' reports that the use of ICT brings a number of benefits in teaching and learning and present open universities as examples of successful models [5, 68]. This group of scholars reasoned that ICT brings together both the students and the teachers/professors from different societies for an educational interaction and thus, plays a crucial role for innovation in the teaching and learning processes. There are arguments that ICT is a transformation in teaching and learning systems and a transition from teacher-assisted learning to the self-learning system; the concerns of equity also can be addressed through ICT. Toro and Joshi [6] reasoned that ICT can contribute to the knowledge growth society with implications of extending the education processes from the use of technologies to the key components of access and pedagogical efficiency.

The other group of scholars cautiously reason that the use of ICT in teaching and learning processes are important but the weak ICT infrastructure at homes and schools in low- and middle-income countries like India and Nepal, ICT untrained students and teachers; and gender-based concerns of online teaching and learning are the key challenges. Therefore, special considerations and deliberations are required to bridge the gaps of digital and gender-based divide for implementing ICT-supported teaching and learning systems [7–10, 69. Some of the studies also identified a host of caveats [7, 8] such as: (i) ICT tools being used only for the teacher talk; (ii) students not having quality Internet access and not possessing ICT tools; (iii) privileges not being equalized among the students, and d) the prevalence of new forms of bullying and inappropriate behavior. Purshothaman [70] highlighted the barriers in the context of India, which were no proper infrastructures in schools and universities, less consideration on students' having technophobia, less trained teachers, lack of motivation for female learners, and existing prejudices towards inappropriateness in villages and semi-urban areas. There has been long-standing evidence suggesting that gender and digital divide gaps have contributed to differentiated access to digital tools, thereby resulting in learning inequities [9, 10, 69].

In China, against the backdrop of the COVID-19 outbreak, the Chinese government launched an emergency policy initiative called "Suspending Classes without Stopping Learning" to continue teaching and learning activities as schools and universities across the country were closed to contain the virus. However, there have been ambiguities, challenges, and disagreements about what contents are to teach, what pedagogy is to be used to teach, how the workload of teachers and students are calculated, how the teaching environment be made sound, how assessment be made robust and all-encompassing, and how the implications for equity with new teaching pedagogy be maintained. Possible difficulties that the Chinese emergency teaching and learning policy faces include: the weakness of the online teaching infrastructure, the inexperience of teachers including unequal learning outcomes caused by teachers' varied experience, the information gap, the complex environment at home, and so forth [11]. Recent studies conducted in the South Asian region also show that the use of ICT in education has greater prospects for educational innovation across different levels of education, however, infrastructure including connectivity and power backup, human resource, e-content, language, technological support, security, and digital divide are the major challenges particularly in low- and middle-income countries like India and Nepal [10, 69]. Likewise, the persistence challenge of teacher preparation presents the education system at risk of losing relatively improved educational equity [71] as a result of lacking digital competencies among teachers. Given these gaps and COVID-19 contexts, the use of ICT as transformative education [12, 72] requires a deeper level of analysis to understand its overall effectiveness, the voices of children of the marginalized communities, thereby looking into the possibilities of empowering solutions. Research suggests that there is also a possibility of morphing teacher centered and didactic learning approaches to participatory educational processes through the use of ICTs [13]. Given this background, the chapter proceeds with education in emergencies (EiE) as an analytical framework to discuss how the transition has been planned, responses have been sequenced, resources have been provisioned, connections between the pandemic and post-pandemic interventions have been ensured.

21.3   ANALYTICAL DISCUSSION: PANDEMICS AND ALTERNATIVE PATHWAYS FOR EDUCATIONAL CONTINUITY

Owing to the nature of the pandemic, the chapter is developed on the conceptual framework of responding to the educational needs in emergencies. Broadly known as EiE, this conceptual and pragmatic orientation proposes educational provisions in emergencies by aligning the plan with national/institutional priorities, taking equity as the key perspective, sequencing the responses, provisioning investment and resources, and making sure that there will be the continuation of education in emergency activities in post-emergency contexts [14].

21.4   NATIONAL ICT CONTEXT AND PRIORITIES

The use of ICT in education has been considered as one of the strategies to achieve the broader goals of education such as EFA and the government of Nepal (GoN) has given it high national priority [15]. The GoN aimed to apply ICT in the education sector for its full-fledged development in order to help achieve the goal of 'no one is left behind' and to promote gender equality for achieving the overall educational goals [16]. For this, the GoN implemented the SSRP (school sector reform plan), which introduced new reforms characterized by strategic intervention such as the restructuring of school education, improvement in the quality of education, and institution-alization of performance accountability, putting priorities on ICT. Ministry of Education (MOE) also prepared a Master Plan [15] for implementing ICT in education sector. MOE has already implemented some of the programs related to ICT in school education sector this far. Some of them are: one laptop per child (OLPC) pilot project, Lab model (computer sharing mecha-nism) Project, Internet connectivity to district education offices (DEOs) and schools and computer labs with the Internet connection from local ISPs. Furthermore, the Department of Education (DOE), with the involvement of some NGOs working in the education sector, has developed interac-tive digital learning materials for the students of grades 2 to 6 in subjects like Nepali, Mathematics, English, and Science [15]. The GoN, through the Ministry of Information and Communication, developed "National Information and Communication Technology Policy" in 2015 to build the foundational groundwork for 'Digital Nepal.' The policy aimed at enhancing overall national ICT readiness with the objective of being at least in the top second quartile of the international ICT development index and government rankings by 2020. It also targeted for at least 75% of the population to have digital literacy skills by the end of 2020. The recent school sector develop-ment plan (SSDP) 2016–2023 of GoN aims to use ICT as a significant tool to improve classroom delivery; to maximize access to teaching-learning materials; and to enhance the effectiveness and efficiency of educational governance and management (*The Kathmandu Post* 7-Nov-2018). Owing to the ongoing crisis, these initiatives provide necessary grounds for initiating ICT-based learning in school education in Nepal. However, the major ques-tion lies in the access, equity, and inclusion as only 20% of students are found to have been using ICT-based teaching during the pandemic [73].

Moving beyond school education to university education, Kathmandu University was the first university, which started its online and distance learning programs in 2011 through PGDE (Post-graduate Diploma in Educa-tion) program. The open distance learning (ODL) program was extended in 2015 with a Master degree in Mathematics Education, English Language Teaching, Leadership, and Management, and Master in Sustainable Development. Likewise, Tribhuvan University started a similar program in Mathematics Education and English Language Teacher. In the same year, TU established Open and Distance Education Center (ODEC) to cater services to more students through online. Though Nepal Open University Infrastruc-ture Development Board was established in 2012 under the chairmanship of

MoE, it launched its programs in online distant mode from 2018, starting with Master and MPhil programs. Besides these major universities of Nepal, there are various contact centers of different foreign universities, which enroll students in different programs through online and distance mode. The educational continuation in the neo-education context could be attributed to this preparation of TU, KU, and Nepal Open Universities.

Although the preceding paragraphs demonstrated that Nepali school education and universities have long been mulling to exploit modern online based teaching and learning system, the question of their preparedness and readiness come in the forefront now. Provided that the authors of this chapter are themselves university faculty members with sound understanding of the digital plight of the schools and universities and the reports of their readiness show that most of these institutions are not yet prepared to run classes online fulfilling the needs and essence of teaching and learning practices. Only a few private schools and Kathmandu University have been able to run classes online using synchronous and asynchronous measures although they also encountered several challenges while doing so. Since there have been inadequate preparation in Nepal and a higher range of inaccessibility to the Internet and devices among the population, the online mode of education is in inequitable implementation. Though there were efforts from GoN [17], such as launching the unitary e-education postal under MOE, it was not sufficient to provide service to the most disadvantaged sections of the population [18].

21.5   EQUITY AND DIGITAL DIVIDE IN ICT BASED EDUCATION

ICT has helped in bridging various gaps in the society, but at the same time, it has also widened the digital gap. ICT has differently impacted women, children, and vulnerable communities and their lives. They do not only have access but are not able to use it for learning [19]. It has reinforced the traditional discrimination and are tangible in computer mediated education [74]. In contrary, ICT can empower women like men. It can promote gender equality through change in their social roles access in education, provide job opportunities and develop capacity for their empowerment [21, 22]. However, women/girls still have lesser access to ICT compared to male counterparts, and while accessing to digital platforms, they may face gender harassment, which ultimately pulls towards the social stigmatization. In essence, technological advancement has also enabled criminals to remain anonymous or use fake identities, and commit crimes without any physical contact and from anywhere in the world, without any major repercussions [23]. This could also put women, children, and vulnerable groups at risk whilst bringing education in virtual platforms.

There is an increasing revolution of the ICT in every field in the techno-based society today, but low access of girls and women in digital devices and platforms has hampered their learning and other activities that can be done through the use of ICT. Gender-based empowerment commonly refers to the process by which women, children, and vulnerable groups augment their power to educate themselves and understand the social system, take control over decisions that shape their lives, including in relation to access to resources, partaking in decision making and control over distribution of benefits [24]. There are five key empowerment components of marginal-ized groups like women, children, and vulnerable groups. They are: sense of self-worth; their right to have and to decide choices; their right to have access to chances and resources; their right to have the power to control their own lives, both within and outside the home; and their aptitude to influence the direction of social conversion to create a more just social and economic order, nationally, and universally [24]. Right to have access on resources like ICT by their own choices without any socio-cultural barriers help empower women, children, and vulnerable groups and in pandemic situations, it is important that equity be taken care of to help women and girls not miss the learning opportunities for their future growth and contribution to the society. Else, as always, women, children, and vulnerable groups are trapped in the circle of poverty, illiteracy, and cultural traditions that function as barriers to computer related technologies, which are expensive, literacy dependent, man defined as a male realm [25, 26].

The faces of the digital divide are multiple inclusive of, inter alia, being male and female, boys, and girls, rich, and poor, urban, and rural, educated, and illiterate and the digital divide is of the major concerns in developing countries like Nepal. For examples, the residents in the cities often have access to massive information system while the residents of the rural areas do not seem to have access to information system and rely heavily in conventional modes of communication. There is uneven distribution of technological and the Internet opportunities based on level of education, geographical location of the residents and their economic status. Our social norms, gender roles, class, and stereotypes influence the use of technology and its benefits distribution [22]. Therefore, despite the significant growth of ICT, there remains a gender and class imbalance in access resources in digital era [27, 28]. This imbalance is an extension of gendered stereotyped embedded in patriarchal norms. The global digital divide has been a constant concern for more than two decades [29], and it has come to be the crux of debate now when schools and universities need to turn towards a digital system of teaching, learning, and research.

21.6   EDUCATION IN EMERGENCY AND IN POST-EMERGENCY CONTEXT

It is very important to discuss how the response can be sequenced from the perspective of making a transitional plan during the pandemic and a long-term vision for post-pandemic situation ensuring education in EiE and post-emergency context. The novel coronavirus seems to exist for about 2-year time since its first mutation and similar pandemic may appear in the future due to the impacts of globalization of trade, economy, food, culture, and transport system. Unless any new innovations happen to exist, the global education system cannot turn its face from going digital, and it is especially true when the fight against the disease is lockdown, social, and physical distancing. It is in this context that there is a need to ensure that pre-COVID and during COVID-19 intervention is connected well with the post-COVID education context. Considering ICT-based as one of the alternatives during these times, digital literacy is one of the attributes to be developed among the learners, teachers, and administrators.

Digital literacy began with the birth of the Internet in 1982, and the development of the World Wide Web in 1989. Digital literacy became popular terminology after the global expansion of the Internet and its expanded use. The first wave of digital literacy was classified as distance learning, which provided instructions through print or electronic communications media to persons engaged in planned learning in a place or time different from that of the instructor or instructors and the learners [30]. It is a sequential and step by step delivery system that connects learners, regardless of their location, with educational resources provided to them. The resources and a step-by-step guide are provided to the learners for keeping in touch with normal regular attending students [31]. Online education is a revolutionary step forward from distance learning as it includes a broader range of services and provides comprehensive and constructive learning experiences [32]. It is a form of distributed learning made possible by the Internet; therefore, online delivery goes beyond traditional computer learning as it makes full use of the Internet and other digital technologies [33]. Online learning can now be understood as a wide range of electronically distributed learning and training materials which are accessible anytime from anywhere [31] and it comprises of both synchronous and asynchronous modes.

Digital literacy needs a number of careful preparations. It requires the ability to understand and use information which are presented through computers and various technologies through navigation and interpreting of the information [34, 35]. According to UNESCO [36] *"digital literacy is the ability to access, manage, understand, integrate, communicate, evaluate, and create information safely and appropriately through digital technologies for employment, decent jobs and entrepreneurship, including competences that are variously referred to as computer literacy, information literacy or ICT literacy."* The tools of ICTs are audio, videos, wireless interfaces, and other hand-held devices, which requires skills to use them practically [37]. Simply, the digital literacy means encompassing traditional literacies and computer literacy due to the invention and diffusion of technologies over time.

Educators, researchers, and students need digital literacy because it helps to access and interpret information to disseminate it for wider community [38].

In the past when teaching and learning was completely dependent on physical presence of teacher and students, there was alternative thinking to make the learning happen with the face-to-face meeting [39] and this gave rise to distance education [40]. Peters [40] have discussed the history of distance education in three periods: the first was when there was a deficiency of vocational training and gap of education among the labors in the industries; the second phase was education was mainly focused to reduce the number of school dropouts and to combine the need of work and study; the third phase was when there was integration of technology which become more significant in teaching and learning. Besides this, many other scholars have divided the phases of emergence of distance education such as the first phase was after the invention of the internet, the second had more advancement in technology and expanded through online education; the third wave was the phase of MOOC (massive open online courses) and the 4th phase focused on the development of new tools for innovative pedagogies to engage students in personalized learning [75]. Online learning system demands students to have additional ICT skills and take responsibility for their learning [20, 41].

It needs to be highlighted that the use of digital technology is not only a means for delivering literacy skills but also an essential part of an information-literate knowledge society and economy. Individual's participation in this digital society does not only involve text digital skills but also equips the participant to create new knowledge products for the benefit of the individual and society today and in the future [42]. ICT can be used for various purposes, from teaching and learning, researching, and disseminating information. In today's digital society, where everyone has easy access to information through the Internet, it has made the teachers and mentors feel that students who are tech-savvy knows more about the digital world [43]. Thus, using the ICT, teachers can overcome the individual challenges and improve the teaching practices [44] on the hand while students can equip them better by accessing to learning materials, taking advantage of good practices of teaching and learning. There are asynchronous and synchronous forms of online education. The asynchronous form refers to the learning of materials at different times by downloading them from the web without real-time interaction, whereas the synchronous form refers to learning online that happens in real time interactions. Today, in the time of COVID-19 pandemic, educational institutions, going beyond distance learning, can utilize hybrid/ blended models of teaching and learning by incorporating the features of asynchronous and synchronous online learning and this will deepen and widen the opportunities of teaching and learning in pandemic and post-pandemic situations.

21.7   EDUCATION CONTEXT OF NEPAL AND PREPAREDNESS FOR EIE

Historically, ever since the Gurukul system, students, and teachers have been sharing and generating knowledge in the presence of one another—face to face in Nepal. However, teaching-learning methods have been changing over time from traditional 'Gurukul' system to 'Chalk Duster' to 'Projectors and PowerPoint slides'—from master model to student centered approaches [45]. Yet, the primary method of academic teaching and learning has been the traditional system in which the teachers and students do not have any reliable choice except the use chalk/marker blackboard/whiteboard and textbooks. The utilization of this primary method of teaching and learning in school and higher education institutions even after having the increased access to computers, the Internet and smart technology suggests the importance, popularity, and mindset about face-to-face teaching and learning mode. Although technologies have long been available, until now, a few universities and schools all over the world, including Nepal, have started to employ online platforms for facilitating the process of teaching and learning, calling themselves open schools and open universities. The actual methods these open schools and open universities used were not and are not entirely ICT based rather a mixed method of teaching and learning utilizing mostly asynchronous resources and a few face-to-face opportunities. Now, the situation has changed drastically—from normalcy to COVID-19 pandemic. The outbreak and prolonged existence of the novel coronavirus has forced all the education institutions and systems to find alternative path of teaching, learning, and evaluation/assessment. Although there are a number of challenges in actually going online, we now have multiple potential and proven options to conduct classes online combine both synchronous and asynchronous methods. Teachers from schools and professors from universities can design the courses and plan their lessons as per their needs, situation, and contexts by accessing to all possible teaching-learning materials through Internet/Web tools, smart board, software tools, audio, and videos.

The COVID-19 has immensely affected the global education system and Nepal's education system cannot keep itself in isolation from what is happening in the world. We have already discussed the cursory history of digital/online learning and the challenges and opportunities they have brought in front of us. Use of radio, television, and homeschooling can be some of the options which have long been used in teaching and learning in Nepal and beyond however if we plan to continue our education system in real-time interactions, there is no alternative to 'going online'—a full-fledged digital system capturing the characteristics of both synchronous and asynchronous modes. As a result, the global education system, including academic institutions of Nepal are mulling and trying to 'go online.' However, there are a number of issues that need to be considered to 'go online' for teaching and learning, and these considerations are especially salient in the case of Nepal. These considerations include preparation and enactment of national education policy on online teaching and learning and ICT readiness of students, teachers, parents, schools, and universities. National digital education policy with codes of conduct needs to be adopted for not only conducting classes online but also encompassing the processes of evaluation mainly for school education. Based on national digital education policy, universities also need to develop their own online teaching and learning policy with codes of conduct using their autonomy, which can provide detailed guidelines for conducting classes and iterative evaluations of students through various assignments and tests. Systemic resiliency is essential for school and higher education systems to cope with such a shift from face-to-face mode of delivery to online and ICT-driven delivery. The relevant ministry and the government of the day need to support online initiatives as all schools and universities cannot be kept in the black and white boxes rather in mosaic with different contexts and needs in Nepal. One of the most crucial points that need to be understood from equity and the digital divide is that in one world, there are multiple worlds, and in Nepal also there is diversity between schools and universities. For example, in the global context, the first world, the second world and the third world or in different way, global south/east (developing countries) or global north/west (developed countries). These countries have different levels of development and human development index, which shows that some people are more equal than others. Likewise, there is diversity among government schools, community schools, and private schools, and huge differences do exist within and between each of these categories, and so is the case of existing universities of Nepal.

In this mosaic of digital divide and inequity, many of the educational institutions, particularly in developed countries, have been running their classes online however a large number of students in middle- and low-income countries including Nepal are not able to attend virtual classes because of hardware and software technologies inaccessibility, online teaching and evaluation skills of teachers/professors and the home environment of students. In this changed context, novelty needs to be innovated instead of only prioritizing the traditional/conventional methods of teaching and learning. Having said these, however, all the schools and universities must consolidate and strengthen their existing online/digital system to fully benefit all the stakeholders and educational processes right from admission to teaching, learning, evaluation to graduation. To consolidate and strengthen the digital system, four key factors must be considered, which include: (1) schools' readiness for conducting ICT classes; (2) teachers/professors' readiness for conducting ICT classes; (3) students' equitable readiness for ICT assisted classes, and (4) home environment readiness for ICT classes [45].

Schools' readiness for conducting classes refers to schools and universities ICT infrastructure to run classes online without any interruption. It may include robust server system, high speed Internet, permanent power supply and audio video supported computer system. Teachers/professors readiness for conducting ICT classes also refers to the availability of ICT devices such as computers, laptops, online course materials and syllabus development, high speed Internet, and sound training about using ICT tools and techniques for teaching, learning, and research activities. Students' equitable readiness for ICT classes refers to sound training of how to use the ICT devices, availability of them in the hands of students, the capacity of the students or parents to pay for high-speed Internet and ICT devices so that students can use them for online classes, working on their assignments, exams, and submissions, etc. The concern of equity must be taken good care of because all the parents may not be equally able to afford ICT readiness preparedness for their children. State can introduce progressive policies to address such issues. And the home environment readiness for ICT classes refers to home atmosphere. Usually, home is unlike office and when students and teachers start taking and giving classes from home, there can be disturbances and distractions, which affect the whole teaching and learning process, therefore, special care needs to be taken about the environment in which we conduct our classes. Ensuring these four pillars keeping equity at the center can help the educational system to resume by going fully online right from admission to graduation in Nepal and many other countries of the world.

21.8 MYTHS ABOUT ONLINE AND DISTANCE EDUCATION

Since traditional teaching and learning has been a long-established culture globally, setting up of physical institutions and management for face-to-face teaching and learning with physical materials have been embedded globally. In formal education history, teaching, and learning means going to schools, colleges, and universities; carrying a bag with some books and interacting or listening to teachers and professors. Against this traditional practice, online teaching and learning practices have been evolving to promote knowledge-based society and 'leave no one behind' from the access of education. However, there exist some myths/stereotypes against online/ digital education. Some of these frequently heard myths are: (a) Online teaching and learning is cheaper so there is doubt on its quality education. But in reality, the initial set up cost of online education such as training to faculties and student support (b) Disappearance of teachers can allow more time for them to do research, but it is also a myth because online teaching does not only involve asynchronous materials as in distance learning rather it demands virtual face to face class enabling the faculties to run classes online by exploiting audio-video technologies through platforms like 'Google meet and the Moodle.' Successful online faculty requires enhanced regular support for designing courses and conducting classes. c) Digital native is another myth which believes that young people are tech-savvy but the students come from diverse background and all of them may not have equally got opportunity to use ICT right from their early age. Due to different factors such as poverty, remote place and no accessibility of modern facilities, the preference often goes to the traditional system of teaching and learning. However, the reality is that the learners do not need to complete computer engineering courses to be able to use ICT assisted classes as recent interventions in two Nepali universities confirms the case (Carm, Johanssen, Luitel, Øgrim, and Phyak, in press). A few hours of orientation can suffice to attend these classes, but successful online learning demands active participation. d) Diminished quality of online courses is another myth because online learning can be of very high quality or at least comparable to the quality of traditional classroom-based teaching and learning activities because online classes offer virtual classes incorporating synchronous and asynchronous materials and the assignments and exams are not regular parroting like rather focus is on critical and advanced thinking. Thus, the use of online classes during pandemic and beyond pandemic can be boon in EIE sector.

21.9   CONCLUSION

Educational continuity in the context of ongoing pandemic can be viewed from the perspective of EiE. The COVID-19, the most dangerous and widespread pandemic, has forced global shut down, impacting the social, cultural, transport, economic, and educational systems. Schools, colleges, and universities have been shut down for several months, halting the normal face-to-face classroom practices. There is a need to bring the education system into new normal through adaptation, which can fight against the novel coronavirus and its measures such as physical and social distancing and lockdowns. In such a context, education/academic sector can opt for online/digital mode of education system for now and for future if there is recurrence of pandemic like the novel coronavirus. However, the educational process and systems are less prepared in adopting ICT and online-driven education in many countries of the world, including Nepal. Likewise, the widespread assumptions of what counts as teaching and learning has made it difficult to implement ICT and online-based educational processes. Due to the lack of adequate preparation of both human and non-human infrastructures, and the digital divide, educators, and learners are likely to suffer from gaining access to quality educational processes and outcomes. Finally, reimagining educational processes during COVID-19 and post-COVID contexts require addressing a host of hardware and software challenges and myths associated with alternative modes of educational processes in general and online/digital education in particular.

KEYWORDS

- **COVID-19**
- **department of education**
- **education for all**
- **information and communication technology**
- **massive open online courses**
- **one laptop per child**

REFERENCES

1. WHO, (2020). *WHO Director-General's Opening Remarks at the Mission Briefing on COVID-19.* https://www.who.int/director-general/speeches/detail/who-director-general-s-opening-remarks-at-the-mission-briefing-on-covid-19---16-april-2020 (accessed on 28 June 2021).
2. UNESCO, (2020). *COVID-19: Impact on Education.* UNESCO. Available at: https://en.unesco.org/covid19/educationresponse (accessed on 28 June 2021).
3. Viner, R., Russell, S., Croker, H., Packer, J., Ward, J., Stansfield, C., Mytton, O., et al., (2020). School closure and management practices during coronavirus outbreaks including COVID-19: A rapid systematic review. *Lancet Child Adolescent Health, 4*, 397–404.
4. Ferguson, N. M., Laydon, D., & Nedjati-Gilani, G., (2020). *Report 9: Impact of Non-Pharmaceutical Interventions (NPIs) to Reduce COVID-19 Mortality and Healthcare Demand.* London: Imperial College.
5. Sangrà, A., & González-Sanmamed, M., (2010). The role of information and communication technologies in improving teaching and learning processes in primary and secondary schools. *ALT-J, 18*(3), 207–220.
6. Toro, U., & Joshi, M., (2012). ICT in higher education: Review of literature from the period 2004–2011. *International Journal of Innovation, Management and Technology, 3*(1), 20–23.
7. Shields, R., (2011). ICT or I see tea? Modernity, technology and education in Nepal. *Globalization, Societies and Education, 9*(1), 85–97.
8. Kindsiko, E., & Türk, K., (2017). Detecting major misconceptions about employment in ICT: A study of the myths about ICT work among females. *International Journal of Social, Behavioral, Educational, Economic, Business and Industrial Engineering, 11*(1), 107–114.
9. Brynin, M., (2006). Gender, technology and jobs. *British Journal of Sociology, 57*(3), 437–453.
10. Pandey, C. L., (2020). Post COVID 19 scenarios: Implication for Nepal amidst changing dynamics of global power relations. In: Rajesh, S., Rupak, S., & Madhavji, S., (eds.), *Green Governance for Sustainability in Context of COVID-19 Pandemic.* Kathmandu: Institute of Foreign Affairs, Government of Nepal.

11. Zang, W., Wang, Y., Yang, L., & Wang, C., (2020). Suspending classes without stopping learning: China's education emergency management policy in the COVID-19 outbreak. *Journal of Risk and Financial Management, 13*(55). doi: 10.3390/jrfm13030055.

12. Luitel, B. C., & Taylor, P. C., (2019). Introduction: Research as transformative learning for sustainable futures. In: Taylor, P. C., & Luitel, B. C., (eds.), *Research as Transformative Learning for Sustainable Futures* (pp. 1–16). Leiden, The Netherlands: Brill|Sense.

13. UNESCO, (2011). *Transforming Education: The Power of ICT Policies.* Paris: UNESCO.

14. Versmesse, I., Derluyn, I., Masschelein, J., & De Haene, L., (2017). After conflict comes education? Reflections on the representations of emergencies in 'education in emergencies. *Comparative Education, 53*(4), 538–557.

15. Ministry of Education, (2013). *Information & Communication Technology (ICT) in Education: Master Plan 2013–2017.* Kathmandu: Government of Nepal. Available: https://www.moe.gov.np/assets/uploads/files/ICT_MP_2013_(Final)_.pdf (accessed on 28 June 2021).

16. Unwin, T., (2004). ICT and education in Africa: Partnership, practice and knowledge sharing. *Review of African Political Economy, 31*(99), 150–160.

17. Government of Nepal, (2018). *2018 Digital Framework Nepal: Unlocking Nepal's Growth Potential.* Nepal: Ministry of Communication and Information Technology.

18. Dawadi, S., Giri, R., & Simkhada, P., (2020) *Impact of COVID-19 on the Education Sector in Nepal - Challenges and Coping Strategies.* Sage Submissions. Preprint. https://doi.org/10.31124/advance.12344336.v1.

19. Purushothaman, A., & Zhou, C., (2014). Change towards a society in developing contexts- women barriers to learning by information and communication technology. *Gender, Technology and Development, 18*(3), 363–386.

20. Kim, M., & Zhang, W., (2007). Does gender matter in computer mediated communication based distance education? *International Journal of Diversity in Organizations, Communities & Nations, 7*(1), 49–54.

21. Spence, N., (2010). Gender, ICTs, human development, and prosperity. *Information Technologies & International Development, 6*(SE), 69.

22. Buskens, I., & Webb, A., (2009). *African Women and ICTs: Creating New Spaces with Technology.* Ottawa: IDRC.

23. Raj, Y., (2019). Cybercrimes against women in India. *FEMICIDE Cyber Crimes Against Women & Girls, 11,* 37–43.

24. Arrawatia, M. A., & Meel, P., (2010). Information and communication technologies & woman empowerment in India. *International Journal of Advanced Research in Computer Engineering & Technology (IJARCET), 1*(8), 99–104.

25. Haddad, W. D., & Jurich, S., (2002). *ICT for Education: Prerequisites and Constraints* (pp. 42–57). WA: UNESCO.

26. Volman, M., & Van, E. E., (2001). Gender equity and information technology in education: The second decade. *Review of Educational Research, 71*(4), 613–634.

27. Hashim, J., (2008). Learning barriers in adopting ICT among selected working women in Malaysia. *Gender in Management: An International Journal, 23*(5), 317–336.

28. Adya, M., & Kaiser, K. M., (2005). Early determinants of women in the IT workforce: A model of girls' career choices. *Information Technology & People, 18*(3), 230–259.

29. Pande, R., & Weide, T. V., (2012). *Globalization, Technology, Diffusion and Gender Disparity: Social Impacts of ICTs.* PA: IGI Global.

30. Moore, L. W., (1991). U.S. Patent No. 5,068,850. WA: U.S. Patent and Trademark Office.

31. Sehra, S., Sunakshi, M., & Bhardawaj, A., (2014) Comparative analysis of e-learning and distance learning techniques. *International Journal of Information & Computation Technology, 4*(8), 823–828.

32. Bejjar, M. A., & Boujelbene, Y., (2014). E-learning and web 2.0: A couple of the 21st century advancements in higher education. In: Gard, A., (ed.), *E-Learning 2.0 Technologies and Web Applications in Higher Education* (pp. 1–21). Hershey, PA: Information Science Reference.

33. Volery, T., & Lord, D., (2000). Critical success factors in online education. *International Journal of Educational Management, 14*(5), 216–223. https://doi.org/10.1108/09513540010344731.

34. Gilster, P., & Glister, P., (1997). *Digital Literacy.* New York: Wiley.

35. Brazelton, G. B., (2016). *Adult Learners at Community Colleges: Influence of Technology on Feelings of Marginality and Mattering.* MI: Michigan State University.

36. UNESCO, (2018). *Building Tomorrow's Digital Skills- What Conclusions Can We Draw from International Comparative Indicators?* Paris: UNESCO.

37. Skudowitz, J., (2009). *Research Report: A Case Study of the Digital Literacy Practices in a Grade 10 English Classroom at a Private School.* Unpublished Master Thesis, University of the Witwatersrand, Johannesburg, South Africa. Available: http://wiredspace.wits.ac.za/handle/10539/5938 (accessed on 28 June 2021).

38. Yazon, A. D., Ang-Manaig, K., Buama, C. A. C., & Tesoro, J. F. B., (2019). Digital literacy, digital competence, and research productivity of educators. *Universal Journal of Educational Research, 7*(8), 1734–1743.

39. Holmberg, B., (2005). *Theory and Practice of Distance Education.* Routledge.

40. Peters, O., (2003). *Distance Education in Transition: New Trends and Challenges.* Oldenburg: BIS Verlag.

41. Blackmon, S. J., & Major, C., (2012). Student experiences in online courses: A qualitative research synthesis. *Quarterly Review of Distance Education, 13*(2).

42. Wagner, A. D., & Kozma, R., (2005). *New Technologies for Literacy and Adult Education: A Global Perspective.* Paris: UNESCO.

43. Kavanagh, A., & O'Rourke, K. C., (2016). *Digital Literacy: Why it Matters.* Available: http://arrow.dit.ie/cgi/viewcontent.cgi?article=1036&context=ltcart (accessed on 28 June 2021).

44. Vieluf, S., Kaplan, D., Klieme, E., & Bayer, S., (2012). *Teaching practices and pedagogical innovation: Evidence from TALIS.* Retrieved from: https://www.oecd.org/education/school/TalisCeri%202012%20(tppi)--Ebook.pdf (accessed on 28 June 2021).

45. Pandey, C. L., (2020). *Education Should go Online Amid COVID-19.* Online Khabar English Edition. Available: https://english.onlinekhabar.com/education-should-go-online-amid-covid-19-here-are-points-to-be-noted-for-shift.html (accessed on 28 June 2021).

46. Bhattacharjee, B., & Deb, K., (2016). Role of ICT in 21st century's teacher education. *International Journal of Education and Information Studies, 6*(1), 1–6.

47. Carlson, S., & Gadio, C. T., (2002). Teacher professional development in the use of technology. *Technologies for Education*, 118–132. UNESCO, Paris.

48. Carm, E., Johanssen, M., Luitel, B. C., Øgrim, L., & Phyak, P. B., (In Press). Reflections and culminations. In: Carm, E., Johanssen, M., Luitel, B. C., Øgrim, L., & Phyak, P. B., (eds.), *Transforming Nepali Higher Education Through Open and Distance Learning: A Case of Eight Year Long Project.* Leiden, The Netherlands: Brill | Sense.

49. Dhungel, S., (2018). Provincial comparison of development status in Nepal: An analysis of human development trend for 1996 to 2026. *Journal of Management and Development Studies, 28*, 53–68.

50. Dube, B., (2020). Rural online learning in the context of COVID 19 in South Africa: Evoking an inclusive education approach. *Multidisciplinary Journal of Educational Research, 10*(2), 135–157. doi: 10.4471/remie.2020.5607.

51. Government of Nepal, (2009). *School Sector Reform Plan 2009–2015*. Kathmandu: Ministry of Education.

52. Hussain, S., Guangju, W., Jafar, R. M. S., Ilyas, Z., Mustafa, G., & Jianzhou, Y., (2018). Consumers' online information adoption behavior: Motives and antecedents of electronic word of mouth communications. *Computers in Human Behavior, 80*, 22–32.

53. Ismail, S. A. M. M., Jogezai, N. A., & Baloch, F. A., (2020). Hindering and enabling factors towards ICT integration in schools: A developing country perspective. *Elementary Education Online, 19*(3), 1537–1547.

54. Katz, R., (2010). Scholars, scholarships and the scholarly enterprise in the digital age. *Educause, 45*(2), 44–56.

55. Ministry of Education, (2007). *Communication Strategy for Education 2063*. Available: https://www.moe.gov.np/assets/uploads/files/NFEC_Policy_English1.pdf (accessed on 28 June 2021).

56. Ministry of Education, (2007). *Open and Distance Learning (ODL) Policy, 2063*. Available: http://www.moe.gov.np/assets/uploads/files/Distance_learning_policy_20631.pdf (accessed on 28 June 2021).

57. Ministry of Education, (2016). *School Sector Development Plan (2016–2023)*. Kathmandu: Ministry of Education. Available: https://moe.gov.np/article/535/school-sector-development-plan.html (accessed on 28 June 2021).

58. Ministry of Information and Communication, (2003). *Long-term Policy of Information and Communication Sector 2059*. Kathmandu: Ministry of Information and Communication. Available: http://www.moic.gov.np/ (accessed on 28 June 2021).

59. Ministry of Information and Communication, (2004). *Telecommunication Policy, 2060*. Kathmandu: Ministry of Information and Communication. Available: http://www.moic.gov.np/ (accessed on 28 June 2021).

60. Ministry of Information and Communication, (2015). *Broadband Policy, 2071*. Kathmandu: Ministry of Information and Communication.

61. Ministry of Information and Communication, (2015). *National Information and Communication Technology Policy*. Kathmandu: Ministry of Information and Communication. Available: http://www.youthmetro.org/uploads/4/7/6/5/47654969/ict_policy_nepal.pdf (accessed on 28 June 2021).

62. Nayyar, T., Aggarwal, S., Khatter, D., Kumar, K., Goswami, S., & Saini, L., (2019). *Opportunities and Challenges in Digital Literacy: Assessing the Impact of Digital Literacy Training for Empowering Urban Poor Women*. New Delhi: Ministry of Women and Child Development, Government of India.

63. Noskova, T., Pavlova, T., Yakovleva, O., Esteban, P. G., Espada, R. M., & Díaz, R. Y. T., (2017). Contemporary teacher competencies development: A study of ICT tools for professional activities in Russia and Spain. *International Journal of Research in E-Learning IJREL, 3*(1), 91–108.

64. Roberts, E., Anderson, B. A., Skerratt, S., & Farrington, J., (2017). A review of the rural-digital policy agenda from a community resilience perspective. *Journal of Rural Studies, 54*, 372–385.

65. Shohel, M. M. C., (2012). *Childhood Poverty and Education in Bangladesh: Policy Implications for Disadvantaged Children.* Florence: NICEF Office of Research.

66. Thakral, P., (2015). Role of ICT in professional development of teachers. *Learning Community-an International Journal of Educational and Social Development, 6*(1), 127–133.

67. Tiwari, A., Das, A., & Sharma, M., (2015). Inclusive education a "rhetoric" or "reality"? Teachers' perspectives and beliefs. *Teaching and Teacher Education, 52*, 128–136.

68. Asian Development Bank (2017). Innovative Strategies for Accelerated Human Resource Development in South Asia: Information and Communication Technology for Education—Special Focus on Bangladesh, Nepal and Sri Lanka. Manila, Philippines: ADB.

69. Pangeni, S. K., (2016). Open and distance learning: cultural practices in Nepal. *European Journal of Open, Distance and E-Learning (EURODL), 19*(2), 32–45.

70. Purshothaman. A., (2011). Role of ICT in the educational upliftment of women—Indian scenario. In: *Proceedings of the 2011 World Congress on Information and Communication Technologies, 6*, 268–273. Mumbai, India: IEEE Publisher. Link: https://vbn.aau.dk/ws/portalfiles/portal/62866817/Role_of_ICT_in_the_Educational_Upliftment_of_Women_Indian_ScenarioIEEEXplore.pdf (accessed on 21 July 2021)

71. MOE., (2015). Nepal in figures 2015 at a glance. Ministry of education, Singhadurbar, Kathmandu.

72. Taylor, E. W., & Cranton, P. (2012). *The handbook of transformative learning: Theory, research, and practice.* John Wiley & Sons.

73. Tulashi Thapalia, (2020). September 12, 2020, Personal Communication.

74. Susan C. Herring, (1994). "Politeness in computer culture: Why women thank and men flame." In M. Bucholtz, A. Liang, & L. Sutton (eds.), Cultural Performances: Proceedings of the Third Berkeley Women and Language Conference, 278–294. Berkeley: Berkeley Women and Language Group.

75. Nayyar, A., Puri, V., & Le, D. N. (2017). Internet of nano things (IoNT): Next evolutionary step in nanotechnology. *Nanoscience and Nanotechnology, 7*(1), 4–8.

Index

For Product Safety Concerns and Information please contact our EU
representative GPSR@taylorandfrancis.com
Taylor & Francis Verlag GmbH, Kaufingerstraße 24, 80331 München, Germany

www.ingramcontent.com/pod-product-compliance
Lightning Source LLC
Chambersburg PA
CBHW060422220326

41598CB00021BA/2259

* 9 7 8 1 7 7 4 6 3 8 6 5 1 *